Critical Care Emergencies

Editors

EVIE MARCOLINI
HANEY MALLEMAT

EMERGENCY MEDICINE
CLINICS OF NORTH AMERICA

www.emed.theclinics.com

Consulting Editor
AMAL MATTU

November 2014 • Volume 32 • Number 4

ELSEVIER

1600 John F. Kennedy Boulevard • Suite 1800 • Philadelphia, Pennsylvania, 19103-2899

http://www.theclinics.com

EMERGENCY MEDICINE CLINICS OF NORTH AMERICA Volume 32, Number 4
November 2014 ISSN 0733-8627, ISBN-13: 978-0-323-32369-7

Editor: Patrick Manley

Developmental Editor: Casey Jackson

Emergency Medicine Clinics of North America (ISSN 0733-8627) is published quarterly by Elsevier Inc., 360 Park Avenue South, New York, NY, 10010-1710. Months of issue are February, May, August, and November. Business and Editorial Offices: 1600 John F. Kennedy Boulevard, Suite 1800, Philadelphia, PA 19103-2899. Customer Service Office: 6277 Sea Harbor Drive, Orlando, FL 32887-4800. Periodicals postage paid at New York, NY, and additional mailing offices. Subscription prices are $155.00 per year (US students), $315.00 per year (US individuals), $523.00 per year (US institutions), $220.00 per year (international students), $450.00 per year (international individuals), $642.00 per year (international institutions), $220.00 per year (Canadian students), $385.00 per year (Canadian individuals), and $642.00 per year (Canadian institutions). International air speed delivery is included in all *Clinics*' subscription prices. All prices are subject to change without notice. **POSTMASTER:** Send address changes to *Emergency Medicine Clinics of North America*, Elsevier Periodicals Customer Service, 11830 Westline Industrial Drive, St. Louis, MO 63146. Customer Service (orders, claims, online, change of address): Elsevier Periodicals Customer Service, 11830 Westline Industrial Drive, St. Louis, MO 63146. Tel: 1-800-654-2452 (U.S. and Canada); 314-453-7041 (outside U.S. and Canada). Fax: 314-453-5170. E-mail: journalscustomerservice-usa@elsevier.com (for print support); journalsonline support-usa@elsevier.com (for online support).

Reprints. For copies of 100 or more of articles in this publication, please contact the Commercial Reprints Department, Elsevier Inc., 360 Park Avenue South, New York, NY 10010-1710. Tel.: 212-633-3874; Fax: 212-633-3820; E-mail: reprints@elsevier.com.

Emergency Medicine Clinics of North America is covered in *MEDLINE/PubMed (Index Medicus), Current Contents/Clinical Medicine, EMBASE/Excerpta Medica, BIOSIS, SciSearch, CINAHL, ISI/BIOMED,* and *Research Alert.*

Printed in the United States of America.

Contributors

CONSULTING EDITOR

AMAL MATTU, MD, FAAEM, FACEP
Professor and Vice Chair, Department of Emergency Medicine, University of Maryland School of Medicine, Baltimore, Maryland

EDITORS

EVIE MARCOLINI, MD, FACEP, FAAEM
Assistant Professor, Divisions of Neurocritical Care and Emergency Neurology and Surgical Critical Care, Departments of Emergency Medicine and Neurology, Yale University School of Medicine, New Haven, Connecticut

HANEY MALLEMAT, MD
Assistant Professor of Emergency Medicine, University of Maryland School of Medicine, Baltimore, Maryland

AUTHORS

ROBERT T. ARNTFIELD, MD, FRCPC, FCCP
Assistant Professor, Divisions of Emergency Medicine and Critical Care Medicine, London Health Sciences Centre, Western University, London, Ontario, Canada

NEERAJ BADJATIA, MD, MSc
Associate Professor, Departments of Neurology, Anesthesiology and Neurosurgery, University of Maryland School of Medicine, Baltimore, Maryland

KIMBERLY BOSWELL, MD
Assistant Professor, Department of Emergency Medicine, University of Maryland School of Medicine; R Adams Cowley Shock Trauma Center, Baltimore, Maryland

WAN-TSU W. CHANG, MD
Assistant Professor, Department of Emergency Medicine, University of Maryland School of Medicine, Baltimore, Maryland

ILENE CLAUDIUS, MD
Associate Professor of Clinical Emergency Medicine, Keck School of Medicine of the University of Southern California, University of Southern California, Los Angeles, California

PETER DeBLIEUX, MD
Section of Emergency Medicine, LSU Health Sciences Center, New Orleans, Louisiana

SEAN K. GORMAN, BSc(Pharm), PharmD
Regional Coordinator, Clinical Quality and Research; Clinical Pharmacy Specialist, Critical Care, Pharmacy Services, Interior Health Authority, Clinical Associate Professor, Faculty of Pharmaceutical Sciences, The University of British Columbia, Kelowna, British Columbia, Canada

ROBERT S. GREEN, MD, FRCPC, FRCP(Edin)
Departments of Critical Care Medicine and Emergency Medicine; Professor, Faculty of Medicine, Dalhousie University; Medical Director, Trauma Nova Scotia, Halifax, Nova Scotia, Canada

JOHN C. GREENWOOD, MD
Division of Pulmonary and Critical Care Medicine, University of Maryland School of Medicine, Baltimore, Maryland

DANIEL L. HERR, MD
Chief, Critical Care Service; Medical Director, Cardiac Surgery ICU; Associate Professor of Medicine, Shock Trauma Center, University of Maryland School of Medicine, Baltimore, Maryland

JOE KANTER, MD, MPH
Section of Emergency Medicine, LSU Health Sciences Center, New Orleans, Louisiana

JOSHUA KEEGAN, MD
Department of Emergency Medicine, Yale School of Medicine, New Haven, Connecticut

HANEY MALLEMAT, MD
Assistant Professor of Emergency Medicine, University of Maryland School of Medicine, Baltimore, Maryland

EVIE MARCOLINI, MD, FACEP, FAAEM
Assistant Professor, Divisions of Neurocritical Care and Emergency Neurology and Surgical Critical Care, Departments of Emergency Medicine and Neurology, Yale University School of Medicine, New Haven, Connecticut

JAY MENAKER, MD
Associate Professor, Department of Surgery; Associate Professor, Department of Emergency Medicine (Secondary), University of Maryland School of Medicine; R Adams Cowley Shock Trauma Center, Baltimore, Maryland

ANTHONY NOTO, MD
Department of Neurology, University of Rochester, Rochester, New York

TARA ANN PATERSON, MD
Anesthesia Critical Care Fellow, Department of Anesthesiology, R Adams Cowley Shock Trauma Center, Baltimore, Maryland

DANIEL PETERSON, BSc, MD, PhD, FRCPC
University of Calgary, Calgary, Alberta, Canada

EMILY ROSE, MD, FAAEM, FAAP
Pediatric Emergency Medicine Medical Student Elective Director, Assistant Professor of Clinical Emergency Medicine, Keck School of Medicine of the University of Southern California, University of Southern California, Los Angeles, California

MICHAEL C. SCOTT, MD
Fellow, Emergency Medicine/Internal Medicine/Critical Care Program, University of Maryland Medical Center, Baltimore, Maryland

ASHLEY SHREVES, MD
Assistant Professor, Department of Emergency Medicine and Brookdale Department of Geriatrics and Palliative Medicine, Icahn School of Medicine at Mt. Sinai, New York, New York

DEBORAH MICHELLE STEIN, MD, MPH, FACS, FCCM
Associate Professor, Department of Surgery, University of Maryland School of Medicine; Chief of Trauma, R Adams Cowley Shock Trauma Center, Baltimore, Maryland

DAVID A. WACKER, MD, PhD
Fellow, Emergency Medicine/Internal Medicine/Critical Care Program, University of Maryland Medical Center, Baltimore, Maryland

MICHAEL E. WINTERS, MD, FACEP, FAAEM
Associate Professor of Emergency Medicine and Medicine, Co-Director, Emergency Medicine/Internal Medicine/Critical Care Program, University of Maryland School of Medicine, Baltimore, Maryland

CHARLES R. WIRA III, MD
Department of Emergency Medicine, Yale School of Medicine, New Haven, Connecticut

BRIAN J. WRIGHT, MD, MPH, FACEP
Departments of Emergency Medicine and Surgery, Stony Brook University School of Medicine, Stony Brook, New York

Contents

EMERGENCY MEDICINE CLINICS OF NORTH AMERICA

FORTHCOMING ISSUES

February 2015
Management of Hazardous Material Emergencies
Stephen Borron, and
Ziad Kazzi, *Editors*

May 2015
Orthopedic Emergencies
David Della-Giustina, and
Katja Goldflam, *Editors*

August 2015
Cardiovascular Emergencies
Semhar Tewelde, and
Joshua Reynolds, *Editors*

RECENT ISSUES

August 2014
Hematology/Oncology Emergencies
John C. Perkins, and
Jonathan E. Davis, *Editors*

May 2014
Endocrine and Metabolic Emergencies
George C. Willis, and
M. Tyson Pillow, *Editors*

February 2014
Clinical Toxicology
Silas W. Smith, and
Daniel M. Lugassy, *Editors*

RELATED INTEREST

Critical Care Clinics, July 2014 (Vol. 30, No. 3)
Cardiac Emergencies in the ICU
Shashank S. Desai, and Nitin Puri, *Editors*

PROGRAM OBJECTIVE

The goal of *Emergency Medicine Clinics of North America* is to keep practicing emergency medicine physicians and emergency medicine residents up to date with current clinical practice in emergency medicine by providing timely articles reviewing the state of the art in patient care.

TARGET AUDIENCE

All practicing physicians and healthcare professionals who provide patient care utilizing findings from *Emergency Medicine Clinics of North America*.

LEARNING OBJECTIVES

Upon completion of this activity, participants will be able to:

1. Discuss the assessment and treatment of the trauma patient in shock.
2. Review pediatric considerations in the emergency setting.
3. Discuss neurotrauma and neurocritical care.

ACCREDITATION

The Elsevier Office of Continuing Medical Education (EOCME) is accredited by the Accreditation Council for Continuing Medical Education (ACCME) to provide continuing medical education for physicians.

The EOCME designates this enduring material for a maximum of 15 *AMA PRA Category 1 Credit*(s)™. Physicians should claim only the credit commensurate with the extent of their participation in the activity.

All other health care professionals requesting continuing education credit for this enduring material will be issued a certificate of participation.

DISCLOSURE OF CONFLICTS OF INTEREST

The EOCME assesses conflict of interest with its instructors, faculty, planners, and other individuals who are in a position to control the content of CME activities. All relevant conflicts of interest that are identified are thoroughly vetted by EOCME for fair balance, scientific objectivity, and patient care recommendations. EOCME is committed to providing its learners with CME activities that promote improvements or quality in healthcare and not a specific proprietary business or a commercial interest.

The planning committee, staff, authors and editors listed below have identified no financial relationships or relationships to products or devices they or their spouse/life partner have with commercial interest related to the content of this CME activity:

Robert T. Arntfield, MD, FRCPC, FCCP, RDMS; Neeraj Badjatia, MD, MSc; Kimberly A Boswell, MD; Ilene A. Claudius, MD; Peter DeBlieux, MD; Sean K. Gorman, BSc.Pharm., Pharm.D.; Robert Green, MD, FRCPC; John C. Greenwood, MD; Kristen Helm; Daniel L. Herr, MD; Brynne Hunter; Joe Kanter, MD, MPH; Joshua Keegan, MD; Indu Kumari; Sandy Lavery; Haney A. Mallemat, MD; Patrick Manley; Evie G. Marcolini, MD, FACEP, FAAEM; Amal Mattu, MD, FAAEM, FACEP; Jill McNair; Jay Menaker, MD; Anthony G. Noto, MD; Tara Ann Paterson, MD; Daniel Peterson, BSc, MD, PhD; Emily A. Rose, MD, FAAEM, FAAP, FACEP; Michael C. Scott, MD; Ashley E. Shreves, MD; Deborah Michelle Stein, MD, MPH, FACS; Dave Wacker, MD, PhD; Michael E. Winters, MD, FACEP, FAAEM; Charles R. Wira, III, MD; Brian Wright.

The planning committee, staff, authors and editors listed below have identified financial relationships or relationships to products or devices they or their spouse/life partner have with commercial interest related to the content of this CME activity:

UNAPPROVED/OFF-LABEL USE DISCLOSURE

The EOCME requires CME faculty to disclose to the participants:

1. When products or procedures being discussed are off-label, unlabelled, experimental, and/or investigational (not US Food and Drug Administration [FDA] approved); and
2. Any limitations on the information presented, such as data that are preliminary or that represent ongoing research, interim analyses, and/or unsupported opinions. Faculty may discuss information about pharmaceutical agents that is outside of FDA-approved labelling. This information is intended solely for CME and is not intended to promote off-label use of these medications. If you have any questions, contact the medical affairs department of the manufacturer for the most recent prescribing information.

TO ENROLL

To enroll in the *Emergency Medicine Clinics* Continuing Medical Education program, call customer service at 1-800-654-2452 or sign up online at http://www.theclinics.com/home/cme. The CME program is available to subscribers for an additional annual fee of $235 USD.

METHOD OF PARTICIPATION

In order to claim credit, participants must complete the following:

1. Complete enrolment as indicated above.
2. Read the activity.
3. Complete the CME Test and Evaluation. Participants must achieve a score of 70% on the test. All CME Tests and Evaluations must be completed online.

CME INQUIRIES/SPECIAL NEEDS

For all CME inquiries or special needs, please contact elsevierCME@elsevier.com.

Foreword
Critical Care Emergencies

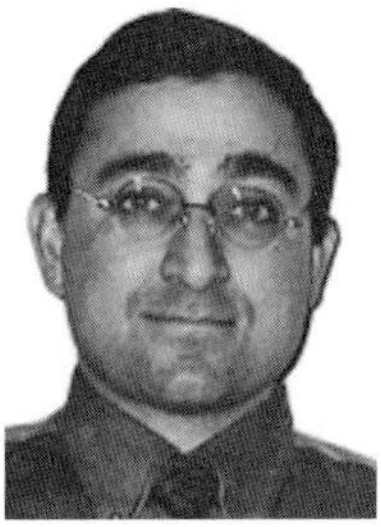

Amal Mattu, MD, FAAEM, FACEP
Consulting Editor

Although critical care medicine has always been a significant part of the specialty of emergency medicine, its practice in the Emergency Department (ED) has never been as prevalent before as it is today. There are several reasons for this evolving change. First, overcrowding continues to be a pervasive and increasing problem in EDs throughout the United States as well as numerous other countries. As a result, critically ill patients are boarded in the ED, awaiting beds in intensive care units that are already filled, and care of these boarded patients falls on emergency care providers. Another reason for the increase in critical care practice in the ED is related to the aging population. First-world countries around the world are reporting a steady increase in their geriatric population, and those patients are bringing their acute medical needs to the ED in increasing numbers. Because of their multiple comorbidities, they tend to have more complicated disease and arrive much sicker than their younger counterparts. A third consideration is that the national increase in outpatient clinics and urgent care centers is pulling the less sick patients away from EDs, leaving a relative increase in critically ill patients in the EDs. These are only just a few of the reasons for the increase in critical care medicine being practiced in the ED.

The increased need for emergency care providers to have a sound knowledge in critical care medicine is now well-recognized. Educational conferences in emergency medicine have increased the amount of teaching that is dedicated to caring for the critically ill. In fact, there are many new conferences over the past five years that have arisen that are focused specifically on teaching critical care to emergency physicians. Many critical care ultrasound and critical care procedures courses have been developed. New textbooks focused on critical care-emergency medicine have been published. Residencies in emergency medicine are increasing their critical care training and ICU rotations, and the number of emergency physicians doing fellowships in critical care has skyrocketed in recent years.

Drs Evie Marcolini and Haney Mallemat have now stepped forward by providing an issue of *Emergency Medicine Clinics of North America* that is sure to be recognized as

Emerg Med Clin N Am 32 (2014) xv–xvi
http://dx.doi.org/10.1016/j.emc.2014.09.002 emed.theclinics.com

another invaluable, cutting-edge resource for emergency health care providers that are interested in increasing their critical care knowledge and skills. Both of these guest editors are emergency physicians that have obtained additional fellowship training and board certification in critical care. They intimately know the challenges of caring for all of these types of critically ill patients in the ED.

Drs Marcolini and Mallemat have created a list of topics that are pertinent to ED providers caring for critically ill patients, and they have assembled an outstanding group of authors to discuss the topics. Authors include physicians experienced in all aspects of critical care—medical, surgical, neurologic, and trauma. They address bread-and-butter topics such as the approach to shock, approach to trauma and neurotrauma, sepsis, pressors and inotropes, ventilator management, antimicrobials, and pediatric critical care. They also cover more in-depth "hot" topics such as managing coagulopathies, critical care ultrasound, lung-protective ventilation strategies, and advanced techniques in assessment of volume status and hemodynamics. Throughout all of the articles, however, they go beyond the basics and address recent advances and controversies.

This issue of *Emergency Medicine Clinics of North America* is an invaluable addition to emergency medicine education. This issue should be considered must-reading not only for practicing emergency physicians but also for emergency medicine trainees and for any other health care providers that are responsible for caring for critically ill patients. Knowledge and practice of the concepts that are discussed in the following pages are certain to save lives. Our sincere thanks go to the guest editors and the authors for their time and commitment to this important issue.

Amal Mattu, MD, FAAEM, FACEP
Department of Emergency Medicine
University of Maryland School of Medicine
Baltimore, MD 21201, USA

E-mail address:
amattu@smail.umaryland.edu

Preface

Critical Care

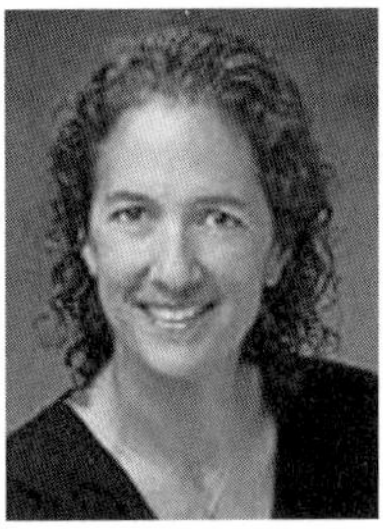

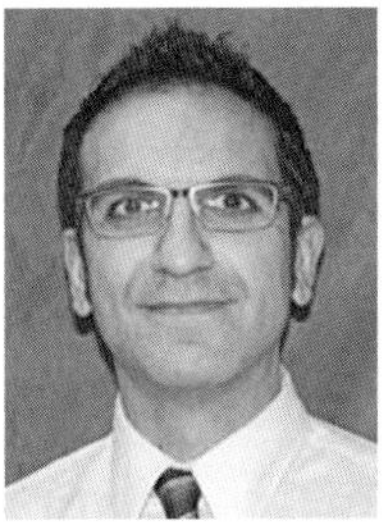

Evie Marcolini, MD Haney Mallemat, MD
Editors

Emergency medicine physicians have been practicing critical care in the emergency department ever since our specialty was recognized more than 40 years ago. We are no strangers to critically ill patients, and we are trained to resuscitate and stabilize the sickest of them. Because of the exceptional care we are able to provide to critically ill patients, we have gained recognition and respect within the critical care community, including opportunities to become fellowship trained with board certification through the specialties of internal medicine, surgery, anesthesia, and neurology.

The prevalence of critically ill patients in the emergency department population is on the rise. Several factors are contributing to this increase, including the aging of the population, our access to more advanced technology, and, subsequently, the complexity of patients' presentations (eg, following organ transplantation or insertion of a left ventricular assist device). In addition, constraints on the health care system are limiting the number of available ICU beds, forcing critically ill patients to remain in the emergency department for extended periods of time. Therefore, emergency physicians have had to become experts in delivering complex care that once was traditionally managed "upstairs" in the ICU (eg., weaning patients from ventilators and providing palliative care).

Like emergency medicine, critical care is a constantly evolving specialty with a rapidly advancing literature and continuous technological advancements. Emergency medicine physicians must change with the times and keep up with the new knowledge in this field. The most recent *Emergency Medicine Clinics of North America* issue devoted to critical care was published in 2008. During the 6 years since then, much has changed. Our goals for this *Emergency Medicine Clinics of North America* issue were to cover the "bread and butter" of critical care delivered in the emergency department as well as to update you on recent changes in the field that will enhance your practice. This issue presents articles on assessing fluid responsiveness, the use of ultrasound during initial resuscitation and evaluation, providing cardiopulmonary mechanical support, and helping patients and families address end-of-life issues.

Emerg Med Clin N Am 32 (2014) xvii–xviii
http://dx.doi.org/10.1016/j.emc.2014.09.001 emed.theclinics.com
0733-8627/14/$ – see front matter

We are grateful to the highly qualified authors whose hard work has created an outstanding *Emergency Medicine Clinics of North America* issue that we hope will serve as a critical care reference for emergency physicians. We also thank the consulting editor, Dr Amal Mattu, for giving us the opportunity to edit this issue of *Emergency Medicine Clinics of North America*. We are very proud of this issue, and we hope you will learn as much from it as we did during the editing process.

Evie Marcolini, MD
Divisions of Neurocritical Care and Emergency Neurology and Surgical Critical Care
Departments of Emergency Medicine and Neurology
Yale University School of Medicine
464 Congress St. Suite 260
New Haven, CT 06519, USA

Haney Mallemat, MD
University of Maryland School of Medicine
110 South Paca Street, 6th Floor, Suite 200
Baltimore, MD 21201, USA

E-mail addresses:
emarcolini@gmail.com (E. Marcolini)
haney.mallemat@gmail.com (H. Mallemat)

Shock

David A. Wacker, MD, PhD[a], Michael E. Winters, MD[b,*]

KEYWORDS

• Shock • Massive pulmonary embolism • Cardiac tamponade
• Tension pneumothorax • Hypovolemia • Hemorrhage • Anaphylaxis
• Acute myocardial infarction

KEY POINTS

- Critically ill patients with undifferentiated shock are complex and challenging cases in the emergency department.
- A systematic approach to patients assessment and management is essential to prevent unnecessary morbidity and mortality.
- The simplified, systematic approach described in this article focuses on determining the presence of a pump, tank, or pipe problem.

INTRODUCTION

Shock is defined as a state of insufficient perfusion and oxygen delivery to the tissues. Regardless of the cause, mortality rates of patients with shock remain high, ranging from 40% to 60% for those with septic shock and approaching 40% for those with hemorrhagic shock.[1,2] Patients with shock commonly present to the emergency department (ED) and require rapid assessment and initiation of treatment to prevent unnecessary increases in morbidity and mortality. As a result, it is imperative that the emergency physician be expert in the rapid identification, assessment, and treatment of patients with shock. This article describes a systematic approach to the evaluation and management of the ED patient with undifferentiated shock, with attention to rapidly identifying conditions that require time-sensitive therapy.

PATHOPHYSIOLOGY

Although the circulatory system is complex and depends on a multitude of variables, it can be simplified to three main components: cardiac function (the pump), intravascular

---

Disclosures: None.
The article was copyedited by Linda J. Kesselring, MS, ELS, the technical editor-writer in the Department of Emergency Medicine at the University of Maryland School of Medicine.
[a] Emergency Medicine/Internal Medicine/Critical Care Program, University of Maryland Medical Center, 110 South Paca Street, 6th Floor, Suite 200, Baltimore, MD 21201, USA; [b] Emergency Medicine/Internal Medicine/Critical Care Program, University of Maryland School of Medicine, 110 South Paca Street, 6th Floor, Suite 200, Baltimore, MD 21201, USA
* Corresponding author.
E-mail address: mwinters@umem.org

Emerg Med Clin N Am 32 (2014) 747–758
http://dx.doi.org/10.1016/j.emc.2014.07.003 **emed.theclinics.com**
0733-8627/14/$ – see front matter

volume (the tank), and systemic vascular resistance (the pipes). In normal conditions, intravascular volume is adequate to maintain cardiac preload, stroke volume and heart rate are adequate to maintain cardiac output, and systemic vascular resistance is preserved to maintain sufficient perfusion to the tissues. In shock, malfunction occurs with the pump, tank, or pipes, such that perfusion and oxygen delivery are impaired. Acute pump malfunction can be caused by arrhythmias, conditions that result in a sudden decrease in cardiac contractility or by extracardiac conditions that obstruct cardiac output.[3] Acute tank malfunction primarily results from a decrease in intravascular volume due to hemorrhage or volume loss. Significant volume loss leads to decreases in venous return and impaired left ventricular preload. Acute tank dysfunction can also result from conditions that mechanically obstruct venous return. Malfunction of the pipes is commonly seen in septic shock and is generally caused by cytokine-induced vasodilation.[4] Alteration in vascular tone is also a common feature of anaphylactic shock, caused by the release of histamine and other immune mediators.[5] Regardless of the underlying mechanism of shock, if impaired perfusion and oxygen delivery are not recognized and reversed, organ dysfunction, tissue necrosis, and death rapidly ensue.

CAUSES

The causes of shock are innumerable and difficult to remember at the bedside of a critically ill patient. Notwithstanding, they can be categorized into conditions that result in pump, tank, or pipe dysfunction. Critical conditions that require time-sensitive therapy and should be considered early in the evaluation of ED patients with shock are listed in **Box 1**.

Box 1
Critical causes of shock

- Pump dysfunction
  - Mechanical obstruction
    - Pericardial tamponade
    - Massive pulmonary embolus
  - Acute myocardial infarction
  - Acute valvular insufficiency
  - Arrhythmia
- Tank dysfunction
  - Hemorrhage
  - Hypovolemia
  - Tension pneumothorax
  - Abdominal compartment syndrome
- Pipe dysfunction
  - Anaphylaxis
  - Sepsis
  - Vascular catastrophes
    - Ruptured abdominal aortic aneurysm
    - Aortic dissection

CLINICAL PRESENTATION

Signs and symptoms of shock reflect impaired oxygen delivery and decreased organ perfusion. In mild shock, physiologic compensation might mask these deficits, resulting initially in nonspecific symptoms such as malaise, weakness, and fatigue. As shock progresses and the patient becomes decompensated, more classic signs and symptoms emerge, including alterations in mental status, tachycardia, hypoxemia, mottled skin, decreased urine output, and hypotension. Importantly, the absence of hypotension should not be used to exclude shock. Inadequate perfusion can occur despite a normal blood pressure reading, especially in patients with preexisting hypertension.

INITIAL ED ASSESSMENT

General

A focused history and physical examination should be performed to guide the diagnostic evaluation in identifying a pump, tank, or pipe problem. An ECG and portable chest radiograph (CXR) should be obtained as soon as possible. Laboratory studies that should be requested in the assessment of ED patients with undifferentiated shock include a comprehensive metabolic panel, complete blood count, coagulation profile, troponin, type and screen, beta-human chorionic gonadotropin for women of reproductive age, and serum lactate concentration (venous or arterial).[6,7] In recent years, emergency ultrasound has emerged as a critical tool in evaluating the ED patient with undifferentiated shock and should be used early in the evaluation.[8]

Pump Assessment

When evaluating the patient with undifferentiated shock, focus first on assessing pump function. Acute pump dysfunction can be caused by mechanical obstruction of cardiac output (eg, tamponade, massive pulmonary embolism [PE]), acute valvular insufficiency, or arrhythmia. Ultrasound is critical in evaluating the pericardial space, the relative size of the left and right ventricles, and overall left ventricular function. The ultrasound examination should be performed systematically to decrease the probability of errors. Although many systematic approaches have been described in the literature, the authors prefer to start with a parasternal long-axis view to assess left ventricular contractility. This is followed by an apical four-chamber view to assess right ventricular contractility and size in relation to the left ventricle. Finally, a subxiphoid view is used to assess the pericardial space for the presence of an effusion.

Pericardial effusion with tamponade must be diagnosed promptly. The physical examination findings with the highest sensitivity for tamponade are pulsus paradoxus (82%), tachycardia (77%), and elevated jugular venous pressure (76%).[9] Less specific findings are Beck triad (hypotension, muffled heart sounds, elevated jugular venous pressure) and Kussmaul sign.[10,11] ECG findings associated with tamponade include tachycardia, low-voltage QRS complexes, and electrical alternans. Though the sensitivity of electrical alternans is only 25%, it is highly specific for tamponade.[9,12] Cardiomegaly may be seen on CXR in patients with tamponade but its specificity is poor; this finding is more reflective of a chronic pericardial effusion.[9] Ultimately, ultrasound remains the gold standard for detecting pericardial effusion with tamponade. Emergency physicians trained in ultrasound can reliably detect the presence of pericardial effusion and evaluate the degree of tamponade.[13,14] Classic ultrasound findings of tamponade include an anechoic space (ie, pericardial fluid), collapse of the right atrium in systole, collapse of the right ventricle in early diastole, and lack of respiratory variation in the inferior vena cava (**Fig. 1**).

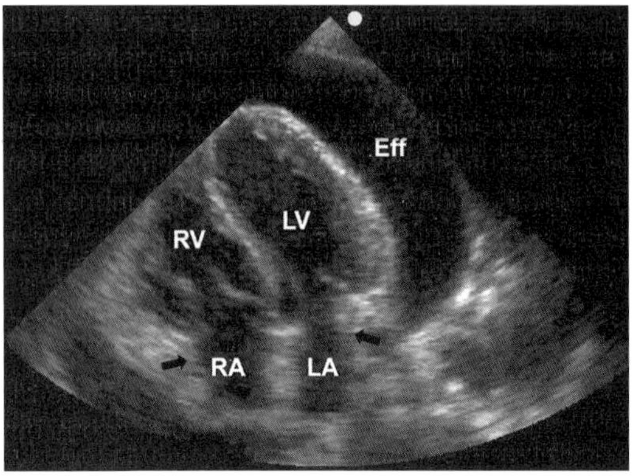

Fig. 1. Ultrasound findings associated with tamponade. Four-chamber apical view of the heart demonstrates a large pericardial effusion (Eff) associated with collapse of both the left atrium (LA) and right atrium (RA) in late diastole (*black solid arrows*). Other signs of tamponade include collapse of the right ventricle (RV) during early diastole and loss of respiratory variation of inferior vena cava (IVC) diameter. LV, left ventricle. (*Courtesy of* H. Mallemat, MD, Baltimore, MD.)

Similar to tamponade, massive PE is another cause of obstructive pump dysfunction that must be diagnosed rapidly. Classic physical examination findings of massive PE include tachycardia, tachypnea, and hypoxemia. Unfortunately, these signs are insensitive and nonspecific for PE.[15,16] An important ECG abnormality suggestive of PE is the presence of T-wave inversion in leads V1 through V4.[17] Emergency ultrasound can provide important clues to the diagnosis of massive PE. In normal conditions, the right ventricle is approximately 60% of the size of the left ventricle. Any increase in the ratio of the right ventricle to the left ventricle indicates right ventricular strain and suggests the presence of PE. Additional ultrasound findings associated with massive PE include hypokinesis of the right ventricle, paradoxic movement of the intraventricular septum toward the left ventricle, and tricuspid valve regurgitation (**Fig. 2**).

In addition to considering tamponade and massive PE, it is important to assess for primary cardiac failure. Acute myocardial infarction (AMI) remains the most common cause of acute left ventricular dysfunction and must be excluded early in the evaluation of patients with undifferentiated shock.[18] Physical examination findings commonly associated with cardiogenic shock due to AMI include cool extremities, jugular venous distention, and pulmonary edema.[19] The presence of ST-segment elevation on the ECG should be detected immediately. The absence of ST-segment elevation on the ECG does not exclude the diagnosis of cardiogenic shock. Ultrasound can be used to assess for acute wall motion abnormalities of the left ventricle, which indicates AMI. Importantly, the emergency physician should also assess the global function of the left ventricle, which can be described as normal, reduced, or hyperdynamic. This delineation is vital in planning the treatment of patients with undifferentiated shock. Mild elevations in troponin are frequently seen in shock patients and generally indicate impaired organ perfusion. Large elevations indicate AMI and a primary cardiac cause of shock.

Tank Assessment

Tank dysfunction is caused primarily by the depletion of intravascular volume. Hypovolemia and hemorrhage, the most common causes of intravascular volume

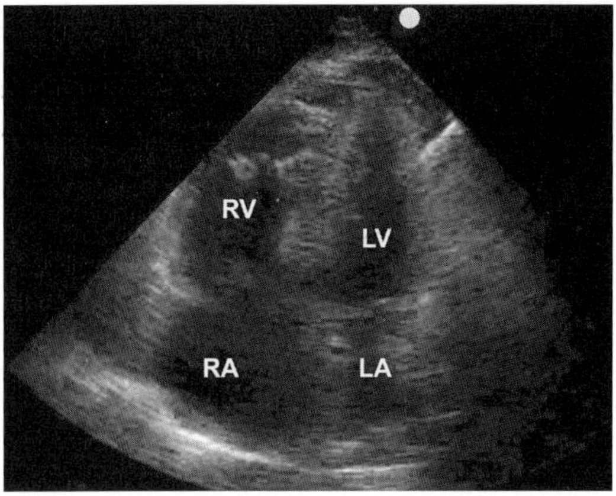

Fig. 2. Ultrasound findings associated with right ventricular strain. Four-chamber apical view of the heart demonstrates enlargement of right ventricle (RV) relative to the left ventricle (LV), as in the setting of RV strain. Usually, the RV is less than 60% the size of the LV. Enlargement of the RV to equal to or exceeding the size of the LV is suggestive of abnormally high RV pressures. Here the right atrium (RA) is also dilated, suggesting elevated RA pressure. LA, left atrium. (*Courtesy of* H. Mallemat, MD, Baltimore, MD.)

depletion, are usually suggested by the history of present illness. Physical examination findings associated with hemorrhagic shock include tachycardia, tachypnea, mental status change, and hypotension.[20] A rectal examination should be performed in the initial assessment of patients with undifferentiated shock to assess for the presence of massive gastrointestinal hemorrhage. As in the assessment of pump dysfunction, ultrasound plays a central role in the initial assessment of tank dysfunction. Though limitations exist, ultrasound measurements of the inferior vena cava can provide valuable information in determining a patient's responsiveness to intravenous fluid therapy. For example, a small diameter of the inferior vena cava that changes significantly with respirations suggests marked intravascular volume depletion. In contrast, a large diameter of the inferior vena cava that has minimal variation with respirations may indicate adequate intravascular volume status or acute pump dysfunction (eg, tamponade, massive PE). The reliability and reproducibility of inferior vena cava measurements depend on whether the patient is intubated and ventilated or spontaneously breathing. The predictive value of inferior vena cava variation unfortunately is less reliable in patients who are breathing spontaneously.[21]

In addition to these assessments of intravascular volume status and fluid responsiveness, ultrasound should be used to look for fluid in the abdominal and chest cavities, suggestive of a traumatic intra-abdominal injury, ruptured ectopic pregnancy, or hemothorax.[22–25]

Acute tank dysfunction can also be caused by mechanical compression of the great vessels, resulting in impaired venous return, and decreased cardiac output. Two conditions that should be considered and excluded during the initial assessment of patients with undifferentiated shock are tension pneumothorax and abdominal compartment syndrome. Physical examination findings associated with tension pneumothorax include tachypnea, decreased breath sounds, and hypertympany on the affected side. When a CXR is delayed or not immediately available, ultrasound can be used to detect pneumothorax and initiate needle decompression. Abdominal compartment syndrome impairs venous return by directly compressing the inferior vena cava,[26] which usually occurs when the intra-abdominal pressure exceeds 15 mm Hg.[27] Unfortunately, physical examination is ineffective for detecting elevations in intra-abdominal pressure. Intravesicular pressure measurement is currently the gold standard for diagnosing abdominal compartment syndrome and should be obtained when the diagnosis is considered. An intra-abdominal pressure greater than 20 mm Hg associated with new organ dysfunction confirms the diagnosis of abdominal compartment syndrome.[27]

Pipe Assessment

Following an assessment of the pump and tank, the emergency physician should assess the patient for pipe dysfunction. Loss of arterial tone decreases perfusion throughout the body and leads to impaired oxygen delivery despite a normal, or elevated, cardiac output. Two conditions that result in loss of arterial tone and should be considered in the initial assessment of ED shock patients are anaphylaxis and sepsis. Anaphylaxis is a clinical diagnosis and should be suspected when any of the following criteria are met: (1) skin or mucosal involvement with acute onset of respiratory distress or hypotension following exposure to a known antigen, (2) any involvement of two or more organ systems (respiratory, skin or mucosa, gastrointestinal, cardiovascular) following exposure to a possible, or (3) hypotension following exposure to a known antigen.[28] If sepsis is suspected, the initial assessment should be directed toward identifying the source of infection. Common locations are the pulmonary and genitourinary tracts, the abdomen, skin and soft tissue, and indwelling catheters and devices.

Aortic catastrophes, namely aortic dissection and ruptured aortic aneurysm, should be considered as a cause of pipe dysfunction. In addition to the traditional risk factors of hypertension, male gender, smoking, and advanced age, cocaine use and pregnancy are also risk factors for aortic dissection. Physical examination findings commonly associated with aortic dissection include hypertension, blood pressure differentials between extremities, pulse deficits, and neurologic deficits. Unfortunately, the sensitivity of these findings is less than 30%.[29] The most common CXR finding in thoracic aortic dissection is an abnormality of the mediastinum, which has a sensitivity of approximately 90%.[29] For assessment of abdominal aortic catastrophes, ultrasound is an important tool. The presence of an abdominal aortic aneurysm in the setting of undifferentiated shock should be considered a rupture until proven otherwise. Although ultrasound is excellent at revealing the presence of an enlarged abdominal aorta, it is less sensitive and cannot be used to exclude abnormalities of the thoracic aorta.

INITIAL ED MANAGEMENT

Regardless of the cause, the initial steps in the management of patients with undifferentiated shock are similar. Airway and breathing should be assessed, keeping a low threshold for intubation and mechanical ventilation. Patients with continued evidence of tissue hypoxia should be intubated, even in the absence of acute respiratory failure. This will reduce the work of breathing, decrease the amount of oxygen needed by the respiratory muscles, and increase oxygen delivery to other vital organs. Large-bore intravenous access should be established, and fluid resuscitation with an isotonic crystalloid infusion should be started. In all patients with shock, accurate monitoring of urine output is essential; therefore, a Foley catheter should be placed early in the assessment. Additional therapy in the ED depends on the cause of the shock.

Pump Dysfunction

Pericardiocentesis remains the definitive treatment of shock caused by cardiac tamponade. Importantly, there are no contraindications to this emergent procedure.[30] When performing this procedure blindly, elevate the head of the bed so that fluid accumulates inferiorly. Insert the needle between the xyphoid process and left costal margin. Advance the needle at a 30° to 45° angle. Once it is under the costal margin, decrease the angle to 15° to 30° and advance the needle toward the left shoulder.[12,30] When possible, perform pericardiocentesis using ultrasound guidance. With ultrasound, the physician can choose the shortest route toward the largest fluid pocket and follow the needle into the pericardial sac. With ultrasound guidance, the complication rate of pericardiocentesis drops to 1% to 3.5%.[30]

Acute pump dysfunction resulting from massive PE is associated with a mortality rate approaching 60%.[31] The American College of Chest Physicians (ACCP) and the American Heart Association (AHA) both recommend the use of either fibrinolytic therapy or invasive methods to remove the clot.[32,33] Though large randomized studies are lacking, meta-analyses of reports of the use of fibrinolytic therapy for massive PE indicate a number needed to treat of just 10.[34] Alteplase is the most common fibrinolytic agent administered; however, there are no studies to demonstrate its superiority to other agents in the setting of massive PE. Both the ACCP and AHA recommend brief intravenous infusion times (2 hours) for fibrinolytic therapy.[32,33] For patients with contraindications to that approach, invasive methods to remove the clot should be pursued. Catheter-directed techniques include removal of the embolus by aspiration or fragmentation of the clot by direct mechanical disruption.[33] To date, no large randomized studies have evaluated these techniques. A clot can also be removed directly by surgical embolectomy. Available data on embolectomy (primarily limited to case series) indicate long-term survival rates ranging from 83% to 93%.[35–37] Some investigators recommend surgical embolectomy as the first-line treatment of patients with massive PE who fail fibrinolytic therapy.[36]

Patients with acute pump dysfunction secondary to ST-segment myocardial infarction require emergent revascularization with percutaneous coronary intervention (PCI).[38] If PCI is unavailable or if access to it will be prolonged, fibrinolytic therapy is indicated.[38] Mechanical support with an intra-aortic balloon pump (IABP) has long been considered a mainstay of therapy as a bridge to PCI in patients with cardiogenic shock. A recent randomized trial of more than 600 subjects with cardiogenic shock failed to demonstrate an improvement in the mortality rate with the use of an IABP.[39] Therefore, an IABP should not be used routinely in cardiogenic shock patients awaiting emergent PCI.

Tank Dysfunction

An isotonic crystalloid solution should be administered to patients with shock associated with intravascular volume depletion. Crystalloid solutions are commonly divided into saline and balanced solutions. Importantly, normal saline is not a true physiologic solution and will reliably induce hyperchloremic metabolic acidosis when given in large quantities. Balanced solutions are more physiologic, including lactated Ringer, Plasma-Lyte, Isolyte-E, and Hartmann solution. Although no randomized controlled study has demonstrated superiority of balanced solutions over saline, the authors prefer to administer a balanced solution to patients with severe or worsening acidosis. Colloid solutions, such as hetastarch, are popular in some regions of the world. Recent studies on colloids, however, demonstrated an increased incidence of acute kidney injury and failed to demonstrate a decrease in the mortality rate.[40–42] As a result, crystalloid solutions remain the resuscitation fluid of choice for patients with hypovolemic shock. The total amount of fluid administered depends on the type of shock and the patient's response to treatment. For patients with septic shock, current international guidelines recommend 30 mL/kg of crystalloid fluid as an initial dose.[43] Additional fluid administration is guided by the use of dynamic markers of fluid responsiveness, such as inferior vena cava variation. In general, intravenous fluids should be administered with targets of a mean arterial blood pressure of at least 65 mm Hg and a urine output greater than 0.5 mL/kg/h.

The management of patients with tank dysfunction caused by hemorrhage hinges on replacement of blood components and source control. For patients receiving more than 10 units of packed red blood cells (PRBCs), improved outcomes have been demonstrated when receiving PRBCs, fresh frozen plasma, and platelets in a 1:1:1 ratio.[44] Source control depends on the cause of the bleeding and can include emergency surgery, vascular embolization, or other invasive procedures. Additional pharmacologic therapies have proven valuable in mitigating bleeding in some patients awaiting intervention. Tranexamic acid (TXA) is an amino acid derivative that binds plasminogen and prevents conversion to its active fibrinolytic form. Recent studies suggest that the early administration of TXA to patients with severe traumatic hemorrhage reduces the mortality rate.[45,46] Prothrombin complex concentrate (PCC) is a mixture of purified vitamin-K-dependent clotting factors designed for use in patients taking vitamin K antagonists (VKAs) (eg, warfarin) with significant bleeding. Early studies suggest that PCC reverses VKA-induced coagulopathy efficiently and significantly faster than fresh frozen plasma.[47] Its use is recommended for patients with VKA-associated major bleeding.[48] Similar effects have been noted in patients with non-VKA–induced coagulopathy.[49] Recombinant activated factor VII has also been proposed for treating patients with life-threatening hemorrhage, particularly intracranial bleeding. Early studies have not convincingly shown an improvement in outcome with this therapy. In addition, it is associated with a significant increase in the rate of arterial thromboembolism.[50,51] Therefore, its use cannot be recommended at this time.

The management of tank dysfunction resulting from tension pneumothorax centers on decompression of the pleural space with tube thoracostomy. Needle decompression is often used as a temporizing measure while preparing for tube thoracostomy. Traditionally, the needle is inserted into the second intercostal space in the midclavicular line of the affected side. Recent evidence suggests that the fifth intercostal space in the midaxillary line might provide more reliable decompression.[52–54] Regardless of the space used, needle decompression must be followed by tube thoracostomy to provide a stable and reliable route for evacuation of air from the pleural space.

Pipe Dysfunction

See the article elsewhere in this issue for further exploration of the treatment of patients with pipe dysfunction related to septic shock.

For patients with anaphylaxis, epinephrine remains the drug of choice.[28] Epinephrine, at a dose of 0.5 mg, should be given intramuscularly into the anterolateral thigh as soon as the diagnosis is suspected. This can be repeated at 5-minute intervals as needed. Patients with anaphylaxis can rapidly extravasate up to one-third of their circulating volume into the tissues within minutes after the onset of disease.[28] Therefore, aggressive fluid resuscitation with an isotonic crystalloid solution should be undertaken as soon as possible. Second-line medications, namely antihistamines and corticosteroids, should never be given in lieu of epinephrine to patients with anaphylaxis. For patients who do not respond to repeated doses of intramuscular injections of epinephrine, an infusion should be started at 1 μg/min. The dosage can be titrated by 1 μg/min every 5 minutes to a maximum of 10 μg/min, based on the patient's clinical response.

SUMMARY

Critically ill patients with undifferentiated shock are complex and challenging cases in the ED. A systematic approach to their assessment and management is essential to prevent unnecessary morbidity and mortality. The simplified, systematic approach described in this article focuses on determining the presence of a pump, tank, or pipe problem. With this approach, the emergency physician can detect select life-threatening conditions and implement time-sensitive therapy.

REFERENCES

1. Martin GS. Sepsis, severe sepsis and septic shock: changes in incidence, pathogens and outcomes. Expert Rev Anti Infect Ther 2012;10:701–6.
2. Heckbert SR, Vedder NB, Hoffman W, et al. Outcome after hemorrhagic shock in trauma patients. J Trauma 1998;45:545–9.
3. Reynolds HR, Hochman JS. Cardiogenic shock: current concepts and improving outcomes. Circulation 2008;117:686–97.
4. Angus DC, van der Poll T. Severe sepsis and septic shock. N Engl J Med 2013;369:2063.
5. De Bisschop MB, Bellou A. Anaphylaxis. Curr Opin Crit Care 2012;18:308–17.
6. Weil MH, Michaels S, Rackow EC. Comparison of blood lactate concentrations in central venous, pulmonary artery, and arterial blood. Crit Care Med 1987;15:489–90.
7. Gallagher EJ, Rodriguez K, Touger M. Agreement between peripheral venous and arterial lactate levels. Ann Emerg Med 1997;29:479–83.
8. Perera P, Mailhot T, Riley D, et al. The RUSH exam: rapid ultrasound in shock in the evaluation of the critically Ill. Emerg Med Clin North Am 2010;28:29–56.
9. Roy CL, Minor MA, Brookhart MA, et al. Does this patient with a pericardial effusion have cardiac tamponade? JAMA 2007;297:1810–8.
10. Cooper JP, Oliver RM, Currie P, et al. How do the clinical findings in patients with pericardial effusions influence the success of aspiration? Br Heart J 1995;73:351–4.
11. Guberman BA, Fowler NO, Engel PJ, et al. Cardiac tamponade in medical patients. Circulation 1981;64:633–40.
12. Spodick DH. Acute cardiac tamponade. N Engl J Med 2003;349:684–90.
13. Mandavia DP, Hoffner RJ, Mahaney K, et al. Bedside echocardiography by emergency physicians. Ann Emerg Med 2001;38:377–82.
14. Manasia AR, Nagaraj HM, Kodali RB, et al. Feasibility and potential clinical utility of goal-directed transthoracic echocardiography performed by noncardiologist intensivists using a small hand-carried device (SonoHeart) in critically ill patients. J Cardiothorac Vasc Anesth 2005;19:155–9.
15. Stein PD, Beemath A, Matta F, et al. Clinical characteristics of patients with acute pulmonary embolism: data from PIOPED II. Am J Med 2007;120:871–9.
16. Pollack CV, Schreiber D, Goldhaber SZ, et al. Clinical characteristics, management, and outcomes of patients diagnosed with acute pulmonary embolism in the emergency department: initial report of EMPEROR (Multicenter Emergency Medicine Pulmonary Embolism in the Real World Registry). J Am Coll Cardiol 2011;57:700–6.

17. Vanni S, Polidori G, Vergara R, et al. Prognostic value of ECG among patients with acute pulmonary embolism and normal blood pressure. Am J Med 2009; 122:257–64.
18. Goldberg RJ, Spencer FA, Gore JM, et al. Thirty-year trends (1975 to 2005) in the magnitude of, management of, and hospital death rates associated with cardiogenic shock in patients with acute myocardial infarction: a population-based perspective. Circulation 2009;119:1211–9.
19. Klein T, Ramani GV. Assessment and management of cardiogenic shock in the emergency department. Cardiol Clin 2012;30:651–64.
20. Gutierrez G, Reines HD, Wulf-Gutierrez ME. Clinical review: hemorrhagic shock. Crit Care 2004;8:373–81.
21. Heenen S, De Backer D, Vincent JL. How can the response to volume expansion in patients with spontaneous respiratory movements be predicted? Crit Care 2006;10:R102.
22. Patel NY, Riherd JM. Focused assessment with sonography for trauma: methods, accuracy, and indications. Surg Clin North Am 2011;91:195–207.
23. Quinn AC, Sinert R. What is the utility of the focused assessment with sonography in trauma (FAST) exam in penetrating torso trauma? Injury 2011;42: 482–7.
24. Rose JS. Ultrasound in abdominal trauma. Emerg Med Clin North Am 2004;22: 581–99.
25. Sisley AC, Rozycki GS, Ballard RB, et al. Rapid detection of traumatic effusion using surgeon-performed ultrasonography. J Trauma 1998;44:291–7.
26. Hedenstierna G, Larsson A. Influence of abdominal pressure on respiratory and abdominal organ function. Curr Opin Crit Care 2012;18:80–5.
27. Al-Mufarrej F, Abell LM, Chawla LS. Understanding intra-abdominal hypertension: from the bench to the bedside. J Intensive Care Med 2012;27:145–60.
28. Simons FE, Ardusso LR, Bilo MB, et al. World allergy organization guidelines for the assessment and management of anaphylaxis. World Allergy Organ J 2011; 4:13–37.
29. Klompas M. Does this patient have an acute thoracic aortic dissection? JAMA 2002;287:2262–72.
30. L'Italien AJ. Critical cardiovascular skills and procedures in the emergency department. Emerg Med Clin North Am 2013;31:151–206.
31. Goldhaber SZ, Visani L, De Rosa M. Acute pulmonary embolism: clinical outcomes in the International Cooperative Pulmonary Embolism Registry (ICOPER). Lancet 1999;353:1386–9.
32. Kearon C, Akl EA, Comerota AJ, et al. Antithrombotic therapy for VTE disease: Antithrombotic Therapy and Prevention of Thrombosis, 9th ed: American College of Chest Physicians Evidence-Based Clinical Practice Guidelines. Chest 2012;141:e419S–94S.
33. Jaff MR, McMurtry MS, Archer SL, et al. Management of massive and submassive pulmonary embolism, iliofemoral deep vein thrombosis, and chronic thromboembolic pulmonary hypertension: a scientific statement from the American Heart Association. Circulation 2011;123:1788–830.
34. Wan S, Quinlan DJ, Agnelli G, et al. Thrombolysis compared with heparin for the initial treatment of pulmonary embolism: a meta-analysis of the randomized controlled trials. Circulation 2004;110:744–9.
35. Fukuda I, Taniguchi S, Fukui K, et al. Improved outcome of surgical pulmonary embolectomy by aggressive intervention for critically ill patients. Ann Thorac Surg 2011;91:728–32.

36. Meneveau N, Seronde MF, Blonde MC, et al. Management of unsuccessful thrombolysis in acute massive pulmonary embolism. Chest 2006;129:1043–50.
37. Leacche M, Unic D, Goldhaber SZ, et al. Modern surgical treatment of massive pulmonary embolism: results in 47 consecutive patients after rapid diagnosis and aggressive surgical approach. J Thorac Cardiovasc Surg 2005;129:1018–23.
38. O'Gara PT, Kushner FG, Ascheim DD, et al. 2013 ACCF/AHA guideline for the management of ST-elevation myocardial infarction: a report of the American College of Cardiology Foundation/American Heart Association Task Force on Practice Guidelines. Circulation 2013;127:e362–425.
39. Thiele H, Zeymer U, Neumann FJ, et al. Intraaortic balloon support for myocardial infarction with cardiogenic shock. N Engl J Med 2012;367:1287–96.
40. Myburgh JA, Finfer S, Bellomo R, et al. Hydroxyethyl starch or saline for fluid resuscitation in intensive care. N Engl J Med 2012;367:1901–11.
41. Guidet B, Martinet O, Boulain T, et al. Assessment of hemodynamic efficacy and safety of 6% hydroxyethylstarch 130/0.4 vs. 0.9% NaCl fluid replacement in patients with severe sepsis: The CRYSTMAS study. Crit Care 2012;16:R94.
42. Perner A, Haase N, Guttormsen AB, et al. Hydroxyethyl starch 130/0.42 versus Ringer's acetate in severe sepsis. N Engl J Med 2012;367:124–34.
43. Dellinger RP, Levy MM, Rhodes A, et al. Surviving Sepsis Campaign: international guidelines for management of severe sepsis and septic shock, 2012. Crit Care Med 2013;41:580–637.
44. Holcomb JB, Zarzabal LA, Michalek JE, et al. Increased platelet:RBC ratios are associated with improved survival after massive transfusion. J Trauma 2011;71:S318–28.
45. Roberts I, Shakur H, Afolabi A, et al. The importance of early treatment with tranexamic acid in bleeding trauma patients: an exploratory analysis of the CRASH-2 randomised controlled trial. Lancet 2011;377:1096–101.
46. Roberts I, Perel P, Prieto-Merino D, et al. Effect of tranexamic acid on mortality in patients with traumatic bleeding: prespecified analysis of data from randomised controlled trial. BMJ 2012;345:e5839.
47. Sarode R, Milling TJ Jr, Refaai MA, et al. Efficacy and safety of a 4-factor prothrombin complex concentrate in patients on vitamin K antagonists presenting with major bleeding: a randomized, plasma-controlled, phase IIIb study. Circulation 2013;128:1234–43.
48. Holbrook A, Schulman S, Witt DM, et al. Evidence-based management of anticoagulant therapy: Antithrombotic Therapy and Prevention of Thrombosis, 9th ed: American College of Chest Physicians Evidence-Based Clinical Practice Guidelines. Chest 2012;141:e152S–84S.
49. Schick KS, Fertmann JM, Jauch KW, et al. Prothrombin complex concentrate in surgical patients: retrospective evaluation of vitamin K antagonist reversal and treatment of severe bleeding. Crit Care 2009;13:R191.
50. Mayer SA, Brun NC, Begtrup K, et al. Efficacy and safety of recombinant activated factor VII for acute intracranial hemorrhage. N Engl J Med 2008;358:2127–37.
51. Simpson E, Lin Y, Stanworth S, et al. Recombinant factor VIIa for the prevention and treatment of bleeding in patients without haemophilia. Cochrane Database Syst Rev 2012;(3):CD005011.
52. Inaba K, Ives C, McClure K, et al. Radiologic evaluation of alternative sites for needle decompression of tension pneumothorax. Arch Surg 2012;147:813–8.

53. Inaba K, Branco BC, Eckstein M, et al. Optimal positioning for emergent needle thoracostomy: a cadaver-based study. J Trauma 2011;71:1099–103.
54. Martin M, Satterly S, Inaba K, et al. Does needle thoracostomy provide adequate and effective decompression of tension pneumothorax? J Trauma Acute Care Surg 2012;73:1412–7.

Early Identification and Management of Patients with Severe Sepsis and Septic Shock in the Emergency Department

Joshua Keegan, MD*, Charles R. Wira III, MD

KEYWORDS

- Sepsis • Shock • Early goal-directed therapy • Organ dysfunction • Sepsis bundles

KEY POINTS

- Severe sepsis and septic shock have high prevalence and mortality.
- Treatment is time-sensitive and depends on early identification and risk-stratification.
- Treatment must include antibiotics and targeted therapies designed to optimize oxygen delivery.
- Adherence to a treatment algorithm decreases mortality.

EPIDEMIOLOGY

Severe sepsis and septic shock have great relevance to Emergency Medicine physicians because of their high prevalence, morbidity, and mortality. In some series, these conditions account for 10% of all intensive care unit (ICU) admissions and 750,000 patients yearly[1,2]; the most common source for these admissions is the Emergency Department (ED).[3] Septic shock is the most common cause of death in the ICU,[4] and the frequency of hospitalization for severe sepsis is climbing rapidly, having doubled between 1993 and 2003.[5] Despite significant advances in treating this common condition, mortality for severe sepsis remains at 15% to 40%,[6–8] with over one-third of patients discharged to a long-term care facility.[8] Outcomes are predictably worse for septic shock, with a mortality of 20% to 72%.[7,9,10] Overall, sepsis is

The authors have no conflicts of interest to disclose.
Disclosure: None.
Department of Emergency Medicine, Yale School of Medicine, 464 Congress Avenue, Suite 260, New Haven, CT 06450, USA
* Corresponding author.
E-mail address: josh.keegan@gmail.com

Emerg Med Clin N Am 32 (2014) 759–776
http://dx.doi.org/10.1016/j.emc.2014.07.002 emed.theclinics.com
0733-8627/14/$ – see front matter

responsible for 9% of the deaths in the United States,[11] ranking it third after heart disease and cancer among leading causes of death.[2] Twenty percent of this critically ill patient population remains in the ED for longer than 6 hours.[12]

DEFINITIONS

Definitions from the surviving sepsis campaign were modified and expanded in 2013.[13] Sepsis is defined as the suspected or documented presence of infection with evidence of a systemic inflammatory state.[14] This definition may prove challenging in the ED, as the culture results required to confirm infection are often unavailable, and laboratory evidence of a systemic inflammatory state may take hours to obtain. Nevertheless, in the proximal phase of presentation, ED providers are able to determine if a patient with suspected infection exhibits an abnormal physiologic response to a likely infectious insult. Traditionally, this has been defined by the vital sign criteria for the systemic inflammatory response syndrome (SIRS), although this has changed with the updated guidelines. Moving further along the severity spectrum, severe sepsis is defined as sepsis plus organ dysfunction or tissue hypoperfusion, and septic shock is defined as persistent sepsis-induced hypotension despite adequate volume resuscitation. Although more comprehensive than the SIRS criteria, the strict definitions include variables unavailable at presentation, such as urine output and fluid balance; adapted criteria more appropriate for use in the ED can be found in **Box 1**.

PATHOPHYSIOLOGY

Although the inciting event for severe sepsis is infectious, the pathophysiology is driven as much by a susceptible host's immune response as by the infection itself[15]; this is particularly apparent when considering the similarity of host responses to noninfectious severe illnesses such as burns and trauma.[14] Classically, this immune response has been considered an overly aggressive pro-inflammatory state causing collateral damage to the host via a variety of mechanisms. However, recent studies have found increasing evidence for a balance of pro-inflammatory and anti-inflammatory mechanisms,[16] with depletion of dendritic cells,[17] prolonged lymphopenic states, and high levels of immunosuppressive T cells,[18] causing increased susceptibility to secondary infections, difficulty clearing existing infections, and reactivation of latent viral infections.[19,20]

In the context of this systemic immune response, a variety of mechanisms are responsible for the end-organ dysfunction that is the hallmark of severe sepsis. The most important is a mismatch between tissue oxygen demand and delivery whereby the cellular need for oxygen exceeds its availability. Oxygen delivery depends on adequate cardiac output (dependent on preload and contractility), afterload, oxygenation, and oxygen-carrying capacity. The inadequate oxygen delivery resulting from septic shock is classically considered distributive from the vasodilatory effects of bacterial endotoxin,[21,22] endogenous vasopressin deficiency,[23] and central downregulation of vasomotor tone.[24] However, a cardiogenic component secondary to cytokine-mediated myocardial suppression and impaired sarcoplasmic reticulum calcium release[25] has been elucidated; reversible, isolated systolic and diastolic dysfunction have both been described.[26] The contributory effects at initial presentation of inadequate preload due to loss of endothelial integrity,[27] increased insensible losses, and impaired access to hydration in elderly or debilitated hosts should not be overlooked. Last, impaired oxygen delivery is possible despite normal or high blood pressure,[28] and failure of oxygen uptake at a cellular level can occur despite adequate delivery.[29] There are also mechanisms for end-organ dysfunction independent of

Box 1
Criteria for sepsis, severe sepsis, and septic shock

Sepsis: documented or suspected infection plus greater than or equal to 1 of the following indicating an abnormal physiologic response:

- Vital sign abnormalities
  - Abnormal temperature (>38.3°C or <36°C)
  - Tachycardia (range of HR >90–130 considered abnormal)[a]
  - Tachypnea (RR >20 or PCO_2 <32 Torr)
  - Elevated shock index (HR/SBP >0.8)[b]
- Evidence of systemic inflammatory state
  - WBC greater than 12,000 or less than 4000, or greater than 10% immature forms

Severe sepsis: sepsis plus organ dysfunction or tissue hypoperfusion as evidenced by at least one of:

- Lactate greater than 2 mmol/L
- Altered mental status (range from any change in baseline to GCS <12)[a]
- Respiratory failure (range from new onset hypoxia <90% on ambient air to Pao_2: Fio_2 <300)[a]
- Acute kidney injury (increase in Cr >0.5 mg/dL above baseline or oliguria)
- Signs of disseminated intravascular coagulation (INR >1.5, aPTT >60, or platelets <100,000)
- Liver failure (bilirubin >2 to >4 mg/dL)[a]
- Troponin elevation[b]
- Transient hypotension (SBP <90 mm Hg or MAP <65 responsive to IVF bolus of 30 mL/kg)[b]
- Unexplained acidosis (serum bicarbonate <20 mmol/L)[b]

Septic shock: sepsis plus any of the following

- Hypotension (SBP <90, MAP <70, or >40 mm Hg SBP decrease from baseline) refractory to IVF
- Lactate greater than 4 mmol/L

Abbreviations: aPTT, activated partial thromboplastic time; GCS, Glasgow Coma Scale; HR, heart rate; INR, international normalized ratio; IVF, intravenous fluids; RR, respiratory rate; SBP, systolic blood pressure; WBC, white blood cells.

[a] Illustrates the variable definitions of organ failure in the literature.

[b] Newer variables in the literature associated with higher risk for mortality or escalation of care.

Adapted from Dellinger RP, Levy MM, Rhodes A, et al. Surviving sepsis campaign: international guidelines for management of severe sepsis and septic shock: 2012. Critical Care Med 2013;41:585–6; and Angus DC, van der Poll T. Severe sepsis and septic shock. New Engl J Med 2013;369:842.

oxygen demand/delivery mismatch, including microvascular thrombosis,[14] mitochondrial damage from oxidative stress,[30] direct injury by activated neutrophils,[31] and apoptotic cell death.[32]

EARLY IDENTIFICATION AND RISK STRATIFICATION

Importance of Early Identification

Early identification and risk-stratification of patients with this sepsis physiology are essential for prompt initiation of treatment and adequate resource allocation. Unlike other conditions necessitating immediate high-resource interventions, such as trauma and acute myocardial infarction, rapid identification of sepsis can be quite difficult, given that inciting events are less clear, disease progression can be more gradual, and the laboratory evidence proving a systemic inflammatory state may require hours to obtain.[33] The necessary interventions are no less emergent, however, and delays to definitive treatment are associated with worse outcomes. For instance, in one multivariate analysis of inpatients with sepsis, the strongest predictor of mortality was duration of hypotension before administration of appropriate antibiotics, with an average delay of 6 hours and an absolute survival decrease of 7.6% for every hour of delay.[34] Despite the importance of early antibiotics, a recent study found that only 61% of ED patients admitted with a diagnosis of sepsis received any antibiotics in the ED.[35] To more rapidly identify and treat such patients, a set of screening criteria based primarily on vital signs may be used; although this approach has limited specificity, it has a high sensitivity,[36] desirable of a screening system to identify patients requiring further evaluation. Some institutions have created rapid response criteria that are based on more extreme vital sign abnormalities and are therefore more specific. Once patients with severe sepsis or septic shock are identified, appropriate interventions and level of care may be determined using a variety of risk-stratification tools.

Vital Sign Abnormalities

The risk-stratification process begins with consideration of the patient's triage assessment and vital signs; even brief abnormalities must not be minimized, as transient hypotension carries a 2.8-fold increased risk of mortality.[37] The shock index, defined as abnormal if heart rate divided by systolic blood pressure is greater than 0.8, predicts mortality, correlates with laboratory markers of poor prognosis,[38] and has prognostic value for ICU admission and likelihood of vasopressor dependence within 72 hours even when heart rate and blood pressure are independently normal.[39] After evaluation of vital sign abnormalities, laboratory testing will more clearly define a patient's prognosis.

Screening for Lactate Elevation

One of the most common risk-stratification laboratory tests is the serum lactate, an independent predictor of mortality and in some cases of more prognostic value than hypotension itself.[40–43] Although the level traditionally considered indicative of a worse prognosis has been 4 mmol/L, studies have found worse outcomes with intermediate (2–4 mmol/L) and even high-normal (1.4–2.3 mmol/L) lactate levels.[41,44] In a survey of Emergency Medicine and ICU providers, both ranked lactate as the most important resuscitation parameter, outranking all vital sign abnormalities and level of consciousness.[45] Lactate clearance is also associated with mortality,[46] with some authors reporting an 11% decrease in mortality risk for every 10% decrease from initial lactate at 6 hours.[47] The sensitivity of other laboratory values such as anion gap to predict lactate is only moderate, mandating measurement of lactate levels specifically.[48] Bicarbonate level and pH are also inadequate surrogates for lactate level, and reliance on them may underestimate illness severity.[49]

Organ Dysfunction

Although lactic acidosis is strongly correlated with prognosis and an excellent marker of global hypoperfusion, organ dysfunction is possible without global hypoperfusion and still portends a worse outcome, especially if cumulative organ failure is present. The sequential organ failure assessment (SOFA) score quantifies the function of multiple organs and predicts ED[50] and ICU[51] mortality, suggesting a role for including liver function tests as risk-stratification laboratory tests. Disseminated intravascular coagulation scores also correlate with mortality,[52] so prothrombin times and fibrin split products may yield additional prognostic information. Beyond the SOFA score, other organ failure scores reveal variability in the organs evaluated and thresholds considered to be abnormal,[53–59] as illustrated in **Box 1**.

Screening for Global Tissue Hypoxia

A final commonly used tool for risk-stratification is the central venous oxygen saturation ($ScvO_2$), measured from the superior vena cava as a surrogate for the mixed venous oxygen saturation. Inadequate oxygen delivery to the tissues or increased oxygen extraction by the tissues results in lower venous oxygen saturation, whereas failure of oxygen extraction causes abnormally high venous oxygen saturation; both abnormalities correlate with mortality.[60,61] However, utilization of $ScvO_2$ to risk-stratify patients has only been validated in septic shock, not normotensive patients with severe sepsis and lactate levels less than 4 mmol/L.

TREATMENT

Antibiotics and Source Control

The main purpose of risk stratification is not merely to identify high-risk patients, but to facilitate timely delivery of interventions that will improve outcomes. The single most important intervention is prompt administration of broad-spectrum antibiotics.[34] In some cases, viral and fungal infections drive sepsis physiology, and consequently, antivirals or antifungals may be necessary to adequately treat a patient's underlying infection. In addition, interventions aimed at source control are essential for surgical sources of sepsis and should proceed as quickly as possible, with concomitant antibiotic administration and hemodynamic optimization.

Early Goal-Directed Therapy

After antimicrobial initiation, many other interventions have been shown to decrease mortality in severe sepsis and septic shock. Perhaps the most well-known is early goal-directed therapy (EGDT), described by Rivers and colleagues[62] in 2001. Mortality for septic shock had previously been minimally changed[63] in undifferentiated studies of goal-directed therapy. EGDT provided an early systematic approach to mitigating the oxygen demand/delivery mismatch from macrocirculatory failure via the rapid, sequential optimization of multiple hemodynamic parameters: preload, afterload, cardiac contractility, and oxygen-carrying capacity. Implementation of this algorithm reduced mortality by 16%. A key difference was increased fluid administration in the treatment group (5 L vs 3.5 L), suggesting patients may have previously been systematically underresuscitated. Because of the significant mortality reduction, EGDT forms the cornerstone of septic shock treatment in the ED at many institutions.

Preload Optimization

The first critical step of EGDT in patients with shock refractory to 30 mL/kg of crystalloid is resuscitation targeted to a central venous pressure (CVP) of 8 to 12 mm Hg. Studies investigating crystalloid versus various colloids demonstrated no mortality benefit of hydroxyethyl starches (HES) but increased rates of renal failure,[64–69] and in some cases higher mortality.[70] The SAFE study of albumin versus saline found a nonsignificant trend toward decreased mortality with albumin in the severe sepsis subgroup, encouraging further study. Current recommendations are that crystalloid be preferred, HES be avoided, and albumin only be considered in certain rare circumstances.[13] Regardless of fluid type, the goal of CVP-based resuscitation is recruitment of cardiac output through preload optimization. However, this static target has been criticized for reasons including poor correlation of CVP with pulmonary capillary wedge pressure[71] and poor ability of either to predict volume-responsiveness.[72–76] Nevertheless, although a low CVP is very informative, an elevated CVP does not preclude volume-responsiveness and may result from tricuspid regurgitation, mechanical ventilation, or the abnormalities in right ventricular function or left ventricular compliance found in critically ill patients. More recently, dynamic methods for characterizing volume responsiveness have been described, including response of pulse pressure[77,78] and cardiac output[78–80] to passive leg raising, respiratory variation of radial artery pulse pressure,[81] peak aortic blood flow velocities measured by transesophageal echocardiography or esophageal Dopplers,[82,83] and ultrasonographically measured brachial artery velocities.[84] These diverse methods share the same objective: quantifying changes in cardiac output resulting from transient preload variations. When they are integrated into the care of patients with septic shock, assessment of preload ceases to be the binary, "is this patient hypovolemic?," and becomes the more sophisticated, "to what degree does this patient have additional preload-recruitable cardiac output?" This evaluation can and should be repeated frequently because sepsis-induced myocardial dysfunction evolves. However, as suggested by their low initial CVP,[62] most patients at ED presentation are hypovolemic, do have preload-recruitable cardiac output, and will benefit from empiric volume expansion before detailed measurement of physiologic parameters.

Afterload Optimization

Following preload optimization, the next step is afterload optimization with vasopressors via a central line, targeting a mean arterial pressure (MAP) of greater than or equal to 65 mm Hg to optimize systemic organ perfusion. A common pitfall is the false belief that, if the patient is awake and alert, then perfusion is adequate. However, cerebral autoregulation can augment cerebral blood flow in the setting of systemic hypoperfusion. In the MUST trial, Shapiro and colleagues[85] reduced mortality by 9% in shock patients while increasing the use of vasopressors by 35%, supporting the importance of this critical intervention. For vasopressor selection, a pivotal trial found that mortality was similar but dopamine caused more arrhythmias than norepinephrine,[86] which is the recommended first-line agent.[13] The VASST trial found no overall mortality difference with norepinephrine versus vasopressin.[87] However, in the prospectively defined subgroup of less severe septic shock (patients requiring <15 μg/min of norepinephrine or the equivalent), mortality was lower with vasopressin than norepinephrine, arguing for its consideration in this group. Patients were already receiving vasopressors before randomization, in 85% of cases, including norepinephrine, suggesting that vasopressin should be added to, rather than substituted for, norepinephrine. A small trial of phenylephrine versus norepinephrine found no significant differences in pulmonary artery catheter or hemodynamic parameters between the two,[88] and phenylephrine is recommended in very limited circumstances.[13]

Reversal of Global Tissue Hypoxia

The final physiologic target in EGDT is maintaining $ScvO_2$ greater than 70% through a combination of blood transfusion and inotropes. As a result of more recent data,[89] the recommended transfusion threshold has been changed to a hemoglobin level of 7 g/dL, but clinical correlation is required.[13] Should cardiac contractility be low or perfusion inadequate despite optimization of preload and blood pressure, dobutamine is the recommended inotrope.

Sepsis Bundles

In an overarching movement, there is mounting evidence that compliance with sepsis bundles based on the sentinel EGDT trial improves outcomes.[85,90–92] A sample sepsis bundle is shown in **Box 2**.

In one study, noncompliance with 6-hour bundles was associated with a more than 2-fold increase in hospital mortality.[90] Despite this, compliance rates are quite low at 16% to 52%.[90,93] Consequently, the National Quality Forum has adopted compliance with sepsis bundles as a process measure for quality of care,[94] and as a result, these bundles in combination with other literature form the framework for sepsis litigation. Multiple barriers to implementation have been identified, including a shortage of nursing staff, difficulty in identifying patients, lack of specialty monitoring equipment, and excessively high resource utilization.[95,96] This lack of compliance may be worse in the ED than the ICU, with 32% less ED providers using CVP monitoring under optimal circumstances, and 33% less ED providers starting vasopressors.[45] Fifty-one percent of ED providers versus 19% of ICU providers thought that ED workload was a barrier to implementation of the surviving sepsis campaign guidelines in the ED, suggesting a fundamentally different view of ED workflow between the 2 specialties. Nevertheless, similar to Emergency Medicine's adaptation to create interdisciplinary systems of care models for trauma, STEMI, and stroke, a systems of care model is required for patients with severe sepsis and septic shock to reduce mortality and optimize outcomes.

Glycemic Control

Although EGDT in the form of sepsis bundles forms the basis of treatment of septic shock, other beneficial supportive therapies can be initiated in the ED, one of which is glycemic control. Tight glycemic control with target glucose of 80 to 110 mg/dL was initially demonstrated to have a 3.4% mortality benefit in the surgical ICU.[97] Replication in the medical ICU yielded mixed results, with mortality increased in patients admitted for less than 3 days, but decreased in those staying longer.[98] In one of the largest studies, with greater than 6000 patients in a mixed ICU, tight glycemic control resulted in a 2.6% increase in mortality.[99] Subgroup analysis of the 22% admitted with severe sepsis did not reveal any differences; the 24% admitted from the ED were not analyzed separately. This study's control group forms the basis for the current recommendation to initiate insulin therapy for a patient with a glucose level greater than 180 md/dL.[13]

Lung-Protective Ventilation

Sepsis frequently leads to and is the most common cause of acute respiratory distress syndrome (ARDS).[100] There have been varying definitions of ARDS,[101,102] but the current one includes onset of noncardiogenic bilateral opacities within a week of an inciting event and a Pao_2:Fio_2 ratio less than 300. Lung-protective ventilation is a supportive therapy recommended by the surviving sepsis campaign that improves mortality of patients with ARDS by 9%.[103] Septic patients with ARDS should be ventilated with a tidal volume of no greater than 6 mL/kg and plateau pressures less than 30 cm H_2O to decrease mortality.[13]

Steroid Replacement

A final recommended supportive therapy is corticosteroid replacement at 200 mg hydrocortisone per day for patients with vasopressor-dependent shock at high risk for adrenal insufficiency.[13] Inconsistent mortality effects have been demonstrated,[104–107] but earlier discontinuation of vasopressors is made possible.[104,108,109] Some studies

Box 2
Sample sepsis bundle

2-h targets: early identification and initial therapies

- Lactate level obtained
- Appropriate cultures sent as indicated (blood, urine, CSF, body fluid)
- Risk-stratification laboratory tests sent for screening for end-organ failure
- Initial crystalloid resuscitation (30 mL/kg bolus)
- Initiation of broad-spectrum antibiotics
- Optimization of oxygenation (supplemental O_2, mechanical ventilation as indicated)

4-h targets: aggressive intervention for septic shock patients

- Central line placement for shock (MAP <65) refractory to 30 mL/kg bolus
  - Consider immediately for hemodynamic extremis (SBP <70 or recurrent SBP <80)
- Preload optimization
  - CVP measured and documented
  - Ongoing IVF resuscitation to target CVP 8–12
- Afterload optimization
  - Vasopressors initiated and titrated for MAP greater than 65 (norepinephrine preferred)
  - Should be initiated sooner in conjunction with IVF for hemodynamic extremis
- Tissue perfusion optimization
  - $ScvO_2$ measured and documented
  - Decreasing serial lactate levels
  - RBCs and dobutamine as indicated to achieve $ScvO_2$ greater than 70%
- Admission to ICU (septic shock) or step-down unit (severe sepsis)

6-h targets: achieving goal-directed endpoints to resuscitation

- Documented attainment of hemodynamic and tissue perfusion targets:
  - CVP 8–12, MAP greater than 65, $ScvO_2$ greater than 70%, lactate clearance demonstrated

Supplemental guidelines:

- Glycemic control for patients with serum glucose greater than 180
- Lung protective ventilation strategy (low Vt) for intubated patients
- Consider steroids for vasopressor-dependent patients at high risk for adrenal insufficiency
- Source control management
  - Bedside removal of source of infection; if applicable (ie, pull PICC line)
  - Acquire definitive imaging within 2 h (ie, CT abdomen)
  - Establish a definitive treatment plan with surgical specialist within 4 h
  - Admit patient to service capable of definitive source control (ie, OR or SICU)

Abbreviations: CSF, cerebrospinal fluid; CT, computed tomography; IVF, intravenous fluids; OR, operating room; PICC, peripherally inserted central catheter; RBC, red blood cells; SBP, systolic blood pressure; SICU, surgical intensive care unit; Vt, tidal volume.

enrolled patients several days after admission[109] and, in others, patients receiving etomidate were excluded,[104] potentially limiting ED generalizability. ACTH stimulation tests were not predictive of response to steroid administration[104,105] and are not recommended for patients with refractory septic shock.[13]

FUTURE DIRECTIONS

Novel Risk-Stratification Methods

It has been shown that serum procalcitonin levels correlate with bacterial infection[110] and predict sepsis.[111,112] However, levels vary considerably early in the course of disease,[113] may be elevated for other reasons,[114,115] and are of inconsistent prognostic value,[116–119] especially when not measured serially.[118,120–122] Consequently, although studies are increasingly prevalent in the critical care literature and procalcitonin may play a larger future role, its current value in initial ED screening and risk stratification remains unclear.

Noninvasive Monitoring

There has been a long-standing trend, driven by the desire to avoid mechanical and infectious complications, toward less invasive treatments, beginning with a 60% decline in pulmonary artery catheterization rates between 2002 and 2006.[123] There is currently no validated noninvasive pathway for septic shock patients, but new noninvasive approaches may benefit normotensive patients with severe sepsis and may complement and enhance the management of patients with septic shock. Among the most powerful of these is the use of ultrasonography to assess hemodynamic parameters and cardiac function. Several studies regarding the size and collapsibility of the inferior vena cava and their correlation with right atrial pressures[124–129] have yielded mixed results. Many were limited by small sizes or methodologic concerns, and most examined patients with primary cardiac dysfunction, limiting generalizability to septic patients. One study specifically examining critically ill septic patients found that tissue Doppler measurements of the tricuspid valve predicted a CVP greater than 10 mm Hg with higher discriminant value than IVC measurements[127]; this technique may become increasingly common in the future but is limited if there is underlying primary or secondary diastolic dysfunction. Ultimately, a review of numerous studies concluded that there is no single ideal parameter or technique for determining right atrial pressures,[130] highlighting the absence of a gold standard for volume status despite decades of research and the need to combine information from a variety of sources, including ultrasonographic measurements of aortic[82,83] and brachial[84] flow velocities, as previously discussed. Last, independent of volume status, echocardiography can contribute by characterizing sepsis-induced myocardial dysfunction,[131] potentially directing earlier administration of inotropes to reverse the shock state. Overall, although the role of ultrasound is being clarified, it promises tremendous ability to guide management noninvasively, particularly in the ED setting, where early and aggressive ultrasound-guided volume resuscitation may obviate central venous access and vasopressors.

However, despite its promise, ultrasound fundamentally does little beyond supplementing or replacing current invasive methods of monitoring macrocirculatory parameters. New technologies allowing characterization of microcirculatory failure and tissue-level imbalances between oxygen demand and delivery are being tested, including near-infrared spectroscopy (NIRS). NIRS noninvasively assesses tissue oxygenation levels (StO_2) via reflectance of infrared light waves from hemoglobin. Additional information is provided by the slope of deoxygenation[132,133] when vascular flow is interrupted, either for a defined period of time or to a defined StO_2.[134] Some studies have found lower StO_2 and an impaired recovery slope in patients with severe sepsis,[135] whereas others demonstrated a more gradual desaturation rate,[136] likely reflecting failure of oxygen uptake. StO_2 measurements may correlate with traditional measurements of oxygen extraction, including both $ScvO_2$[137] and SvO_2,[138] although in some cases this correlation is moderate only.[139] From a more clinical perspective, a recent large, multicenter, ED-based observational study demonstrated lower baseline StO_2 in patients with septic shock versus sepsis, as well as the ability of the StO_2 recovery slope to predict 24-hour organ failure scores and mortality.[140] However, other ED-based studies have not supported an association of StO_2 with septic shock,[141] and it is not yet known whether NIRS adds prognostic information beyond currently available measures.[132] Although further study is needed, particularly in the ED setting and for use as a resuscitation endpoint, this technology has the potential to provide equal or greater physiologic information less invasively than currently accepted modalities.

Novel Therapies

In addition to monitoring technologies, several new therapies are being investigated. Accepted practice largely treats the macrocirculatory failure associated with severe sepsis and provides general supportive care. This accepted practice does not directly address much of the underlying pathophysiology driving cellular oxygen demand:delivery mismatch and end-organ dysfunction. Blood purification is one treatment attempting to address this and includes hemoperfusion, hemofiltration, and plasma exchange. The goal is modulation of the immune response, although inability to individually control pro-inflammatory and anti-inflammatory cytokines makes this a crude instrument. However, a recent meta-analysis concluded that blood purification techniques reduce mortality, an especially prominent effect with polymyxin-B hemoperfusion,[142] and such treatments may become more common in the future. A more specific treatment that has also been demonstrated to reduce mortality, albeit also by meta-analysis only, is anti-tumor necrosis factor therapy, with a relative 7% decrease in mortality.[143] Further study of both therapies in larger trials is needed, and because the immune pathways driving sepsis are further defined, additional targets will likely be examined. Other possible mechanisms for ameliorating end-organ dysfunction include inhibiting apoptosis,[144] mitigating damage caused by reactive oxygen species,[145] and improving oxygen uptake at a mitochondrial level with exogenous cytochrome C.[146] Ultimately, it is likely that increasingly specific and sophisticated therapies targeting the immune response, microcirculatory failure, and cell death associated with sepsis will become available in the future.

SUMMARY

Severe sepsis and septic shock form a continuum of disease that is quite common and associated with high morbidity and mortality. The hallmark of this disease is organ dysfunction and/or shock resulting from the interaction of an infection and the systemic immune response of a susceptible host. Although sometimes challenging, early identification of patients based on screening tools allows rapid delivery of the aggressive interventions that they require. The most important of these is adequate source control with antibiotics and possibly procedural intervention. Next, sequential optimization of hemodynamic parameters via EGDT and with a firm understanding of the underlying physiology described above ameliorates macrocirculatory failure, improving the mismatch between oxygen demand and delivery and decreasing mortality. Compliance with sepsis bundles incorporating these treatments and specific supportive therapies improves patient outcomes. Collectively, these therapies are standard of care and can and should be performed in the ED, especially as some patients have prolonged stays while awaiting ICU beds. In addition to these proven treatments, newer monitoring technologies and pharmacologic therapies are being tested and will have an increasing role in the future. Eventually, specific components of the systemic immune response may be enhanced or suppressed individually as they prove beneficial or harmful, with ongoing noninvasive monitoring to ensure that patients are responding appropriately to treatment. However, the excitement surrounding future treatments should not minimize the value of the basic treatments already available and proven in countless studies to positively impact the outcomes of patients that the emergency physician evaluates and treats in the ED on a daily basis.

REFERENCES

1. Angus DC, Linde-Zwirble WT, Lidicker J, et al. Epidemiology of severe sepsis in the United States: analysis of incidence, outcome, and associated costs of care. Crit Care Med 2001;29:1303–10.
2. Gaieski DF, Edwards JM, Kallan MJ, et al. Benchmarking the incidence and mortality of severe sepsis in the United States. Crit Care Med 2013;41:1167–74.
3. Vincent JL, Sakr Y, Sprung CL, et al. Sepsis in European intensive care units: results of the SOAP study. Crit Care Med 2006;34:344–53.
4. Annane D, Aegerter P, Jars-Guincestre MC, et al. Current epidemiology of septic shock: the CUB-Rea Network. Am J Respir Crit Care Med 2003;168:165–72.
5. Dombrovskiy VY, Martin AA, Sunderram J, et al. Rapid increase in hospitalization and mortality rates for severe sepsis in the United States: a trend analysis from 1993 to 2003. Crit Care Med 2007;35:1244–50.
6. Catenacci MH, King K. Severe sepsis and septic shock: improving outcomes in the emergency department. Emerg Med Clin North Am 2008;26:603–23, vii.
7. Degoricija V, Sharma M, Legac A, et al. Survival analysis of 314 episodes of sepsis in medical intensive care unit in university hospital: impact of intensive care unit performance and antimicrobial therapy. Croat Med J 2006;47:385–97.
8. Kumar G, Kumar N, Taneja A, et al. Nationwide trends of severe sepsis in the 21st century (2000-2007). Chest 2011;140:1223–31.
9. Schrier RW, Wang W. Acute renal failure and sepsis. N Engl J Med 2004;351: 159–69.
10. Freitas FG, Salomao R, Tereran N, et al. The impact of duration of organ dysfunction on the outcome of patients with severe sepsis and septic shock. Clinics (Sao Paulo) 2008;63:483–8.
11. Farcy DA. Critical care emergency medicine. New York: McGraw-Hill Medical; 2012.
12. Wang HE, Shapiro NI, Angus DC, et al. National estimates of severe sepsis in United States emergency departments. Crit Care Med 2007;35:1928–36.
13. Dellinger RP, Levy MM, Rhodes A, et al. Surviving sepsis campaign: international guidelines for management of severe sepsis and septic shock: 2012. Crit Care Med 2013;41:580–637.
14. Angus DC, van der Poll T. Severe sepsis and septic shock. N Engl J Med 2013; 369:840–51.
15. Cerra FB. The systemic septic response: multiple systems organ failure. Crit Care Clin 1985;1:591–607.

16. van der Poll T, Opal SM. Host-pathogen interactions in sepsis. Lancet Infect Dis 2008;8:32–43.
17. Hotchkiss RS, Tinsley KW, Swanson PE, et al. Depletion of dendritic cells, but not macrophages, in patients with sepsis. J Immunol 2002;168:2493–500.
18. Inoue S, Suzuki-Utsunomiya K, Okada Y, et al. Reduction of immunocompetent T cells followed by prolonged lymphopenia in severe sepsis in the elderly. Crit Care Med 2013;41:810–9.
19. Torgersen C, Moser P, Luckner G, et al. Macroscopic postmortem findings in 235 surgical intensive care patients with sepsis. Anesth Analg 2009;108:1841–7.
20. Limaye AP, Kirby KA, Rubenfeld GD, et al. Cytomegalovirus reactivation in critically ill immunocompetent patients. JAMA 2008;300:413–22.
21. Opal SM. The host response to endotoxin, antilipopolysaccharide strategies, and the management of severe sepsis. Int J Med Microbiol 2007;297:365–77.
22. Morrison DC, Bucklin SE. Evidence for antibiotic-mediated endotoxin release as a contributing factor to lethality in experimental gram-negative sepsis. Scand J Infect Dis Suppl 1996;101:3–8.
23. Russell JA. Bench-to-bedside review: vasopressin in the management of septic shock. Crit Care 2011;15:226.
24. Sayk F, Vietheer A, Schaaf B, et al. Endotoxemia causes central downregulation of sympathetic vasomotor tone in healthy humans. Am J Physiol Regul Integr Comp Physiol 2008;295:R891–8.
25. Rudiger A, Singer M. Mechanisms of sepsis-induced cardiac dysfunction. Crit Care Med 2007;35:1599–608.
26. Bouhemad B, Nicolas-Robin A, Arbelot C, et al. Isolated and reversible impairment of ventricular relaxation in patients with septic shock. Crit Care Med 2008;36:766–74.
27. Goldenberg NM, Steinberg BE, Slutsky AS, et al. Broken barriers: a new take on sepsis pathogenesis. Sci Transl Med 2011;3:88ps25.
28. Wo CC, Shoemaker WC, Appel PL, et al. Unreliability of blood pressure and heart rate to evaluate cardiac output in emergency resuscitation and critical illness. Crit Care Med 1993;21:218–23.
29. Levy RJ, Deutschman CS. Cytochrome c oxidase dysfunction in sepsis. Crit Care Med 2007;35:S468–75.
30. Galley HF. Oxidative stress and mitochondrial dysfunction in sepsis. Br J Anaesth 2011;107:57–64.
31. Zhang Q, Raoof M, Chen Y, et al. Circulating mitochondrial DAMPs cause inflammatory responses to injury. Nature 2010;464:104–7.
32. Hotchkiss RS, Tinsley KW, Swanson PE, et al. Endothelial cell apoptosis in sepsis. Crit Care Med 2002;30:S225–8.
33. Funk D, Sebat F, Kumar A. A systems approach to the early recognition and rapid administration of best practice therapy in sepsis and septic shock. Curr Opin Crit Care 2009;15:301–7.
34. Kumar A, Roberts D, Wood KE, et al. Duration of hypotension before initiation of effective antimicrobial therapy is the critical determinant of survival in human septic shock. Crit Care Med 2006;34:1589–96.
35. Filbin MR, Arias SA, Camargo CA Jr, et al. Sepsis visits and antibiotic utilization in U.S. Emergency Departments. Crit Care Med 2014;42:528–35.
36. Sebat F, Musthafa AA, Johnson D, et al. Effect of a rapid response system for patients in shock on time to treatment and mortality during 5 years. Crit Care Med 2007;35:2568–75.

37. Marchick MR, Kline JA, Jones AE. The significance of non-sustained hypotension in emergency department patients with sepsis. Intensive Care Med 2009;35:1261–4.
38. Berger T, Green J, Horeczko T, et al. Shock index and early recognition of sepsis in the emergency department: pilot study. West J Emerg Med 2013;14:168–74.
39. Rady MY, Smithline HA, Blake H, et al. A comparison of the shock index and conventional vital signs to identify acute, critical illness in the emergency department. Ann Emerg Med 1994;24:685–90.
40. Lee SW, Hong YS, Park DW, et al. Lactic acidosis not hyperlactatemia as a predictor of in hospital mortality in septic emergency patients. Emerg Med J 2008;25:659–65.
41. Mikkelsen ME, Miltiades AN, Gaieski DF, et al. Serum lactate is associated with mortality in severe sepsis independent of organ failure and shock. Crit Care Med 2009;37:1670–7.
42. Vitek V, Cowley RA. Blood lactate in the prognosis of various forms of shock. Ann Surg 1971;173:308–13.
43. Shapiro NI, Howell MD, Talmor D, et al. Serum lactate as a predictor of mortality in emergency department patients with infection. Ann Emerg Med 2005;45:524–8.
44. Wacharasint P, Nakada TA, Boyd JH, et al. Normal-range blood lactate concentration in septic shock is prognostic and predictive. Shock 2012;38:4–10.
45. Jiwaji Z, Brady S, McIntyre LA, et al. Emergency department management of early sepsis: a national survey of emergency medicine and intensive care consultants. Emerg Med J 2013. [Epub ahead of print].
46. Arnold RC, Shapiro NI, Jones AE, et al. Multicenter study of early lactate clearance as a determinant of survival in patients with presumed sepsis. Shock 2009;32:35–9.
47. Nguyen HB, Rivers EP, Knoblich BP, et al. Early lactate clearance is associated with improved outcome in severe sepsis and septic shock. Crit Care Med 2004;32:1637–42.
48. Berkman M, Ufberg J, Nathanson LA, et al. Anion gap as a screening tool for elevated lactate in patients with an increased risk of developing sepsis in the Emergency Department. J Emerg Med 2009;36:391–4.
49. Wira CR, Donnino M, Shirazi E, et al. Surrogate markers for lactic acidosis in patients with severe sepsis and septic shock. Crit Care Med 2004;32:A151.
50. Innocenti F, Bianchi S, Guerrini E, et al. Prognostic scores for early stratification of septic patients admitted to an emergency department-high dependency unit. Eur J Emerg Med 2014;21(4):254–9.
51. Janssens U, Graf C, Graf J, et al. Evaluation of the SOFA score: a single-center experience of a medical intensive care unit in 303 consecutive patients with predominantly cardiovascular disorders. Sequential Organ Failure Assessment. Intensive Care Med 2000;26:1037–45.
52. Gando S, Saitoh D, Ogura H, et al. A multicenter, prospective validation study of the Japanese Association for Acute Medicine disseminated intravascular coagulation scoring system in patients with severe sepsis. Crit Care 2013;17:R111.
53. Shapiro NI, Howell MD, Talmor D, et al. Mortality in Emergency Department Sepsis (MEDS) score predicts 1-year mortality. Crit Care Med 2007;35:192–8.
54. Trzeciak S, Dellinger RP, Parrillo JE, et al. Early microcirculatory perfusion derangements in patients with severe sepsis and septic shock: relationship to hemodynamics, oxygen transport, and survival. Ann Emerg Med 2007;49:88–98, 98.e1–2.

55. Dellinger RP, Levy MM, Carlet JM, et al. Surviving Sepsis Campaign: international guidelines for management of severe sepsis and septic shock: 2008. Crit Care Med 2008;36:296–327.
56. Spies C, Haude V, Fitzner R, et al. Serum cardiac troponin T as a prognostic marker in early sepsis. Chest 1998;113:1055–63.
57. Mehta NJ, Khan IA, Gupta V, et al. Cardiac troponin I predicts myocardial dysfunction and adverse outcome in septic shock. Int J Cardiol 2004;95:13–7.
58. Turner A, Tsamitros M, Bellomo R. Myocardial cell injury in septic shock. Crit Care Med 1999;27:1775–80.
59. ver Elst KM, Spapen HD, Nguyen DN, et al. Cardiac troponins I and T are biological markers of left ventricular dysfunction in septic shock. Clin Chem 2000; 46:650–7.
60. Pope JV, Jones AE, Gaieski DF, et al. Multicenter study of central venous oxygen saturation (ScvO(2)) as a predictor of mortality in patients with sepsis. Ann Emerg Med 2010;55:40–6.e1.
61. Varpula M, Tallgren M, Saukkonen K, et al. Hemodynamic variables related to outcome in septic shock. Intensive Care Med 2005;31:1066–71.
62. Rivers E, Nguyen B, Havstad S, et al. Early goal-directed therapy in the treatment of severe sepsis and septic shock. N Engl J Med 2001;345:1368–77.
63. Friedman G, Silva E, Vincent JL. Has the mortality of septic shock changed with time. Crit Care Med 1998;26:2078–86.
64. Guidet B, Martinet O, Boulain T, et al. Assessment of hemodynamic efficacy and safety of 6% hydroxyethylstarch 130/0.4 vs. 0.9% NaCl fluid replacement in patients with severe sepsis: The CRYSTMAS study. Crit Care 2012;16:R94.
65. Bayer O, Reinhart K, Kohl M, et al. Effects of fluid resuscitation with synthetic colloids or crystalloids alone on shock reversal, fluid balance, and patient outcomes in patients with severe sepsis: a prospective sequential analysis. Crit Care Med 2012;40:2543–51.
66. Myburgh JA, Finfer S, Bellomo R, et al. Hydroxyethyl starch or saline for fluid resuscitation in intensive care. N Engl J Med 2012;367:1901–11.
67. Schortgen F, Lacherade JC, Bruneel F, et al. Effects of hydroxyethylstarch and gelatin on renal function in severe sepsis: a multicentre randomised study. Lancet 2001;357:911–6.
68. McIntyre LA, Fergusson D, Cook DJ, et al. Fluid resuscitation in the management of early septic shock (FINESS): a randomized controlled feasibility trial. Can J Anaesth 2008;55:819–26.
69. Brunkhorst FM, Engel C, Bloos F, et al. Intensive insulin therapy and pentastarch resuscitation in severe sepsis. N Engl J Med 2008;358:125–39.
70. Perner A, Haase N, Guttormsen AB, et al. Hydroxyethyl starch 130/0.42 versus Ringer's acetate in severe sepsis. N Engl J Med 2012;367:124–34.
71. Packman MI, Rackow EC. Optimum left heart filling pressure during fluid resuscitation of patients with hypovolemic and septic shock. Crit Care Med 1983;11: 165–9.
72. Diebel LN, Wilson RF, Tagett MG, et al. End-diastolic volume. A better indicator of preload in the critically ill. Arch Surg 1992;127:817–21 [discussion: 821–2].
73. Osman D, Ridel C, Ray P, et al. Cardiac filling pressures are not appropriate to predict hemodynamic response to volume challenge. Crit Care Med 2007;35: 64–8.
74. Bindels AJ, van der Hoeven JG, Graafland AD, et al. Relationships between volume and pressure measurements and stroke volume in critically ill patients. Crit Care 2000;4:193–9.

75. Sakka SG, Bredle DL, Reinhart K, et al. Comparison between intrathoracic blood volume and cardiac filling pressures in the early phase of hemodynamic instability of patients with sepsis or septic shock. J Crit Care 1999;14:78–83.
76. Calvin JE, Driedger AA, Sibbald WJ. Does the pulmonary capillary wedge pressure predict left ventricular preload in critically ill patients? Crit Care Med 1981;9:437–43.
77. Boulain T, Achard JM, Teboul JL, et al. Changes in BP induced by passive leg raising predict response to fluid loading in critically ill patients. Chest 2002;121:1245–52.
78. Lafanechere A, Pene F, Goulenok C, et al. Changes in aortic blood flow induced by passive leg raising predict fluid responsiveness in critically ill patients. Crit Care 2006;10:R132.
79. Monnet X, Rienzo M, Osman D, et al. Passive leg raising predicts fluid responsiveness in the critically ill. Crit Care Med 2006;34:1402–7.
80. Lamia B, Ochagavia A, Monnet X, et al. Echocardiographic prediction of volume responsiveness in critically ill patients with spontaneously breathing activity. Intensive Care Med 2007;33:1125–32.
81. Marik PE, Cavallazzi R, Vasu T, et al. Dynamic changes in arterial waveform derived variables and fluid responsiveness in mechanically ventilated patients: a systematic review of the literature. Crit Care Med 2009;37:2642–7.
82. Michard F, Teboul JL. Predicting fluid responsiveness in ICU patients: a critical analysis of the evidence. Chest 2002;121:2000–8.
83. Feissel M, Michard F, Mangin I, et al. Respiratory changes in aortic blood velocity as an indicator of fluid responsiveness in ventilated patients with septic shock. Chest 2001;119:867–73.
84. Brennan JM, Blair JE, Hampole C, et al. Radial artery pulse pressure variation correlates with brachial artery peak velocity variation in ventilated subjects when measured by internal medicine residents using hand-carried ultrasound devices. Chest 2007;131:1301–7.
85. Shapiro NI, Howell MD, Talmor D, et al. Implementation and outcomes of the Multiple Urgent Sepsis Therapies (MUST) protocol. Crit Care Med 2006;34:1025–32.
86. De Backer D, Biston P, Devriendt J, et al. Comparison of dopamine and norepinephrine in the treatment of shock. N Engl J Med 2010;362:779–89.
87. Russell JA, Walley KR, Singer J, et al. Vasopressin versus norepinephrine infusion in patients with septic shock. N Engl J Med 2008;358:877–87.
88. Morelli A, Ertmer C, Rehberg S, et al. Phenylephrine versus norepinephrine for initial hemodynamic support of patients with septic shock: a randomized, controlled trial. Crit Care 2008;12:R143.
89. Hebert PC, Wells G, Blajchman MA, et al. A multicenter, randomized, controlled clinical trial of transfusion requirements in critical care. Transfusion Requirements in Critical Care Investigators, Canadian Critical Care Trials Group. N Engl J Med 1999;340:409–17.
90. Gao F, Melody T, Daniels DF, et al. The impact of compliance with 6-hour and 24-hour sepsis bundles on hospital mortality in patients with severe sepsis: a prospective observational study. Crit Care 2005;9:R764–70.
91. Focht A, Jones AE, Lowe TJ. Early goal-directed therapy: improving mortality and morbidity of sepsis in the emergency department. Jt Comm J Qual Patient Saf 2009;35:186–91.
92. Kortgen A, Niederprum P, Bauer M. Implementation of an evidence-based "standard operating procedure" and outcome in septic shock. Crit Care Med 2006;34:943–9.

93. Ferrer R, Artigas A, Levy MM, et al. Improvement in process of care and outcome after a multicenter severe sepsis educational program in Spain. JAMA 2008;299:2294–303.
94. Forum NQ. NQF #0500 Severe sepsis and septic shock: management bundle. Last updated date: October 05, 2012. Available at: qualityforum.org. Accessed January 2, 2014.
95. Carlbom DJ, Rubenfeld GD. Barriers to implementing protocol-based sepsis resuscitation in the emergency department–results of a national survey. Crit Care Med 2007;35:2525–32.
96. Stoneking L, Denninghoff K, Deluca L, et al. Sepsis bundles and compliance with clinical guidelines. J Intensive Care Med 2011;26:172–82.
97. van den Berghe G, Wouters P, Weekers F, et al. Intensive insulin therapy in critically ill patients. N Engl J Med 2001;345:1359–67.
98. Van den Berghe G, Wilmer A, Hermans G, et al. Intensive insulin therapy in the medical ICU. N Engl J Med 2006;354:449–61.
99. Investigators NS, Finfer S, Chittock DR, et al. Intensive versus conventional glucose control in critically ill patients. N Engl J Med 2009;360:1283–97.
100. Fein AM, Calalang-Colucci MG. Acute lung injury and acute respiratory distress syndrome in sepsis and septic shock. Crit Care Clin 2000;16:289–317.
101. Bernard GR, Artigas A, Brigham KL, et al. The American-European Consensus Conference on ARDS. Definitions, mechanisms, relevant outcomes, and clinical trial coordination. Am J Respir Crit Care Med 1994;149:818–24.
102. Force AD, Ranieri VM, Rubenfeld GD, et al. Acute respiratory distress syndrome: the Berlin Definition. JAMA 2012;307:2526–33.
103. Ventilation with lower tidal volumes as compared with traditional tidal volumes for acute lung injury and the acute respiratory distress syndrome. The Acute Respiratory Distress Syndrome Network. N Engl J Med 2000;342:1301–8.
104. Annane D, Sebille V, Charpentier C, et al. Effect of treatment with low doses of hydrocortisone and fludrocortisone on mortality in patients with septic shock. JAMA 2002;288:862–71.
105. Sprung CL, Annane D, Keh D, et al. Hydrocortisone therapy for patients with septic shock. N Engl J Med 2008;358:111–24.
106. Annane D, Bellissant E, Bollaert PE, et al. Corticosteroids in the treatment of severe sepsis and septic shock in adults: a systematic review. JAMA 2009;301:2362–75.
107. Sligl WI, Milner DA Jr, Sundar S, et al. Safety and efficacy of corticosteroids for the treatment of septic shock: a systematic review and meta-analysis. Clin Infect Dis 2009;49:93–101.
108. Briegel J, Forst H, Haller M, et al. Stress doses of hydrocortisone reverse hyperdynamic septic shock: a prospective, randomized, double-blind, single-center study. Crit Care Med 1999;27:723–32.
109. Bollaert PE, Charpentier C, Levy B, et al. Reversal of late septic shock with supraphysiologic doses of hydrocortisone. Crit Care Med 1998;26:645–50.
110. Simon L, Gauvin F, Amre DK, et al. Serum procalcitonin and C-reactive protein levels as markers of bacterial infection: a systematic review and meta-analysis. Clin Infect Dis 2004;39:206–17.
111. Uzzan B, Cohen R, Nicolas P, et al. Procalcitonin as a diagnostic test for sepsis in critically ill adults and after surgery or trauma: a systematic review and meta-analysis. Crit Care Med 2006;34:1996–2003.
112. Faix JD. Biomarkers of sepsis. Crit Rev Clin Lab Sci 2013;50:23–36.

113. Brunkhorst FM, Al-Nawas B, Krummenauer F, et al. Procalcitonin, C-reactive protein and APACHE II score for risk evaluation in patients with severe pneumonia. Clin Microbiol Infect 2002;8:93–100.
114. Becker KL, Snider R, Nylen ES. Procalcitonin assay in systemic inflammation, infection, and sepsis: clinical utility and limitations. Crit Care Med 2008;36: 941–52.
115. Billeter A, Turina M, Seifert B, et al. Early serum procalcitonin, interleukin-6, and 24-hour lactate clearance: useful indicators of septic infections in severely traumatized patients. World J Surg 2009;33:558–66.
116. Clec'h C, Ferriere F, Karoubi P, et al. Diagnostic and prognostic value of procalcitonin in patients with septic shock. Crit Care Med 2004;32:1166–9.
117. Claeys R, Vinken S, Spapen H, et al. Plasma procalcitonin and C-reactive protein in acute septic shock: clinical and biological correlates. Crit Care Med 2002; 30:757–62.
118. Karlsson S, Heikkinen M, Pettila V, et al. Predictive value of procalcitonin decrease in patients with severe sepsis: a prospective observational study. Crit Care 2010;14:R205.
119. Lee CC, Chen SY, Tsai CL, et al. Prognostic value of mortality in emergency department sepsis score, procalcitonin, and C-reactive protein in patients with sepsis at the emergency department. Shock 2008;29:322–7.
120. Charles PE, Tinel C, Barbar S, et al. Procalcitonin kinetics within the first days of sepsis: relationship with the appropriateness of antibiotic therapy and the outcome. Crit Care 2009;13:R38.
121. Schuetz P, Maurer P, Punjabi V, et al. Procalcitonin decrease over 72 hours in US critical care units predicts fatal outcome in sepsis patients. Crit Care 2013;17: R115.
122. Magrini L, Travaglino F, Marino R, et al. Procalcitonin variations after Emergency Department admission are highly predictive of hospital mortality in patients with acute infectious diseases. Eur Rev Med Pharmacol Sci 2013;17(Suppl 1): 133–42.
123. Koo KK, Sun JC, Zhou Q, et al. Pulmonary artery catheters: evolving rates and reasons for use. Crit Care Med 2011;39:1613–8.
124. Kircher BJ, Himelman RB, Schiller NB. Noninvasive estimation of right atrial pressure from the inspiratory collapse of the inferior vena cava. Am J Cardiol 1990;66:493–6.
125. Moreno FL, Hagan AD, Holmen JR, et al. Evaluation of size and dynamics of the inferior vena cava as an index of right-sided cardiac function. Am J Cardiol 1984;53:579–85.
126. Jue J, Chung W, Schiller NB. Does inferior vena cava size predict right atrial pressures in patients receiving mechanical ventilation? J Am Soc Echocardiogr 1992;5:613–9.
127. Arbo JE, Maslove DM, Beraud AS. Bedside assessment of right atrial pressure in critically ill septic patients using tissue Doppler ultrasonography. J Crit Care 2013;28(6):1112.e1–5.
128. Nagueh SF, Kopelen HA, Zoghbi WA. Relation of mean right atrial pressure to echocardiographic and Doppler parameters of right atrial and right ventricular function. Circulation 1996;93:1160–9.
129. Brennan JM, Blair JE, Goonewardena S, et al. Reappraisal of the use of inferior vena cava for estimating right atrial pressure. J Am Soc Echocardiogr 2007;20: 857–61.

130. Beigel R, Cercek B, Luo H, et al. Noninvasive evaluation of right atrial pressure. J Am Soc Echocardiogr 2013;26:1033–42.
131. Griffee MJ, Merkel MJ, Wei KS. The role of echocardiography in hemodynamic assessment of septic shock. Crit Care Clin 2010;26:365–82 table of contents.
132. Macdonald SP, Brown SG. Near-infrared spectroscopy in the assessment of suspected sepsis in the emergency department. Emerg Med J 2013. [Epub ahead of print].
133. Creteur J. Muscle StO2 in critically ill patients. Curr Opin Crit Care 2008;14: 361–6.
134. Lipcsey M, Woinarski NC, Bellomo R. Near infrared spectroscopy (NIRS) of the thenar eminence in anesthesia and intensive care. Ann Intensive Care 2012;2:11.
135. Skarda DE, Mulier KE, Myers DE, et al. Dynamic near-infrared spectroscopy measurements in patients with severe sepsis. Shock 2007;27:348–53.
136. Pareznik R, Knezevic R, Voga G, et al. Changes in muscle tissue oxygenation during stagnant ischemia in septic patients. Intensive Care Med 2006;32:87–92.
137. Nardi O, Gonzalez H, Fayssoil A, et al. Masseter muscle oxygen saturation is associated with central venous oxygen saturation in patients with severe sepsis. J Clin Monit Comput 2010;24:289–93.
138. Mulier KE, Skarda DE, Taylor JH, et al. Near-infrared spectroscopy in patients with severe sepsis: correlation with invasive hemodynamic measurements. Surg Infect (Larchmt) 2008;9:515–9.
139. Napoli AM, Machan JT, Forcada A, et al. Tissue oxygenation does not predict central venous oxygenation in emergency department patients with severe sepsis and septic shock. Acad Emerg Med 2010;17:349–52.
140. Shapiro NI, Arnold R, Sherwin R, et al. The association of near-infrared spectroscopy-derived tissue oxygenation measurements with sepsis syndromes, organ dysfunction and mortality in emergency department patients with sepsis. Crit Care 2011;15:R223.
141. Vorwerk C, Coats TJ. The prognostic value of tissue oxygen saturation in emergency department patients with severe sepsis or septic shock. Emerg Med J 2012;29:699–703.
142. Zhou F, Peng Z, Murugan R, et al. Blood purification and mortality in sepsis: a meta-analysis of randomized trials. Crit Care Med 2013;41:2209–20.
143. Qiu P, Cui X, Sun J, et al. Antitumor necrosis factor therapy is associated with improved survival in clinical sepsis trials: a meta-analysis. Crit Care Med 2013;41:2419–29.
144. Harjai M, Bogra J, Kohli M, et al. Is suppression of apoptosis a new therapeutic target in sepsis? Anaesth Intensive Care 2013;41:175–83.
145. Zapelini PH, Rezin GT, Cardoso MR, et al. Antioxidant treatment reverses mitochondrial dysfunction in a sepsis animal model. Mitochondrion 2008;8:211–8.
146. Piel DA, Deutschman CS, Levy RJ. Exogenous cytochrome C restores myocardial cytochrome oxidase activity into the late phase of sepsis. Shock 2008;29: 612–6.

Assessment and Treatment of the Trauma Patient in Shock

Kimberly Boswell, MD[a,*], Jay Menaker, MD[b]

KEYWORDS

• Trauma patient • Shock • Nonoperative management • Solid organ injury

KEY POINTS

- High-volume crystalloid resuscitation is associated with increased length of stay, ICU and ventilator days, and organ failure and infection rates.
- Rapid evaluation of a hemodynamically unstable trauma patient is vital to diagnosis and treatment of the cause of shock.
- CT scanning should be used liberally in trauma patients to effect decreased mortality.
- Nonoperative management (NOM) and catheter-based interventions are becoming the standard of care in appropriately selected patients with solid organ injuries.

INTRODUCTION

The presentation of a critically ill trauma patient demands the quick response and diagnostic savvy of an emergency medicine–trained physician. As with all critically ill or injured patients, the physician should begin an evaluation by addressing airway, breathing, and circulation (ABCs), after which further assessment of a patient's injuries can occur. Advanced Trauma Life Support guidelines establish a specific sequence of events when examining a trauma patient, including the ABCs and primary and secondary surveys. These sequences should be both familiar and routine to every emergency physician.

Trauma patients often present with signs and symptoms of shock, with or without obvious cause. Patients with polytrauma may have more than 1 injury contributing to hemodynamic instability, which may further complicate the picture when attempting to determine the cause of shock.

Disclosure: None.

[a] Department of Emergency Medicine, University of Maryland School of Medicine, 655 West Baltimore Street, Baltimore, MD 21201-1559, USA; [b] Department of Surgery (Primary)/Emergency Medicine (Secondary), University of Maryland School of Medicine, 22 S. Greene Street, Baltimore, MD 21201, USA

* Corresponding author.

E-mail address: drkimb@gmail.com

Emerg Med Clin N Am 32 (2014) 777–795
http://dx.doi.org/10.1016/j.emc.2014.07.004 emed.theclinics.com
0733-8627/14/$ – see front matter

RESUSCITATION

In spite of historic recommendations to administer 1 to 2 L of fluid for resuscitation,[1] recent literature has suggested that high-volume crystalloid resuscitation after injury is associated with significant morbidity, including increased ventilator days, longer ICU and hospital length of stay, development of acute respiratory distress syndrome, and multisystem organ failure and increased infection rates.[2,3] Crystalloid infusion, in the setting on ongoing hemorrhage, promotes bleeding and hemodilution, and perpetuates acidosis, hypothermia, and coagulopathy.[4] This belief has led many centers to use blood products earlier in resuscitation in patients with ongoing hemorrhage. Recent data have suggested benefit from transfusion of red blood cells (RBCs), plasma, and platelets in even ratios.[3,5,6] This practice, often referred to as "1-1-1," has become standard practice in many trauma centers and is currently being studied in a large multicenter prospective trial.[6]

For patients who require resuscitation but do not have ongoing hemorrhage, the ideal fluid for resuscitation remains unknown. Normal saline and lactated Ringer solutions have been the traditional choices. Aggressive resuscitation with crystalloid solutions, however, has been associated with negative clinical outcomes in blunt trauma patients.[2,7,8] When comparing crystalloid and colloid resuscitation, colloids have been associated with a trend toward increased mortality in trauma patients.[9] When the study excluded patients with traumatic brain injury, however, there was no difference in mortality. PlasmaLyte, a crystalloid balance solution, has also been used as a resuscitative fluid. With several different formulations, it is similar to plasma and has been termed, *physiologic solution* or *balanced solution*. PlasmaLyte has some advantages over Ringer lactate and normal saline in that it corrects both volume and electrolyte deficits without causing a hyperchloremic acidosis. Despite these advantages, studies evaluating its use after injury have shown no evidence of superiority to other crystalloids for the management of traumatic hypovolemia.[10]

Hypertonic saline has also been used as a resuscitative fluid. Due to its oncotic quality, it augments perfusion through volume expansion.[11] This is beneficial for patients with traumatic brain injury to help decrease elevated intracranial pressure. Additionally, animal models have shown that hypertonic saline helps minimize the inflammatory response after traumatic and hemorrhagic shock.[11–15] Unfortunately, no clinical trial has demonstrated benefit for the use of hypertonic saline after injury, except possibly for patients with traumatic brain jury[11] (see the neurotrauma chapter elsewhere in this issue).

Permissive hypotension is the practice of targeting a lower systolic blood pressure in the setting of hemorrhagic shock. The landmark study by Bickell and colleagues[16] demonstrated a survival benefit for patients with penetrating torso trauma who received delayed (once in the operating room) resuscitation compared with those who received fluid administration in the field. Due to significant differences in injury and mechanism patterns, subsequent studies have not been able to duplicate this work.[11,17,18] Despite this, permissive hypotension in the setting of hemorrhage, specifically penetrating torso trauma, is practiced at many high-volume trauma centers. A specific blood pressure has not been elucidated in the literature; however, based on the current available studies, a systolic blood pressure goal of 70 to 100 mm Hg is reasonable.[17,18]

ASSESSMENT OF BODY COMPARTMENTS

Head/Neck

Examination

Patients who have sustained head trauma can present with a mental status ranging from severely obtunded and unresponsive to essentially normal, depending on the severity of the brain injury. Patients presenting with head or facial injuries, concerning mechanisms of injury, or any complaints of neck pain should have a hard cervical collar in place until the cervical spine has been appropriately examined, both on physical and radiologic examination, and clinically cleared when able. Clinical clearance of the cervical spine has been studied by several groups. Specifically, the NEXUS criteria and the Canadian Cervical Spine Rule are the most well known. The criteria require that a patient cannot have any of the following: distracting injury, evidence of intoxication, midline cervical spine tenderness on palpation, or altered level of consciousness. If none of these is present, the physician can clear the cervical spine without obtaining imagining. The presence of 1 or more of these criteria dictates the need for imaging prior to clinical clearance.[19] The Canadian Cervical Spine Rule includes patients who are hemodynamically stable, alert and oriented, and have a dangerous mechanism of injury in addition to several other inclusion and exclusion criteria to determine the need for cervical spine imaging.[20]

A full neurologic examination, including determination of a patient's presenting Glasgow Coma Scale (GCS), should be performed in every trauma patient. Neurologic deficit patterns can suggest specific injuries and guide therapy. Injuries to the brain and spine can result in vital signs that are indicative of shock but often are associated with specific examination findings suggestive of neurologic or spinal shock rather than hemorrhagic. Neurogenic shock, which is a true circulatory problem, is considered a form of distributive, or warm, shock secondary to the vasodilation associated with the loss of vascular sympathetic tone after spinal cord injury.[1] It is rare to see the classic findings of hypotension and bradycardia of neurogenic shock but, if suspected, these manifestations should be treated aggressively.[21] Spinal shock is a presentation of acute spinal cord injury occurring within the first 24 hours and is usually a pattern of symptoms that include total loss of reflexes below the level of injury; flaccid paralysis, including loss of rectal tone; and complete loss of sensation. Spinal shock is often accompanied by autonomic dysfunction but is not exclusively a hemodynamic phenomenon.

Facial fractures, scalp lacerations, and hematomas can be significant sources of external hemorrhage; hemostasis should be achieved as quickly as possible. Internally, subarachnoid, subdural, and epidural hematomas are imperative diagnoses to make but do not in isolation cause hemorrhagic shock.

Imaging

CT scans of the head and cervical spine have become routine in trauma patients with abnormal mental status, intoxication, or evidence of lateralizing signs on examination. Patients with a GCS of 13 to 15 can be evaluated, however, using the Canadian CT Head Rule (CCHR) or the New Orleans Criteria (NOC) to determine the need for CT scan (**Boxes 1** and **2**). In a 2012 study comparing the 2 rules for mild traumatic brain injury, researchers found a similar sensitivity but an increased specificity in the use of the CCHR (35% compared with 9.9% in the NOC) in diagnosing an intracranial lesion on CT scan, a clinically significant brain injury, or the requirement for neurosurgical evaluation.[22]

Chest

Examination

Patients with thoracic trauma and hypotension should be immediately assessed for external signs of injury, including evidence of penetrating wounds, tracheal deviation, jugular venous distention, or flail chest/paradoxic breathing patterns. Diminished or absent breath sounds should prompt the urgent placement of a thoracostomy tube,

Box 1
New Orleans criteria

GCS less than 15

Drug or alcohol intoxication

Headache

Age greater than 60 years

Vomiting

Persistent anterograde amnesia

Seizure

Trauma appreciated above the clavicle

especially in a patient with unstable hemodynamics, for the evacuation of a potential tension pneumothorax or hemothorax. Open wounds should be covered to prevent exacerbation of a pneumothorax until a chest tube can be placed. The presence of jugular venous distention, distant cardiac sounds, and hypotension in the setting of blunt chest trauma should raise concern for tamponade and should be assessed as part of the focused assessment with sonography for trauma (FAST) examination. The physician should proceed cautiously when considering endotracheal intubation of patients with evidence of tamponade. Even in a stable patient with early signs of tamponade, sedation and positive pressure ventilation can cause significant hemodynamic instability and cardiac arrest by compromising venous return to the heart.[23] Treatment of the tamponade prior to securing an airway can potentially avert cardiovascular collapse.

The management of patients with chest trauma varies depending on the mechanism. Blunt thoracic trauma and penetrating trauma can both present with significant hemodynamic instability for similar reasons but by different mechanisms. Both blunt and penetrating trauma can lead to pneumothorax, hemothorax, or tamponade.

Resuscitative thoracotomy should be considered in specific patients. Traditionally, it has been used primarily in the setting of penetrating chest trauma, but over the past 2 decades it has been used more often in the setting of blunt trauma as well. Indications include witnessed penetrating trauma with less than 15 minutes of prehospital cardiopulmonary resuscitation (CPR) or witnessed blunt trauma with less than 5 minutes of

Box 2
Canadian CT head rule

High-risk findings—CT required

- GCS less than 15 two hours after injury
- Signs of basal skull fracture
- Suspected open or depressed skull fracture
- Greater than 2 episodes of vomiting
- Age greater than 65 years

Medium-risk findings

- Amnesia prior to impact greater than 30 minutes
- Dangerous mechanism

prehospital CPR. Other indications include severe, persistent hypotension after injury likely due to tamponade, hemorrhage, or air embolism.[24] In 2011, The Western Trauma Association published a prospective study evaluating the survival rate of patients with both blunt and penetrating injuries having received thoracotomy. The investigators concluded that resuscitative thoracotomy should be considered futile when prehospital CPR exceeds 10 minutes without response in patients with blunt trauma and 15 minutes in patients with penetrating injuries. Additionally, if asystole is the presenting cardiac rhythm and there no clear signs of tamponade, thoracotomy should not be performed.[25]

Imaging

A plain chest radiograph for both blunt and penetrating chest trauma should be done as urgently as possible to assess for hemothorax, pneumothorax-associated rib fractures, or an abnormal mediastinal contour. At a minimum, this is a screening examination for an unstable patient. CT evaluation of true, penetrating trauma should be performed in every setting when patients are stable. Unstable patients with penetrating injuries should have surgical exploration.

In the vast majority of patients with blunt chest trauma, a normal chest radiograph predicts an unremarkable chest CT (82%). In a recent study, injuries diagnosed on CT scan after negative chest radiograph included rib fractures, minor pulmonary contusions, and occult pneumothoraces but did not result in changes to management.[26] Brink and colleagues have proposed parameters that can be used to determine the need for chest CT in blunt trauma patients. These parameters include abnormal chest examination; age greater than 55; abnormal radiograph of the chest, spine, or pelvis; abnormalities on the FAST examination; and laboratory abnormalities, including a hemoglobin less than 6 mmol/L or a base deficit greater than 3 mmol/L. Using these parameters, the investigators found that less than 2% of clinically significant injuries are missed.[27] The presence of a normal mediastinal contour does not rule out the possibility of aortic injury. Demetriades demonstrated that 45% of patients with CT diagnosis of aortic rupture had normal chest radiographs. These finding suggest that despite a normal chest radiograph, patients with high-risk mechanisms, including high-speed deceleration, should undergo CT angiography of the chest.[28] Over the past decade, a shift in diagnosis of aortic injury has occurred. Although transesophageal echocardiogram and aortography have been historically the gold standard for diagnosis, they are rarely used since CT angiography has undergone improvements in quality and availability. More than 93% of aortic injuries are diagnosed based on CT angiography.[29]

Abdomen

Examination

Similar to thoracic trauma, abdominal trauma results from blunt or penetrating mechanisms, and has a broad differential. Examining the abdomen for distention or outward signs of trauma, including a seat belt sign or penetrating wounds, should be done quickly. Palpation of the abdomen for tenderness or rigidity can be helpful if a patient is able to participate in the examination. Obvious extrusion of mesentery or evisceration of hollow viscous indicates peritoneal violation and the need for operative intervention.

Establishing pelvic stability through examination and bedside pelvic radiograph assists in rapid diagnosis of pelvic fractures contributing to hemorrhagic shock. A pelvic binder should be placed in the setting of likely or known pelvic fractures associated with hemodynamic instability and should remain in place until definitive stabilization is affected. Specifically, anterior-posterior compression pelvic fractures, or open book fractures, are the most responsive to external pelvic stabilization. Lateral compression fractures are not often associated with hemodynamic instability and in this case caution should be exercised when placing a pelvic binder.

Imaging

Historically, the use of diagnostic peritoneal lavage (DPL) was used to evaluate for intraperitoneal blood after trauma, but over the past 2 decades, DPL has been largely replaced with bedside ultrasound and the FAST examination. An abdominal examination in conjunction with a FAST examination should prove a starting place to determine the acute need for operative intervention in a trauma patient. Hemodynamically unstable patients with a positive FAST examination should be considered for exploratory laparotomy. Many studies exist that support the efficacy of the FAST examination in bedside diagnosis of intraperitoneal free fluid, although there are several limiting factors to their reliability, including operator skills and patient body habitus.[30] The FAST examination can be performed quickly at the bedside, preventing an unstable patient from leaving the emergency department to be evaluated in the CT scanner.

A hemodynamically unstable patient with penetrating trauma to the abdomen should be taken to an operating room for exploration. In recent years, there has been a shift in management of hemodynamically stable patients with penetrating trauma to the abdomen. CT scan with triple contrast is both sensitive and specific in evaluating for peritoneal violation and viscous injury to determine the necessity of operative management.[31–33]

The utility of CT scan in the setting of a patient with blunt abdominal trauma has also been challenged in the past decade, with many proposed diagnostic algorithms.[34] In 2009, a prediction rule, including GCS less than 14, abdominal tenderness or costal margin tenderness, hematuria (>25 RBCs/high-power field), femur fracture, abnormal chest radiograph, and a hematocrit less than 30%, showed 96% sensitivity for any intra-abdominal injury, particularly if it required acute intervention.[35] Overall, however, there is no general consensus about who can safely be monitored and who requires an abdominal CT scan.

The need for oral contrast in the assessment for hollow viscous injury in the setting of blunt abdominal trauma has been questioned. Stuhlfaut and colleagues,[36] in 2004, determined that oral contrast was not necessary for the successful and accurate diagnosis of bowel and mesenteric injury. A prospective randomized study evaluating CT diagnosis of viscous injury in blunt abdominal trauma using oral contrast suggests there is no difference between oral contrast and only intravenous contrast. The investigators of this study also observe that it is unlikely that oral contrast is given enough time to transit the intestinal tract after administration and before CT scanning is performed to be of benefit when assessing for hollow viscous injury.[37]

Compartments

Examination

In a patient with shock, it may be difficult to appreciate pulses in all extremities as a result of low systemic blood pressure. The use of Doppler may be required. Determining the equality of pulses in extremities is important and differences should be concerning for arterial injury. In the evaluation of suspected vascular injury, the presence of hard signs indicates the absolute need for operative investigation and repair (**Box 3**). Soft signs (**Box 4**) can be equally concerning to a physician. In the presence of soft signs and a suspicion of vascular injury, the use of the ankle-brachial index (ABI) can be useful.[38] An ABI of less than or equal to 0.9 should raise suspicion for vascular injury and warrants additional imaging or operative evaluation. An ABI of less than 0.9 has been shown to have a specificity of approximately 97% for identifying arterial

Box 3
Hard signs of vascular injury

Evidence of external bleeding

Hematoma—rapidly expanding

Evidence of arterial occlusion (pain, pallor, pulselessness, parasthesias, or paralysis)

Palpable thrill

Bruit

injury.[39] Compartment syndrome can have devastating effects, including tissue necrosis and rhabdomyolysis; palpation of a tense compartment should trigger direct measurement of compartment pressure. Pain, especially with passive range of motion, is often the initial symptom of compartment syndrome and is frequently out of proportion to what is expected based on physical examination findings. Parasthesias are also common and an early sign. Classic findings of pallor, paralysis, and pulselessness are late findings.

Hemodynamic instability and shock are occasionally related to blood loss due to extremity trauma. Usually, if blood loss in the setting of extremity injury is significant enough to create hemodynamic compromise, partial or total amputation or arterial injury is often appreciable on examination. In these settings, emergent control of bleeding can occur through direct pressure on a bleeding artery or through the application of tourniquets while preparing for operative intervention and definitive control of bleeding and injury.

The use of tourniquets has been extensively studied in the military arena. Up to 20% of combat injuries involve severe trauma to the limb(s), which can result in rapid exsanguination. Tourniquet application has been shown highly effective in both upper and lower extremity trauma with little associated complication. It has been shown an expeditious maneuver that can be performed by even inexperienced personnel with high success rates and improved outcomes.[40]

Imaging

Generally, imaging of extremity injuries should be done with plain radiographs. If concern exists that vascular injury has also occurred in the setting of fracture or other traumatic injury, CT angiography can be performed. Intraoperative angiography of the extremities can be accomplished in most trauma centers and may be more appropriate in patients who require emergent operative intervention for other injuries. Inaba and colleagues[41] found that CT angiography was both 100% sensitive and specific for clinically significant (requiring operative repair) arterial injuries and should be used in patients with soft signs of vascular injury to potentially avoid unnecessary operative exploration.

Box 4
Soft signs of vascular injury

Proximity of penetrating or blunt injury to an artery

Presence of hematoma over an artery

Arterial bleeding at the scene or during transport

Neurologic deficit in the distribution of a named artery

GENERAL TRENDS IN TRAUMA IMAGING

There has been and overall shift in the general imaging practices in trauma care over the past decade. Significant literature has focused on the liberalization of CT scanning in trauma patients whereas the general medicine focus has shifted toward minimizing unnecessary radiation exposure to patients. In patients with polytrauma, whole-body CT (WBCT), including imaging of the head, cervical spine, chest, abdomen, and pelvis, has been shown both cost effective and demonstrating a statistically significant survival benefit when performed early in a patient's resuscitation. Majeed and colleagues[42] noted that 74% of their management plans changed based on WBCT and the cost savings were noted to occur primarily as a result of preventing unnecessary admissions for observation.[43] Also, as a result of the increased WBCT scanning in trauma patients, there has been a significant increase in the number of incidental findings, many of which did not change the evaluation for the presenting problem, but up to 10% of which required urgent follow-up. Recent studies that have evaluated this unintended result of WBCT report upwards of 40% to 45% of patients undergoing CT scan are found to have an unrelated incidental finding.[44,45]

Spleen

The spleen is the most commonly injured solid organ in adults after blunt trauma.[46,47] It can occur in isolation or with other injuries, both intra- and extra-abdominal. The Organ Injury Scaling Committee of the American Association for the Surgery or Trauma describes a graded scale, from 1 to 5, based on radiographic findings on CT or at time of laparotomy.[48] With the development of multidetector CT technology, the grading system of splenic injuries has evolved.[49] Some investigators have subclassified grade IV injuries to differentiate between those with intraparenchymal bleeding, without intraperitoneal bleeding (IVa), and with intraperitoneal bleeding (IVb).

Traditionally injuries to the spleen were managed surgically with splenectomy; however, with the discovery of overwhelming postsplenectomy sepsis (OPSS)[50] and the desire to preserve splenic immune function, paradigms in management began to change. The incidence of OPSS is believed to be 0.05% to 2% of patients with splenectomy.[51] Despite this low rate, surgeons began to attempt splenic salvage. Techniques included partial splenectomy or a splenorrhaphy. It was not until the late 1960s that NOM was first described in the pediatric population.[52] Since that time, NOM and the use of angiography has grown significantly. There are many advantages to NOM, including shorter hospital length of stay, decreased hospital costs, decreased intra-abdominal complication rates, and decreased blood transfusions.[53,54]

The use of CT scan has greatly changed the management of patients with splenic injuries. Over time, with the improvement in CT technology, the information provided has significantly increased. CT has been shown highly accurate (98%) in diagnosing acute splenic injuries.[55] Additionally, angiography can be used to diagnose and treat traumatic splenic vascular injuries with high rates of success.[56–58] As a result, the management of the splenic injuries continues to evolve and change. A 1991 study by Sclafani and colleagues[56] evaluated hemodynamically stable patients with a splenic injury diagnosed using first-generation CT scan technology. All patients subsequently had angiography performed. Those patients demonstrating active extravasation (AE) on angiography had proximal splenic artery embolization whereas those without AE had simple observation. The investigators were able to avoid laparotomy in 94% of the patients selected for NOM. In 2005, Haan and colleagues[59] looked at a 5-year experience in a high-volume trauma center using splenic embolization. The investigators demonstrated that patients selected for observation alone with serial hematocrits (average grade of injury approximately 2) had 100% salvage rate. Patients who had angiography and embolization (average grade of injury approximately 3) had a 90% success rate of NOM. The investigators noted that as the grade of injury increased, the success rate of NOM declined. The investigators concluded, however, that significant hemoperitoneum, AE, and pseudoaneurysm on admission CT were not predictive of NOM failure, which contradicted the EAST (Eastern Association for the Surgery of Trauma) multi-institutional trial.[46] Historically, age over 55 years has been suggested as a risk factor for failure of NOM of splenic injuries and considered a contraindication to NOM.[60–62] Other studies have shown, however, that age alone should not be considered a contraindication and that outcomes are similar between the age groups.[63–65]

The amount of published literature regarding NOM of the spleen continues to grow and evolve as technology and newer treatment techniques are developed. As such, no 2 institutions have the same treatment algorithm. Currently, the authors' management algorithm for stable blunt splenic injuries is as follows:

- Grade I and II splenic injuries are managed with observation, serial complete blood counts, and serial abdominal examinations.
- Grade III injuries, in addition to serial complete blood counts and abdominal examinations, have a nonemergent angiography performed (nonemergent is defined as during the daytime hours).
- Grade IV and V injuries have an emergent angiography performed.

Those patients who have angiography performed, with or without embolization, have a repeat CT performed at 48 to 72 hours after injury. If repeat imaging is stable and patients are otherwise clinically stable, they are discharged. There is considerable debate over the need for repeat imaging after blunt splenic injuries. Lower-grade injuries (I and II) probably do not need repeat imaging.[66] Early studies showed a mean of 2.7 days from admission to failure for those patients who had angiography without embolization and 1 day for those who had embolization.[67] Davis and colleagues[68] demonstrated approximately two-thirds of pseudoaneurysms were present on repeat imaging on day 3 that were not present on the initial CT scan thus advocating serial CT scan.

Liver

As with the spleen, injuries to the liver can occur after both blunt and penetrating trauma. Additionally, a grading system based on injury severity has been developed.[48] Traditionally, operative intervention was the accepted management strategy for blunt liver injury; however, many injuries were found minor without active bleeding.[69–72] Based on these findings and that NOM of liver injures in pediatric patients had very high success rates, the techniques for managing blunt liver injuries began to change.[69,73–76] As a result, there is a growing body of literature supporting the use on NOM for liver injuries with high rates of success.[70,77–79]

Current diagnostic strategies for liver injuries are similar to those of the spleen. DPL and FAST are bedside procedures that can be rapidly performed; however, they do not specifically identify the liver as the source of hemorrhage. CT remains the imaging modality of choice for liver injuries. As with the spleen, as CT technology evolves so does the detail of information provided. This constant evolution of technology creates ever-changing treatment algorithms. Despite new technology, any hemodynamically unstable patient should proceed directly to the operating room. Additionally, any patients with an alternate indication for laparotomy, including peritonitis, should proceed directly for surgical exploration.[80,81]

For those patients who do not have an indication for immediate operative intervention, NOM has become the standard of care for patients who are hemodynamically stable.[81–85] Traditional risk factors thought related to failure of NOM included grade of injury, simultaneous traumatic brain injury, amount of hemoperitoneum, age greater than 55 years, transfusion requirements, or blush on CT scan.[77,82,86] Recent literature, however, questions these risk factors and currently they are not believed absolute contraindications to attempting NOM in hemodynamically stable patients with a liver injury.[65,82,87,88]

Low-grade injuries (I and II) usually can be managed with simple observation and serial laboratory evaluation. A patient's clinical scenario should dictate any further intervention surgical or repeat imaging. Higher-grade injuries without AE, as demonstrated by blush on CT scan, can also typically be managed with simple observation with serial laboratory and clinical examinations. Injuries that demonstrate AE should be considered for angiographic evaluation.[89] Angiographic embolization can be helpful in the NOM treatment of liver injury,[73] and several studies have demonstrated its benefit in controlling hemorrhage.[90,91] Despite these reports, its use remains controversial.[82] Studies have demonstrated that angioembolization of liver injuries is associated with several complications, including major hepatic necrosis, liver abscess, gall bladder necrosis/ischemia, bile leak[92–94] vessel damage at site of arterial cannulation, and renal dysfunction-related contrast injection.[82]

Kidney

The kidney, like the spleen and the liver, has a grading system of injury.[48] Renal injuries occur in up to 3% of all trauma patients and are as high as 10% for those with abdominal trauma.[95] Unlike other intra-abdominal injuries, a renal (genitourinary) injury can be quickly suspected based on a urinalysis. Gross hematuria increases the likelihood of injury.

Prior to the wide availability of CT, intravenous pyelogram (IVP) was used in patients with suspected renal injury. This was most often in the setting of evidence of either frank or microscopic hematuria. A 1987 study by Oakland and colleagues[96] suggested that an IVP should only be performed for naked eye hematuria or prolonged microscopic hematuria. Studies have demonstrated, however, that as many as 20% of significant renal injuries are missed with IVP.[95] As CT has become more widely available, the use of IVP has significantly decreased. CT has many advantages over IVP, including providing better injury-specific detail and demonstrating contrast extravasation more reliably as well as injuries to the collecting system with the use of delayed imaging.[95] Additionally CT can identify other solid organ and hollow viscous injuries at the same time.

Initial diagnostics for patients with suspected renal injuries include the FAST examination and/or, for those patients deemed stable, CT scan. Patients who have a positive FAST and are hemodynamically unstable should have immediate operative exploration. DPL, which has been traditionally used to identify free intraperitoneal blood, may not be as effective in diagnosing a renal injury because the kidney is located in the retroperitoneum.

It is believed that many patients who undergo exploratory laparotomy for a concerned renal injury simply end up with a nephrectomy as opposed to any attempt for renal salvage.[97–99] Because most renal injuries are minor contusions and hematomas, NOM and renal preservation can often be achieved with a minimum of complications.[98–102] Additionally, standard routine follow-up imaging is unnecessary for these low-grade (I–III) injuries.[103] The management of higher-grade injuries remains, however, somewhat controversial, with varying success rates.[102,104] The use of angiography and embolization has been extended to renal injuries, specifically those with AE on CT scan. Indications for angiography include AE on CT scan and high-grade injury.[102] Angiography has been shown safe in terms of not causing nephropathy due to the contrast agent[105]; however, published success rates vary for the prevention of operative intervention and subsequent nephrectomy.[102,104,105]

Damage Control

The concept of "damage control laparotomy" originated in the early 1900s to help manage severe liver injuries.[106,107] The idea is that acute hemorrhage and contamination are surgically controlled; however, definitive repair of injuries is deferred.[108] The idea became popular in the 1980s with the increase in inner-city violence and use of high-velocity, multiple round weapons. For the first time, patients with multiple, severe anatomic injuries were presenting to emergency departments. These constellations of injuries did not seem best managed with a single surgical intervention because it was quickly observed that many of these patients were dying from the physiologic sequelae of their injuries prior to completion of definitive surgical repair.[6,109] As a result, techniques of abbreviated laparotomy began to be used, with increase rates of survival.[110,111] In 1993, a landmark article by Rotondo and colleagues[108] coined the term, *damage control*, and significantly changed the way trauma care is delivered.

It is well known that severely injured trauma patients often die from intraoperative metabolic complications rather than from the inability to repair the injuries.[6] The lethal triad—hypothermia, acidosis, and coagulopathy—once started is difficult and often impossible to reverse in an operating room. As a result, the concept of damage control laparotomy allows for a brief operative intervention, a temporary closure with a vacuum-assisted device, and rapid transfer to an ICU where resuscitation can continue. Once patients have been warmed, coagulopathy treated, and acidosis reversed, they are considered physiologically resuscitated/stable and can better tolerate additional and longer operative interventions for definitive repair. The role of intensivists and the care provided by an ICU is paramount in improving survival and allowing early and safe return to the operating room for definitive surgical management.[6,111] The specific appropriate timing of this reoperation is unknown; however, according to Rotondo and colleagues,[108] aggressive intensive care management can return normal physiology within 48 hours. The goal of the second operation should be removal of any packing, definitive repair of known injuries, evaluation for missed injuries, and planned closure of intestinal wall and skin.[6] If the abdominal cavity is unable to be closed, once again a temporary vacuum-assisted device is placed and planned reoperation is planned. Unfortunately, each time definitive closure is not achieved, the likelihood of complications, including enterocutaneous fistulae, intra-abdominal sepsis, and resultant long-term hernia, increases.[112]

The ideas and principles of damage control have been expanded beyond the abdomen. Similar techniques have been used for thoracic[113,114] and vascular[115,116] trauma. In 2000, Scalea and colleagues[117] applied the principles of damage control surgery to trauma orthopedics and coined the term, *damage control orthopedics*. Just as Rotondo and colleagues revolutionized the surgical management of the abdomen in critically injured trauma patients, the application of damage control to orthopedic trauma has changed the way care is delivered.[118–121] Damage control orthopedics has been shown associated with a lesser systemic inflammatory response than early total care fracture fixation.[122]

Abdominal Compartment Syndrome

As its name implies, abdominal compartment syndrome (ACS) consists of a constellation of clinical findings leading to a diagnosis. The term is believed to have been coined in a 1989 publication by Fietsam and colleagues.[123] The investigators described intra-abdominal hypertension from a ruptured aortic aneurysm causing "increased ventilatory pressure, increased central venous pressure and decreased urinary output."[123,124] The concept of ACS was first suggested in the late 1800s by several investigators who described that the "effects that respiration produces on the thorax are the inverse of those present in the abdomen," and, who seem to have been the first to measure intraabdominal pressures (IAPs).[124,125] In 1874, Wendt was the first to describe an association between elevated intra-abdominal pressure and organ dysfunction.[124–127]

Today, ACS is defines as a sustained IAP greater than 20 mm Hg that is associated with new onset of organ dysfunction or failure.[6,128] IAP is determined by measuring a bladder pressure transmitted through a Foley catheter. It should be measured at end expiration while a patient is supine and relaxed or sedated and the transducer is zeroed at the midaxillary line.[128,129] Even a slight elevation of the head of the bed can cause an erroneous reading. Clinicians should be cognizant of symptoms of organ dysfunction, which can manifest as oliguria, hypoxia, hypercarbia, increased peak airway pressures, persistent hypotension, or increased acidosis from intestinal ischemia. Risk factors for developing ACS include massive crystalloid fluid resuscitation (>5000 mL in 24 h), massive transfusions (>10 unit PRBC in 24 h), hypothermia, base deficit/acidosis (pH<7.2), and a body mass index greater than 30.[6,128,129]

ACS has been classified as primary, secondary, or tertiary. Primary ACS refers to a situation when a primary intra-abdominal cause (ruptured aneurysm, abdominal trauma, or retroperitoneal hematoma) is the cause of ACS. Secondary ACS refers to a condition as a result of massive bowel edema secondary to conditions that required massive volume resuscitation, which most commonly occurs after hemorrhagic shock or severe burns.[129] Decompressive laparotomy is the definitive treatment regardless of whether it is primary or secondary ACS. Tertiary or recurrent ACS is rare and usually occurs after a previous episode of ACS has resolved and there is aggressive attempt at abdominal closure in an edematous patient with an open abdomen.[129] Over the past 10 years, the incidence of ACS has decreased, mostly due to adoption of massive transfusion protocols limiting the volume of crystalloid infusion as well as damage control techniques and temporary abdominal closure methods.[129]

SUMMARY

Rapid evaluation, diagnostics, and intervention of injured patients presenting in shock are paramount for good outcome and improved survival. Over the past 30 to 40 years with advances in technology, including bedside ultrasonography and the multidetector CT technology, the techniques for diagnosing hemorrhage and shock have changed. The basic concept of trauma care, however, has remained the same, which is rapidly identifying sources of hemorrhage and shock, delivering adequate resuscitation, and providing definitive care as quickly and as safely as possible. Over the past 10 years, resuscitation using blood products has replaced large-volume crystalloid infusions in many centers. Specific ratio of blood products transfused remains unknown and is currently an area of ongoing research. Additionally, when used, the ideal crystalloid remains unknown. NOM of many injuries has become standard of care. Correctly identifying patients for NOM is key to its success. Despite the increase in NOM, many patients with multiple injuries require immediate operative intervention.

Damage control techniques are often used to quickly treat life-threatening injuries and allow for physiologic normalization prior to definitive repair. As trauma care continues to evolve, newer techniques and management algorithms, including expanding catheter-based therapies for hemorrhage, will emerge.

REFERENCES

1. American College of Surgeons. Shock. In: American College of Surgeon – Committee on Trauma, editor. ATLS advanced trauma life support for doctors. 8th edition. Chicago: American College of Surgeons; 2008. p. 10–1.
2. Kasotakis G, Sideris A, Yang Y, et al. Aggressive early crystalloid resuscitation adversely affects outcomes in adult blunt trauma patients: an analysis of the Glue Grant database. J Trauma Acute Care Surg 2013;74(5):1215–22.
3. Duchesne JC, Heaney J, Guidry C, et al. Diluting the benefits of hemostatic resuscitation: a multi-institutional analysis. J Trauma Acute Care Surg 2013;75(1): 76–82.
4. Moore FA, McKinley BA, Moore EE. The next generation in shock resuscitation. Lancet 2004;363(9425):1988–96.
5. Holcomb JB, Zarzabal LA, Michalek JE, et al. Increased platelet:RBC ratios are associated with improved survival after massive transfusion. J Trauma 2011;71: S318–28.
6. Stein DM, Lazaridis C, Ling GS. Non-Neurologic trauma, burns and thermal injury. 2013 Neurocritical Care Society Practice update. Available at: www.neurocriticalcare.org. Accessed January 6, 2014.
7. Holcomb JB, Jenkins D, Rhee P, et al. Damage control resuscitation: directly addressing the early coagulopathy of trauma. J Trauma 2007;62:307–10.
8. Deb S, Sun L, Martin B, et al. Lactated Ringer's solution and hetastarch but not plasma resuscitation after rat hemorrhagic shock is associated with immediate lung apoptosis by the up-regulation of the Bax protein. J Trauma 2000;49:47–53.
9. Finfer S, Bellomo R, Boyce N, et al. A comparison of albumin and saline for fluid resuscitation in the intensive care unit. N Engl J Med 2004;350:2247–56.
10. Rizoli S. PlasmaLyte. J Trauma 2011;70:S17–8.
11. Pieracci FM, Biffl WL, Moore EE. Current concepts in resuscitation. J Intensive Care Med 2012;27:79–96.
12. Rizoli SB, Kapus A, Fan J, et al. Immunomodulatory effects of hypertonic resuscitation on the development of lung inflammation following hemorrhagic shock. J Immunol 1998;161:6288–96.
13. Coimbra R, Hoyt DB, Junger WG, et al. Hypertonic saline resuscitation decreases susceptibility to sepsis after hemorrhagic shock. J Trauma 1997;42:602–6.
14. Zallen G, Moore EE, Tamura DY, et al. Hypertonic saline resuscitation abrogates neutrophil priming by mesenteric lymph. J Trauma 2000;48:45–8.
15. Junger WG, Coimbra R, Liu FC, et al. Hypertonic saline resuscitation: a tool to modulate immune function in trauma patients? Shock 1997;8:235–41.
16. Bickell WH, Wall MJ Jr, Pepe PE, et al. Immediate versus delayed fluid resuscitation for hypotensive patients with penetrating torso injuries. N Engl J Med 1994;331:1105–9.
17. Turner J, Nicholl J, Webber L, et al. A randomized controlled trial of prehospital intravenous fluid replacement therapy in serious trauma. Health Technol Assess 2000;4:1–57.
18. Dutton RP, Mackenzie CF, Scalea TM. Hypotensive resuscitation during active hemorrhage: impact on in-hospital mortality. J Trauma 2002;52:1141–6.

19. Hoffman JR, Wolfson AB, Todd K, et al. Selective cervical spine radiography in blunt trauma: Methodology of the National Emergency X-Radiography Utilization Study (NEXUS). Ann Emerg Med 1998;32:461–9.
20. Stiell IG, Wells GA, Vandemheen KL, et al. The Canadian C-spine rule for radiography in alert and stable trauma patients. JAMA 2001;286(15): 1841–8.
21. Mallek JT, Inaba K, Branco BC, et al. The incidence of neurogenic shock after spinal cord injury in patients admitted to a high-volume level I trauma center. Am Surg 2012;78:623–6.
22. Papa L, Stiell IG, Clement CM, et al. Performance of the Canadian CT head rule and the New Orleans criteria for predicting any traumatic intracranial injury on computer tomography in a United States Level I Trauma Center. Acad Emerg Med 2012;19:2–10.
23. Ho AM, Graham CA, Ng CS, et al. Timing of tracheal intubation in traumatic cardiac tamponade: a word of caution. Resuscitation 2009;80:272–4.
24. Cothren CC, Moore EE. Emergency department thoracotomy for the critically injured patient: objectives, indications, and outcomes. World J Emerg Surg 2006;1:4.
25. Moore EE, Knudson MM, Burlew CC, et al. Defining the limits of resuscitative emergency department thoracotomy: a contemporary Western Trauma Association perspective. J Trauma 2011;70:334–9.
26. Kea B, Gamarallage R, Vairamuthu H, et al. What is the clinical significance of chest CT when the chest x-ray result is normal in patients with blunt trauma? Am J Emerg Med 2013;31:1268–73.
27. Brink M, Deunk J, Dekker H, et al. Criteria for the selective use of chest computed tomography in blunt trauma patients. Eur Radiol 2010;20:818–28.
28. Demetriades D, Gomez H, Velmahos GC. Routine helical computed tomographic evaluation of the mediastinum in high-risk blunt trauma patients. Arch Surg 1998;133:1084–8.
29. Demetriades D, Velmahos GC, Scalea TM. Diagnosis and treatment of blunt thoracic aortic injuries: changing perspectives. J Trauma 2008;64: 1415–8.
30. Patel NY, Riherd JM. Focused assessment with sonography for trauma; methods, accuracy, and indications. Surg Clin North Am 2011;91:195–207.
31. Shanmuganathan K, Mirvis SE, Chiu WC, et al. Penetrating torso trauma: triple-contrast helical CT in peritoneal violation and organ injury—a prospective study in 200 patients. Radiology 2004;231:775–84.
32. Velmahos GC, Constantinou C, Tillou A, et al. Abdominal computed tomographic scan for patients with gunshot wounds to the abdomen selected for nonoperative management. J Trauma 2005;59:1155–60.
33. Goodman CS, Hur JY, Adajar MA, et al. How well does CT predict the need for laparotomy in hemodynamically stable patients with penetrating abdominal injury? A review and meta-analysis. Am J Roentgenol 2009;193:432–7.
34. Deunk J, Brink M, Dekker H, et al. Predictors for the selection of patients for abdominal CT after blunt trauma; a proposal for a diagnostic algorithm. Ann Surg 2010;251:512–20.
35. Holmes JF, Wisner DH, McGahan JP, et al. Clinical prediction rules for identifying adults at very low risk for intra-abdominal injuries after blunt trauma. Ann Emerg Med 2009;54:575–84.
36. Stuhlfaut JW, Soto JA, Lucey BC, et al. Blunt abdominal trauma: performance of CT without oral contrast material. Radiology 2004;233:689–94.

37. Stafford RE, McGonigal MD, Weigelt JA, et al. Oral contrast solution and computed tomography for blunt abdominal trauma: a randomized study. Arch Surg 1999;134: 622–7.
38. Feliciano DV. Management of peripheral arterial injury. Curr Opin Crit Care 2010; 16:602–8.
39. Johansen K, Lynch K, Paun M, et al. Non-invasive vascular tests reliably exclude occult arterial trauma in injured extremities. J Trauma 1991;31:515–9.
40. Lakstein D, Blumenfeld A, Sokolov T, et al. Tourniquets for hemorrhage control on the battlefield: a 4-year accumulated experience. J Trauma 2003;54: S221–5.
41. Inaba K, Branco BC, Reddy S, et al. Prospective evaluation of multidetector computed tomography for extremity vascular trauma. J Trauma 2011;70:808–15.
42. Majeed M, Yeo D, Kayani J. Is whole body CT safe and cost effective in managing major trauma patients in the emergency department? J Emerg Med 2012;43:939.
43. Huber-Wagne S, Lefering R, Qvick LM, et al. Effect of whole-body CT during trauma resuscitation on survival: a retrospective, multicentre study. Lancet 2009;373:1455–61.
44. Devine AS, Jackson CS, Lyons L, et al. Frequency of incidental findings on computed tomography of trauma patients. West J Emerg Med 2010;11:24–7.
45. Sierink JC, Saltzherr TP, Russchen MJ, et al. Incidental findings on total-body CT scans in trauma patients. Injury 2014;45(5):840–4.
46. Peitzman AB, Heil B, Rivera L, et al. Blunt splenic injury in adults: multi-institutional Study of the Eastern Association for the Surgery of Trauma. J Trauma 2000;49: 177–87.
47. Cogbill TH, Moore EE, Jurkovich GJ, et al. Nonoperative management of blunt splenic trauma: a multicenter experience. J Trauma 1989;29:1312–7.
48. Moore EE, Cogbill TH, Malangoni MA, et al. Organ injury scaling. Surg Clin North Am 1995;75:293–303.
49. Marmery H, Shanmuganathan K, Alexander MT, et al. Optimization of selection for nonoperative management of blunt splenic injury: comparison of MDCT grading systems. AJR Am J Roentgenol 2007;189:1421–7.
50. King H, Schumacher HB. Splenic studies I: susceptibility to infection after splenectomy performed in infancy. Ann Surg 1952;136:239–42.
51. Shatz DV. Vaccination practices among North American trauma surgeons in splenectomy for trauma. J Trauma 2002;53:950–6.
52. Upadhyaya P, Simpson JS. Splenic trauma in children. Surgery 1968;126: 781–90.
53. Sartorelli KH, Frumiento C, Rogers FB, et al. Non-operative management of hepatic, splenic, and renal injuries in adults with multiple injuries. J Trauma 2000; 49:56–61.
54. Pachter HL, Guth AA, Hofstetter SR, et al. Changing patterns in the management of splenic trauma. Ann Surg 1998;227:708–19.
55. Shanmuganathan K, Mirvis SE, Boyd-Kranis R, et al. Nonsurgical management of blunt splenic injury: use of CT criteria to select patients for splenic arteriography and potential endovascular therapy. Radiology 2000;217:75–82.
56. Sclafani SJ, Weisberg A, Scalea TM, et al. Blunt splenic injuries: nonsurgical treatment with CT, arteriography, and transcatheter arterial embolization of the splenic artery. Radiology 1991;181:189–96.
57. Sclafani SJ, Shaftan GW, Scalea TM, et al. Nonoperative salvage of computed tomography-diagnosed splenic injuries: utilization of angiography for triage and embolization for hemostasis. J Trauma 1995;39(5):818–25.

58. Hagiwara A, Yukioka T, Ohta S, et al. Nonsurgical management of patients with blunt splenic injury: efficacy of transcatheter arterial embolization. AJR Am J Roentgenol 1996;167:159–66.
59. Haan JM, Bochicchio GV, Kramer N, et al. Nonoperative management of blunt splenic injury: a 5-year experience. J Trauma 2005;58:492–8.
60. Godley CD, Warren RL, Sheridan RL, et al. Nonoperative management of blunt splenic injury in adults: age over 55 years as a powerful indicator for failure. J Am Coll Surg 1996;183:133–9.
61. Smith JS Jr, Wengrovitz MA, DeLong BS. Prospective validation criteria, including safe, nonsurgical management of the ruptured spleen. J Trauma 1992;33:363–9.
62. Harbrecht BG, Peitzman AB, Rivera L, et al. Contribution of age and gender to outcome of blunt splenic injury in adults: a multicenter study of the Eastern Association for the Surgery of Trauma. J Trauma 2001;51:887–95.
63. Albrecht RM, Schermer CR, Morris A. Nonoperative management of blunt splenic injuries: factors influencing success in age >55 years. Am Surg 2002;68:227–31.
64. Cocanour CS, Moore FA, Ware DN, et al. Age should not be a consideration for nonoperative management of blunt splenic injury. J Trauma 2000;48:606–12.
65. Sharma OP, Oswanksi MF, Singer D, et al. Assessment of nonoperative management of blunt spleen and liver trauma. Am Surg 2005;71:379–86.
66. Haan JM, Boswell S, Stein D, et al. Follow-up abdominal CT is not necessary in low-grade splenic injury. Am Surg 2007;73(1):13–8.
67. Haan J, Scott J, Boyd-Kranis RL, et al. Admission angiography for blunt splenic injury: advantages and pitfalls. J Trauma 2001;51(6):1161–5.
68. Davis KA, Fabian TC, Croce MA, et al. Improved success in non-operative management of blunt splenic injuries: embolization of splenic artery pseudoaneurysm. J Trauma 1998;44:1008–15.
69. Carrillo EH, Platz A, Miller FB, et al. Non-operative management of blunt hepatic trauma. Br J Surg 1998;85:461–8.
70. Croce MA, Fabian TC, Menke PG, et al. Nonoperative management of blunt hepatic trauma is the treatment of choice for hemodynamically stable patients. Results of a prospective trial. Ann Surg 1995;221:744–55.
71. Pachter HL, Feliciano DV. Complex hepatic injuries. Surg Clin North Am 1996; 76:763–82.
72. Mirvis SE, Whitley NO, Vainwright JR, et al. Blunt hepatic trauma in adults: CT-based classification and correlation with prognosis and treatment. Radiology 1989;171:27–32.
73. Stein DM, Scalea TM. Nonoperative management of spleen and liver injuries. J Intensive Care Med 2006;21:296–304.
74. Karp MP, Cooney DR, Pros GA, et al. The nonoperative management of pediatric hepatic trauma. J Pediatr Surg 1983;18:512–8.
75. Cywes S, Rode H, Millar AJ. Blunt liver trauma in children: nonoperative management. J Pediatr Surg 1985;20:14–8.
76. Oldham KT, Guice KS, Ryckman F, et al. Blunt liver injury in childhood: evolution of therapy and current perspective. Surgery 1986;100:542–9.
77. Pachter HL, Knudson MM, Esrig B, et al. Status of nonoperative management of blunt hepatic injuries in 1995: a multicenter experience with 404 patients. J Trauma 1996;40:31–8.
78. Velmahos GC, Toutouzas K, Radin R, et al. High success with nonoperative management of blunt hepatic trauma: the liver is a sturdy organ. Arch Surg 2003;138: 475–81.

79. Tinkoff G, Esposito TJ, Reed J, et al. American Association for the Surgery of Trauma Organ Injury Scale I: spleen, liver, and kidney, validation based on the National Trauma Data Bank. J Am Coll Surg 2008;207(5):646–55.
80. Meredith JW, Young JS, Bowling J, et al. Nonoperative management of blunt hepatic trauma: the exception or the rule? J Trauma 1994;36:529–35.
81. Brasel KJ, DeLisle CM, Olson CJ, et al. Trends in the management of hepatic injury. Am Surg 1997;174:674–7.
82. Stassen NA, Bhullar I, Cheng JD, et al. Nonoperative management of blunt hepatic injury: an Eastern Association for the Surgery of Trauma practice management guideline. J Trauma Acute Care Surg 2012;73(5 Suppl 4):S288–93.
83. Hellins TE, Morse G, McNabney WK. Treatment of liver injuries at Level I and II centers in a multi-institutional metropolitan trauma system. J Trauma 1997;42:1091–6.
84. Coimbra R, Hoyt DB, Engelhart S, et al. Non-operative management reduces the overall mortality of Grades 3 and 4 blunt liver injuries. Int Surg 2006;91:251–7.
85. Velmahos GC, Toutouzas K, Radin R, et al. Non-operative treatment of blunt injury to solid abdominal organs: a prospective study. Arch Surg 2003;138:844–51.
86. Fang JF, Chen RJ, Wong YC, et al. Pooling of contrast material on computed tomography mandates aggressive management of blunt hepatic injury. Am J Surg 1998;176:315–9.
87. Falimirski ME, Provost D. Nonsurgical management of solid abdominal organ injury in patients over 55 years of age. Am Surg 2000;66:631–5.
88. Archer LP, Rogers FB, Shackford SR. Selective non-operative management of liver and spleen injuries in neurologically impaired adult patients. Arch Surg 1996;131:309–15.
89. Hagiwara A, Murata A, Matsuda T, et al. The efficacy and limitations of transarterial embolization for severe hepatic injury. J Trauma 2002;52:1091–6.
90. Hagiwara A, Yukioka T, Ohta S, et al. Nonsurgical management of patients with blunt hepatic injury: efficacy of transcatheter arterial embolization. AJR Am J Roentgenol 1997;169:1151–6.
91. Carrillo EH, Spain DA, Wohltmann CD, et al. Interventional techniques are useful adjuncts in non-operative management of hepatic injuries. J Trauma 1999;46:619–24.
92. Dabbs DN, Stein DM, Scalea TM. Major hepatic necrosis: a common complication after angioembolization for treatment of high-grade liver injuries. J Trauma 2009;66:621–7.
93. Misselbeck TS, Teicher EJ, Cipolle MD, et al. Hepatic angioembolization in trauma patients: indications and complications. J Trauma 2009;67:769–73.
94. Mohr AM, Lavery RF, Barone A, et al. Angiographic embolization for liver injuries: low mortality, high morbidity. J Trauma 2003;55:1077–81.
95. Coburn M. Genitourinary trauma. In: Feliciano DV, Mattox KL, Moore EE, editors. Trauma. 6th edition. New York: McGraw-Hill; 2008. p. 789–824.
96. Oakland CD, Britton JM, Charlton CA. Renal trauma and the intravenous urogram. J R Soc Med 1987;80:21–2.
97. Wessells H, Suh D, Porter JR, et al. Renal injury and operative management in the Unites States: results of a population study. J Trauma 2003;54:423–30.
98. van der Vlies CH, Olthof DC, Gaakeer M, et al. Changing patterns in diagnostic strategies and the treatment of blunt injury to solid abdominal organs. Int J Emerg Med 2011;4:47.
99. Bergren CT, Chan FN, Bodzin JH. Intravenous pyerlogram results in association with renal pathology and therapy in trauma patients. J Trauma 1987;27:515–8.
100. Goff CD, Collin GR. Management of renal trauma at a rural, level I trauma center. Am Surg 1998;64:226–30.

101. Nguyen HT, Carroll PR. Blunt renal trauma: renal preservation through careful staging and selective surgery. Semin Urol 1995;13:83–9.
102. Menaker J, Joseph B, Stein DM, et al. Angiointervention: high rates of failure following blunt renal injuries. World J Surg 2011;35:520–7.
103. Malcolm JB, Derweesh IH, Mehrazin R, et al. Nonoperative management of blunt renal trauma: is routine early follow-up imaging necessary? BMC Urol 2008;8:11.
104. van der Wilden GM, Velmahos GC, Joseph DK, et al. Successful nonoperative management of the most severe blunt renal injuries: a multicenter study of the research consortium of New England Centers for Trauma. JAMA Surg 2013;148:924–31.
105. Sarani B, Powell E, Taddeo J, et al. Contemporary comparison of surgical and interventional arteriography management of blunt renal injury. J Vasc Interv Radiol 2011;22:723–8.
106. Pringle JH. Notes on the arrest of hepatic hemorrhage due to trauma. Ann Surg 1908;48(4):541–9.
107. Halsted WS. Ligature and suture material: the employment of fine silk in preference to catgut and the advantages of transfixion of tissues and vessels in control of hemorrhage: also an account of the introduction of gloves, gutta-percha tissue and silver foil. JAMA 1913;60(15):1119–26.
108. Rotondo MF, Schwab CW, McGonigal MD, et al. 'Damage control': an approach for improved survival in exsanguinating penetrating abdominal injury. J Trauma 1993;35:375–82.
109. Stone HH, Strom PR, Mullins RJ. Management of the major coagulopathy with onset during laparotomy. Ann Surg 1983;197:532–5.
110. Burch JM, Ortiz VB, Richardson RJ, et al. Abbreviated laparotomy and planned reoperation for critically injured patients. Ann Surg 1992;215:476–84.
111. Sagraves SG, Toschlog EA, Rotondo MF. Damage control surgery–the intensivist's role. J Intensive Care Med 2006;21:215–6.
112. Bradley MJ, Dubose JJ, Scalea TM, et al. Independent predictors of enteric fistula and abdominal sepsis after damage control laparotomy: results from the prospective AAST Open Abdomen registry. JAMA Surg 2013;148:947–54.
113. Caceres M, Buechter KJ, Tillou A, et al. Thoracic packing for uncontrolled bleeding in penetrating thoracic injuries. South Med J 2004;97:637–41.
114. Moriwaki Y, Toyoda H, Harunari N, et al. Gauze packing as damage control for uncontrollable haemorrhage in severe thoracic trauma. Ann R Coll Surg Engl 2013;95:20–5.
115. Oliver JC, Gill H, Nicol AJ, et al. Temporary vascular shunting in vascular trauma: a 10-year review from a civilian trauma centre. S Afr J Surg 2013;51:6–10.
116. Ball CG, Feliciano DV. Damage control techniques for common and external iliac artery injuries: have temporary intravascular shunts replaced the need for ligation? J Trauma 2010;68:1117–20.
117. Scalea TM, Boswell SA, Scott JD, et al. External fixation as a bridge to intramedullary nailing for patients with multiple injuries and with femur fractures: damage control orthopedics. J Trauma 2000;48:613–23.
118. Nowotarski PJ, Turen CH, Brumback RJ, et al. Conversion of external fixation to intramedullary nailing for fractures of the shaft of the femur in multiply injured patients. J Bone Joint Surg Am 2000;82:781–8.
119. Pape HC, Hildebrand F, Pertschy S, et al. Changes in the management of femoral shaft fractures in polytrauma patients: from early total care to damage control orthopedic surgery. J Trauma 2002;53:452–61.

120. Taeger G, Ruchholtz S, Waydhas C, et al. Damage control orthopedics in patients with multiple injuries is effective, time saving, and safe. J Trauma 2005;5:409–16.
121. Parekh AA, Smith WR, Silva S, et al. Treatment of distal femur and proximal tibia fractures with external fixation followed by planned conversion to internal fixation. J Trauma 2008;64:736–9.
122. Harwood PJ, Giannoudis PV, van Griensven M, et al. Alterations in the systemic inflammatory response after early total care and damage control procedures for femoral shaft fracture in severely injured patients. J Trauma 2005;58:446–52.
123. Fietsam R Jr, Villalba M, Glover JL, et al. Intra-abdominal compartment syndrome as a complication of ruptured abdominal aortic aneurysm repair. Am Surg 1989;55:396–402.
124. Schein M. Abdominal compartment syndrome: historical background. In: Ivatury RR, Cheatham ML, Makbrain ML, et al, editors. Abdominal compartment syndrome. Georgetown (TX): Landes Bioscience; 2006. p. 1–7.
125. Emerson H. Intra-abdominal pressures. Arch Intern Med 1911;7:754–84.
126. Atema JJ, van Buijtenen JM, Lamme B, et al. Clinical studies on intra-abdominal hypertension and abdominal compartment syndrome. J Trauma Acute Care Surg 2014;76:234–40.
127. Wendt EC. Ueber den Einfluss des intraabdominalen Druckes auf die Absonderungsgeschwindigkeit des Harnes. Arch Heilkunde 1876;17:527–46.
128. Malbrain ML, Cheatham ML, Kirkpatrick A, et al. Results from the international conference of experts on intra-abdominal hypertension and abdominal compartment syndrome. I. Definitions. Intensive Care Med 2006;32:1722–32.
129. Carr JA. Abdominal compartment syndrome: a decade of progress. J Am Coll Surg 2013;216:135–46.

Hemorrhage and Coagulopathy in the Critically Ill

Tara Ann Paterson, MD[a,*], Deborah Michelle Stein, MD, MPH, FCCM[b]

KEYWORDS

- Hemorrhage • Coagulopathy • Transfusion • Resuscitation
- Massive transfusion protocol

KEY POINTS

- Hemorrhage and coagulopathy in the critically ill, if not intervened upon early, can precipitate a vicious cycle of hypothermia and acidosis that worsens coagulopathy and bleeding.
- Transfusion medicine has come a long way since its origin in 1665, but still has a long way to go.
- Coagulopathy may be induced by trauma, acute blood loss, medications, resuscitation with blood products or crystalloid devoid of coagulation factors, or hypothermia.
- Recent oral anticoagulants complicate coagulopathy and present a new dilemma for treatment, not responding to traditional reversal agents.

INTRODUCTION

The first successful blood transfusion was performed by physician Richard Lower on dogs in 1665 and the first accounts of mass casualties and lifesaving blood transfusions was during World War I.[1] Military transfusion practice continues to influence civilian protocols in emergency and trauma medicine. This is so vital because trauma is a major health issue worldwide and is responsible for more than 5 million deaths annually, projected to be more than 8 million by 2020.[2] Uncontrolled hemorrhage is responsible for 40% of all deaths in trauma. The development of coagulopathy in the setting of hemorrhage occurs frequently and confounds our ability to restore normal

---

Disclosures: None.

[a] Department of Anesthesiology, R Adams Cowley Shock Trauma Center, 22 South Greene Street, Baltimore, MD 21201, USA; [b] Department of Surgery, University of Maryland School of Medicine, R Adams Cowley Shock Trauma Center, 22 South Greene Street, Baltimore, MD 21201, USA
* Corresponding author.
E-mail address: taraannpaterson@gmail.com

Emerg Med Clin N Am 32 (2014) 797–810
http://dx.doi.org/10.1016/j.emc.2014.07.005 emed.theclinics.com

physiology. In an emergency setting, coagulopathy may be a direct result of trauma, ongoing bleeding, traumatic brain injury, upper or lower gastric hemorrhage, cirrhosis, medication effects, or multifactorial. Consumption of clotting factors, hemodilution, acidosis, hypoperfusion, and hypothermia are causes of hypocoagulability that occur within the first 24 hours of admission. One third of patients presenting to the emergency department are coagulopathic, which in turn increases mortality and morbidity.[3]

THE COAGULATION CASCADE

To discuss hemorrhage and coagulopathy, the coagulation cascade must be reviewed (**Fig. 1**). The endothelium normally promotes blood fluidity unless there is an intimal injury. Coagulation is promoted at the site of injury and the response is contained by a series of procoagulating and anticoagulating interactions. Tissue factor is expressed on the surface of injured adventitial vascular walls, after activation by local cytokines. Tissue factor binds to activated factor VII (FVIIa) then activates FX; FX and is the major activator of the extrinsic pathway. The intrinsic pathway is a series of proteolytic reactions, which culminate to activate FIX. The intrinsic and extrinsic pathways converge at the level of FX, the common pathway (see **Fig. 1**).

MONITORING OF COAGULATION

Clotting tests routinely performed in the emergency setting include partial thromboplastin time (PTT), prothrombin time (PT), International Normalized Ratio (INR). Fibrinogen, fibrin split products, and D-dimer are other measured factors that can alter bleeding. PTT is an indicator of the efficacy of both the intrinsic and the common pathway, and is used to monitor therapeutic levels of heparin. PT is a measure of the extrinsic pathway. The INR is a ratio of the PT and the normal mean PT, and

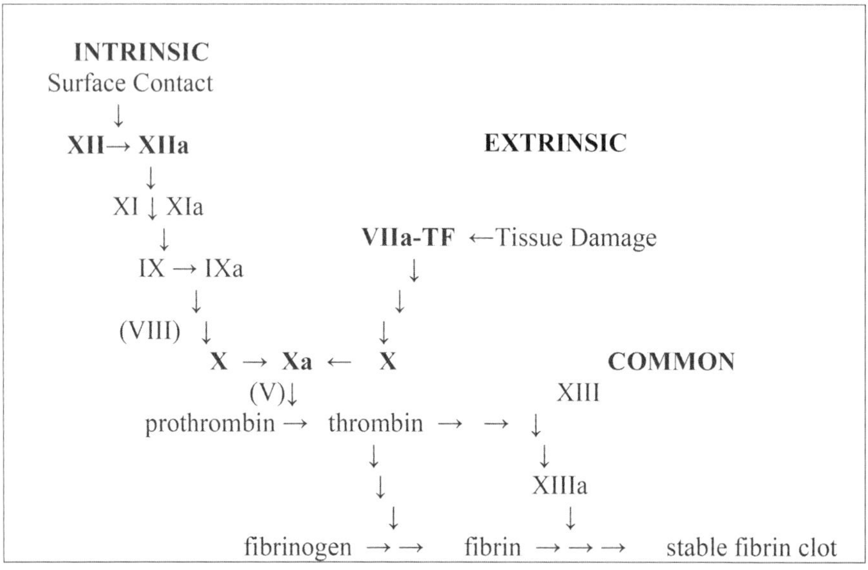

Fig. 1. The coagulation cascade. (*Adapted from* The Classical Blood Coagulation Pathway by Dr Graham Beards under the Creative Commons Attribution-Share Alike 3.0 Unported license.)

measures the extrinsic pathway, monitors warfarin dosing, vitamin K status, and liver function. The PT/INR is more sensitive than the aPTT to low coagulation factor levels in trauma patients. PT and aPTT are poor predictors of bleeding in acquired coagulopathy.[4] An INR greater than 1.5 and PTT greater than 18 seconds are typically considered to denote "coagulopathy."[5] Low platelet counts on admission are associated with increased mortality.[4]

In addition to the traditional coagulation parameters discussed above, point of care testing such as Sonoclot, thromboelastometry, and thrombelastography (TEG) are technologies that measure the viscoelastic changes in whole blood and are widely available. TEG has been used since 1948 and helps to guide resuscitation and early coagulopathy. TEG represents components and quality of the coagulation system and provides a rapid, dynamic bedside evaluation of the initiation and kinetics of clot formation, maximal clot firmness, and clot breakdown.[6] Classic clotting factor laboratory tests are measures in plasma and were developed to monitor anticoagulation therapy rather than coagulation in trauma, focusing on initial thrombin formation or time to clotting. TEG and its newer versions can assess the range of acute coagulopathies in trauma injury, identify the type of coagulopathy early, and guide appropriate therapy.[6] Viscoelastic tracings evaluate the speed of clot formation, the strength of the clot, and the time to initiation of coagulation (**Fig. 2**).

BLOOD AND TRANSFUSION COMPONENTS

Transfusion is a vital element of resuscitation, replacing blood and blood components lost. Blood is composed of red blood cells, white blood cells, plasma, and platelets. Whole blood is referred to as blood with all of its components. Plasma is the liquid portion of blood and comprises 55% of the body's blood volume. It carries red cells, white cells, platelets, albumin, fibrinogen, and globulins. Packed red blood cells (PRBC) are red cells that have been separated from plasma, packaged, processed, and stored in 450 to 500 mL doses for up to 42 days. Platelets are separated from whole blood, stored, and screened for bacteria within the first 48 hours, with a lifespan of 5 days. Fresh frozen plasma (FFP) is the fluid portion of a unit of blood that has been separated, centrifuged, and frozen at -18°C within 8 hours of collection, containing heat-sensitive proteins, FV and FVIII, and is usually 250 mL in volume. FFP contains 80% of the factors contained in whole blood.[7] Cryoprecipitate is a frozen blood product prepared from plasma containing 100 IU of FVIII, 250 mg of fibrinogen, von Willebrand factor, and FXIII.

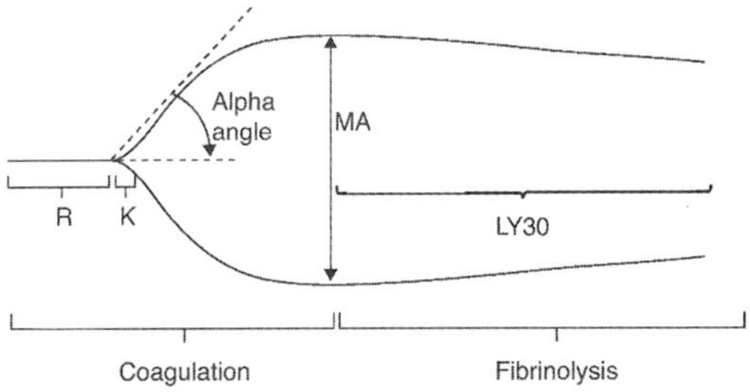

Fig. 2. Thromboelastography (TEG). The R, K, and alpha angles represent the coagulation portion of the TEG. The MA represents the strength of the clot and platelet function. LY30 represents fibrinolysis. (*From* Gempeler FE, Díaz L, Murcia PC. [Evaluating coagulation in prostatectomy]. Rev Colomb Anestesiol 2009;37(3):205; with permission.)

INDICATIONS FOR TRANSFUSION

There are 30 million units of blood transfused in the United States to 4.5 million people annually.[8] The transfusion rate has steadily increased over the past 20 years. One must take into consideration the patient's intravascular volume status, evidence of shock, duration and extent of anemia and coagulopathy, cardiopulmonary physiologic parameters, lactate, and base deficit. These parameters guide management and predict mortality. Trauma-induced coagulopathy, for example, carries a mortality rate of 50%, and is often associated with increased transfusions, greater risk of multiple organ failure, sepsis, and increased intensive care days.[9] Some of our major resources for best practices with respect to transfusion have been and continue to be from military experiences, because the number one cause of preventable death on the battlefield is hemorrhage.[10] To date, there are no validated methods to guide transfusion therapy, only guidelines, which often results in overtransfusion, undertransfusion, increased waste, and risks.

In the setting of acute hemorrhage, transfusion should be initiated when blood loss is estimated at 30% of the blood volume or class III hemorrhage. Advance Trauma Life Support still suggests that patients with hypovolemic shock, failure to respond to 40 to 60 mL/kg of crystalloid, and hemoglobin less than 10 g/dL and hematocrit less than 30 g/dL be transfused. The Eastern Association for the Surgery of Trauma in conjunction with the Society of Critical Care Medicine guidelines recommend limiting transfusions of FFP and platelets by avoiding transfusing at PT and PTT ratios of less than 1.5 and platelet counts above 30,000.[11] Patients in hemorrhagic shock lose blood volume proportionate to clotting factors and platelets.[7] Methods to prevent such occurrences have been established, and fixed ratio resuscitation has improved mortality in both military and civilian contexts.

MASSIVE TRANSFUSION PROTOCOLS AND RATIOS

Acute coagulopathy of trauma is the result of the injury, hypothermia, acidosis, ongoing bleeding, dilution, and decreased activity of clotting factors. Coagulopathy in trauma patients is identified in 25% to 30% of the population upon presentation.[12] The mechanism is not fully understood. Hypoperfusion to tissue increases endothelial thrombomodulin expression that activates protein C, an anticoagulant.[13] Injury causes local tissue factor generation and clotting. However, overwhelming injury can lead to consumption of these clotting factors or disseminated intravascular coagulopathy and overactivation of fibrinolysis. The severity of the injury can cause an imbalance between the capacity of the coagulation system and fibrinolysis, leading to uncontrollable hemorrhage contributing to the degree of coagulopathy.

Hypothermia slows plasma coagulation factor reactions. A drop of 1°C is associated with a drop of 10% in clotting activity. When temperatures fall below 33°C, there is a 50% drop in normal factor activity and platelet function.[12] Platelet activation by the von Willebrand factor–glycoprotein Ib (FIX, FV) interaction is cold sensitive. PRBC has a pH of 7.4 to 6.9 after blood banking. The pH continues to fall as hydrogen ion concentration increases, destabilizing coagulation factor complexes and activity, and lactate level rises with storage time.[12] Coagulopathy also worsens when serum fibrinogen levels fall below 100 mg/dL; therefore, fibrinogen levels should be monitored along with clotting factors and TEG.

Protocols for massive transfusion have been implemented to improve outcomes. The military was the first to initiate plasma:PRBC in 1:1 ratios for massive transfusion, classically defined as greater than 10 units of PRBC within a 24-hour period. Recently, it has also been defined as 5 units transfused over 3 or 4 hours, or 3 units in 1 hour, also known as the new critical administration threshold.[14,15] Massive transfusion protocols are designated fixed ratios of PRBC:FFP:platelets, designed to mimic whole blood transfusions and restore the normal physiologic composition.[9,16] Therefore, expert consensus and US Army Surgeon General guidelines suggest resuscitation that reduces dependence on crystalloid and focuses on repletion in 1:1 proportions.[17–19] Some may argue that these ratios do not actually get close to normal blood composition, resulting in a hematocrit of 29%, platelet count of 85,000, and 60% normal clotting activity.[20] Studies from Baghdad promoted the 1:1 ratio; however, there were survival biases.[21] Holcomb and colleagues[22] showed that higher ratios were associated with decreased mortality within the first 24 hours. Two recent studies have shown no improvement in mortality; instead, there was an increase in complications. The risk for acute respiratory distress syndrome was 12 times greater with higher FFP.[23,24]

TRANSFUSION IN THE CRITICALLY ILL

In the setting of nonhemorrhaging critically ill patients, the National Institutes of Health, the American College of Chest Physicians, the American Society of Anesthesiology, the Society of Thoracic Surgeons, and the American College of Surgeons have published some guidelines that agree transfusion is not beneficial, and may even be harmful, when hemoglobin is greater than 10 g/dL, and may provide benefit if hemoglobin concentration is less than 6 to 8 g/dL.[25,26] It is difficult to define guidelines based on high-quality evidence because transfusion about the critically ill is often based on clinical judgment. In the TRICC trial, no difference in 30-day mortality was seen in liberal verses restrictive transfusion strategies; however, there was a decrease in 30-day mortality in a subgroup with lower APACHE scores and age less than 55 years in the restrictive group.[27] Based on this study, recommendations have been adopted for a hemoglobin goal of 7 to 9 g/dL, with exception to patients with unstable angina or myocardial infarction.[27]

There are special groups in whom more liberal transfusion thresholds may be considered, such as elderly and cardiac patients. The elderly population may have little reserve, and may not tolerate lower hemoglobin and increased cardiac output like younger patients, placing them at high risk for myocardial infarction. In a large study of patients older than 65 years with an acute myocardial infarction and hematocrit less than 24%, higher 30-day mortality rates with no survival improvement was noted at a higher hematocrit.[28] However, Carson and colleagues[29] found no difference in death rates, ability to walk without assistance upon follow-up, acute coronary syndrome, or complications between the liberal and restrictive groups. Therefore, despite cardiac risks, there was no benefit or risk using restrictive transfusion strategies.

RISKS AND REACTIONS

Transfusion-related acute lung injury (TRALI) is the most common transfusion-related reaction and is the leading cause of transfusion-related death in the United States reported to the Food and Drug Administration.[30] In 2012, there were 74 transfusion recipient fatality reports and 17 (45%) were secondary to TRALI.[30] It occurs in approximately 1:6000 transfusions and within 6 hours of administration of blood products. All blood products are implicated in TRALI; however, it is most often associated with FFP.[31] TRALI is noncardiac pulmonary edema after transfusion cause by leukocyte-mediated antibodies within the plasma-releasing granules that disrupt the epithelium, cellular membranes, and lung parenchyma. Pulmonary infiltrates in TRALI, unlike acute respiratory distress syndrome, resolve within 96 hours. Patients receiving higher

FFP:PRBC ratios have a 2-fold greater incidence of TRALI.[8] Inaba and colleagues[23] reported that patients transfused at a high ratio of FFP:PRBC had increased complications, especially acute respiratory distress syndrome, with no improvement in survival. In most cases of TRALI, follow-up donor antibody screens have implicated multiparous females positive for anti-HLA or antigranulocyte antibodies. Palfi and colleagues[32] studied patients receiving FFP from multiparous women and showed impaired pulmonary function. Since this study and others, in 2006 the United States has recommended the exclusion of multiparous females as plasma donors.[33] The American Red Cross demonstrated that plasma donation from men has decreased plasma-related TRALI by 80%.[34]

Transfusion-associated circulatory overload (TACO) is acute pulmonary edema secondary to congestive heart failure precipitated by transfusion in volumes that overwhelm the recipient's circulatory system.[35] It often occurs within 6 hours of administration of products, similar to TRALI. Between 2011 and 2012, there were 74 transfusion recipient fatalities reported to the Food and Drug Administration, and 51% were transfusion related. In 2012, TACO was the second most common cause of these fatalities at 21%.[30] Risk factors for TACO are ill defined, but it is possible that the transfusion rate is more important than the amount of volume given, and extremes of age—younger than 3 years or older than 60 years—are at risk.[36] Preexisting fluid balance, number of blood products administered, renal failure, and preexisting heart conditions are associated with TACO.[36] TACO, although not as prevalent as TRALI, is associated with higher morbidity and mortality and should not be disregarded.

Massive transfusion protocols have increased the overall usage of plasma among trauma and emergency services. A survey of 10 large blood centers in March 2012 showed an increase in plasma demand, a 27% increase in AB plasma usage, and only 3% AB plasma donors.[37] Compatibility of plasma is important; as exposure to ABO-compatible plasma increases, the result is an increase in overall complications.[38] In emergency settings, AB plasma is administered to non-AB plasma recipients as a result of rapid infusion, unavailable valid type and screens, and massive transfusion protocol initiation.[39] ABO and non-ABO hemolytic transfusion reactions have been reported as frequently as 1 in 1.8 million per transfused PRBC units.[40] In 2004, the Food and Drug Administration required that machine readable information be included on blood container labels and by 2006 a reduction in these ABO–hemolytic transfusion reactions avoidable deaths was noted, thought to be secondary to clerical errors.[40]

Transfusion of PRBC after prolonged storage has been shown to result in early immune activation leading to a systemic inflammatory response syndrome, delayed immune suppression, and increased predisposition to infections.[41] A recent metaanalysis demonstrated increased risk of death associated with increased age of blood.[42,43] Risk associated with the transfusion of old blood is thought to be owing to cellular deformation and loss of rheology, increased accumulation of lysophospholipids, and loss of microvascular flow and density. Koch and colleagues[44] demonstrated an increase in mortality in patients receiving PRBCs stored longer than 14 days. Lactate increases 15-fold and pH drops to 6.7 after 3 weeks of storage.[7]

In the early days of transfusion medicine, infectious disease transmission was highly related to the volume and frequency of blood transfused. Currently, steps are taken to reduce these risks, namely, viral inactivation methods. The risk for HIV is 1 in 1 to 2 million, and hepatitis B, hepatitis C, and hepatitis A is 1 in 250 to 500,000.[40] All blood donated now is tested for A blood type (A), B blood type (B), O blood type (O), Rhesus blood group, HIV-1, HIV-2, human T-lymphotropic virus, hepatitis B, hepatitis C, *Treponema pallidum*, *Trypanosoma cruzi*, West Nile virus, and cytomegalovirus within 24 hours of donation.[40]

ANTICOAGULANTS AND REVERSAL OF ANTICOAGULANTS

Warfarin is a direct vitamin K antagonist, preventing the synthesis of FII, FVII, FIX, FX, and proteins C and S. Novel anticoagulation agents are now replacing warfarin. Treatment of coagulopathy owing to these novel agents is complicated owing to lack of reversal methods and agents. Dabigatran is a direct thrombin inhibitor, preventing conversion of fibrinogen into fibrin by thrombin. Compared with warfarin, it showed lower rates of bleeding; however, mortality rates were similar.[45] Dabigatran use in those ages 70 to 80 years, those with renal failure, and increased dosage has been associated with increased risk of major bleeding events.[8] Rivaroxaban is a FXa inhibitor, which inhibits conversion of FII (prothrombin) into thrombin. Compared with warfarin, there were similar bleeding rates but lower rates of intracranial and fatal hemorrhage.[46] Apixaban is another FXa inhibitor, shown to have a mortality benefit compared with warfarin.[47] A variety of methods to reverse theses anticoagulation medications are available; however, it remains a topic of ongoing research.[48]

FFP

FFP is a plasma-derived blood product containing all the clotting factors and fibrinogen. Each unit is about 250 mL so there is volume-associated risk, as well as time to administration constraints owing to thawing requirements, as well as a risk of virus or bacteria transmission because it is a derivative of whole blood.[7] A review investigated the efficacy of FFP in reversing coagulopathy and found no consistent evidence.[49] A small study administered FFP in traumatic brain injury, leading to more adverse events and increased the frequency of delayed traumatic intracranial hematoma.[50] Despite this, it remains the most widely used product for emergent reversal of warfarin. The Society of Thoracic Surgeons recommends plasma transfusion in the context of serious bleeding with multiple coagulation factor deficiencies, massive transfusion, or urgent warfarin reversal with bleeding if prothrombin complex concentrate (PCC) is not available.[51] It may also play a role in reversal of new thrombin inhibitor agents. Recent animal studies show the potential for FFP administered in conjunction with PCC to be efficacious in dabigatran-associated intracranial hemorrhage (**Table 1**).[52] Since 2005, there has been a 23% increase in FFP usage; this is most likely secondary to massive transfusion protocols and the elderly population on warfarin.[30]

VITAMIN K

Vitamin K is a fat-soluble compound administered for reversal of warfarin-induced coagulopathy. Vitamin K orally or IV is recommended for urgent reversal. If given IV, a rate of 1 mg/min is suggested to avoid anaphylactic reactions.[53] The American College of Chest Physicians practice guidelines of 2012 recommend oral vitamin K for an INR greater than 10 without signs of bleeding and IV vitamin K 5 or 10 mg for all major bleeding, regardless of the INR (see **Table 1**).[54] In a recent study, IV administration was compared with oral administration; IV administration demonstrated a significantly lower INR and more rapid onset of action.[53] There is no defined role of vitamin K in the reversal of novel oral anticoagulants.[53]

Table 1
Oral anticoagulants and reversal agents

Anticoagulant	Mechanism of Action	Reversal Agent
Warfarin	Direct vitamin K antagonist	FFP
		PCC (major bleeding, ICH, CHF, liver and renal failure)
		PCC + factor VII (INR > 4.5)
		PCC + vitamin K (increased time of efficacy)
		Vitamin K oral (no evidence bleeding, INR > 9)
		Vitamin K IV (major bleeding, INR irrelevant)
Dabigatran	Direct thrombin inhibitor	Hemodialysis
		Hemoperfusion
		Activated charcoal (ingestion < 2 h)
		4-Factor PCC (case studies, basic science reports)
		Hemodialysis + factor VII (animal studies)
		FFP + PCC (ICH in animal studies)
Rivaroxaban	Xa inhibitor	Activated charcoal (ingestion < 2 h)
		4-Factor PCC (RCT, small study)
Apixaban	Xa inhibitor	Activated charcoal (ingestion < 2 h)
		4-Factor PCC

Abbreviations: CHF, congestive heart failure; FFP, fresh frozen plasma; ICH, intracranial hemorrhage; INR, International Normalized Ratio; PCC, prothrombin complex concentrate; RCT, randomized controlled trial.

FVII

Recombinant FVIIa (rFVIIa; eptacog alfa, NovoSeven, NovoNordisk, Bagsvaerd, Denmark) was first approved in 1999 for treatment of bleeding in hemophiliacs, inhibitors to FVIII or FIX. RFVIIa promotes clotting by activating FIX and FX in the presence of tissue factor, and promotes thrombin generation on the surface of activated platelets, forming a clot at the site of vascular injury.[55] The dose ranges from 20 to 90 μg/kg based on clinical trails and use in hemorrhage and coagulopathy is off label. RFVIIa has been reported to control bleeding in liver disease, liver transplantation, and cardiac surgery.[55] There is also a possible role for rFVIIa to reverse dabigatran-mediated bleeding; animal models and case reports have used rFVIIa in conjunction with hemodialysis (see **Table 1**).[56] In randomized controlled trials, rFVIIa failed to improve outcomes, but decreased expansion of intracerebral hemorrhage in hemorrhagic stroke. Boffard and colleagues[57] showed significant decrease in the number of RBC transfusions in blunt trauma. Another trial attempted to validate these results; however, no difference was noted in mortality and the study was labeled futile.[58] Dutton and colleagues[59] noted retrospectively that rFVIIa was administered when conventional methods of hemorrhage control had been exhausted. Stein and colleagues[60] studied the use of rFVIIa in traumatic brain injury with coagulopathy; time to neurosurgical intervention and the number of plasma units administered before intervention was lower in the rFVIIa group compared with the plasma. No difference was found in the rate of thromboembolic events and mortality.[60] In another study, Stein and colleagues[61] compared the cost of rFVIIa with the cost of FFP in traumatic brain injury. Intensive care unit admissions for the rFVIIa group had a significantly lower total cost, hospital duration of stay, plasma use, and ventilator days. Risk of thrombosis, especially in those older than 65 years, is owing to the procoagulant FVIIa without opposition from proteins C and S. It has been contraindicated in severe disseminated intravascular coagulopathy and crush injuries. Stein and colleagues[62] documented a 15% thromboembolic event rate retrospectively in low-dose rFVIIa and Thomas and colleagues[63] documented 9.4%, with 10 of 14 deaths partially caused by these complications. Criticism of these studies suggests that the quality of data has been inconclusive and underpowered. FVIIa is a heat-sensitive molecule and becomes deactivated or less active in the setting of hypothermia associated with trauma, and therefore does not demonstrate improved outcomes. Although rFVIIa has not been proven to improve survival, it has been proven to significantly decrease transfusions and cost of care.

PCC

PCC is an inactivated concentrate of vitamin K-dependent factors, which has undergone virus removal and viral inactivation. Three-factor PCC contains FII, FIX, FX, and trace amounts of FVII. Four-factor PCC (4-FPCC) contains FII, FIX, FX, FVII, and proteins C and S. It is administered as a weight-based dose, depending on the INR, and is fast acting (see **Table 1**). Rapid infusion of large volumes of FFP may not be tolerated in certain patient populations. PCC is given as 15 to 30 IU/kg and is usually less than 50 mL. Early studies show rapid reversal of postoperative bleeding. Quick and colleagues[64] demonstrated that geriatric patients given PCC received significantly less FFP and had a greater decrease in INR. A recent trial studied 24-hour hemostatic efficacy in nonsurgical hemorrhage, and noninferiority between 4-FPCC and plasma was seen; however, a significant superiority in rapid INR reduction was demonstrated with 4-FPCC.[65] There is debate over the efficacy, safety profile, onset, duration, and overall usage of PCC versus FFP for reversal of warfarin. When comparing the two, there is no difference in overall mortality or hemostatic efficacy, but there is reduction in transfusion needs and INR.[64,65] The definitive dosage of PCC is still being tested and a range dose is suggested based on trials. Risk of thrombosis with PCC is less than 2%.[66] Four-FPCC should conceptually reverse activity of the FXa inhibitors, but there are few case reports of reversal.[67] FFP administered in conjunction with PCC has shown efficacy in animal models in dabigatran-associated intracranial hemorrhage.[52] The Working Group on Perioperative Haemostasis proposed in 2013 treating bleeding in a critical organ secondary to dabigatran or rivaroxaban with activated PCC 30 to 50 U/kg or PCC 50 U/kg.[68] The Thrombosis and Hemostasis Summit of North America in 2012 recommended treatment of major bleeding associated with novel anticoagulants with oral activated charcoal for ingestions within 2 hours. They also recommend hemodialysis, hemoperfusion, and activated charcoal in dabigatran-associated bleeding (see **Table 1**).[69] They discuss the possible benefit from 4-FPCC, uncertain benefits of 3-factor FPCC, and recommend against the use of FFP. The American College of Chest Physicians recommends reversal irrespective to INR with 4-FPCC instead of FFP and vitamin K in the setting of life-threatening or critical hemorrhage (see **Table 1**).[51]

TRANEXAMIC ACID

Tranexamic acid (TXA) is an antifibrinolytic or procoagulant molecule. In the CRASH-2 trial, Shakur and colleagues[70] demonstrated efficacy in reducing mortality in hemorrhage if administered TXA within the first 3 hours after injury.[71] It has also been reported that TXA safely reduced the risk of death.[70,71] Kashuk and colleagues[72] demonstrated primary fibrinolysis in 34% of patients requiring massive transfusion using TEG. He also showed early administration of TXA resulted in reduced all-cause mortality, reduced mortality from bleeding, and a safe side effect profile.

The MATTERs II trial demonstrated a 50% reduction in overall mortality in the massive transfusion subgroup with the early use of TXA.[73] Optimal dosage and timing is still in question and risks include thrombosis and increased incidence of seizures.[74]

SUMMARY

Hemorrhage and coagulopathy in the critically ill, if not intervened upon early, can precipitate a vicious cycle of hypothermia and acidosis that worsens coagulopathy and bleeding. Transfusion medicine has come a long way since its origin in 1665, but still has a long way to go. Coagulopathy may be induced by trauma, acute blood loss, medications, resuscitation with blood products or crystalloid devoid of coagulation factors, or hypothermia. Recent oral anticoagulants complicate coagulopathy and present a new dilemma for treatment, because they do not respond to traditional reversal agents. For now, the basic principles of transfusion are recommended; PCC and hemodialysis are proposed for reversal of dabigatran. The military currently recommends low volumes of resuscitation, increased ratios of 1:1:1, targeting endpoints of resuscitation such as lactate, base deficit, $ScVO_2$, classic coagulation factors, and TEG or thromboelastometry for improved outcomes. Currently most research regarding fixed ratios is retrospective and there is the need for further investigation. Goal hemoglobin should be targeted for 7 g/dL unless there is ongoing hemorrhage or acute coronary syndrome. TEG or thromboelastometry may be used in addition to classic coagulation factors, understanding function as well as quantity to target transfusion. In addition to blood products, replacement of coagulation factors with PCC and rFVIIa is recommended. Transfusions may be necessary and life saving, but they are not benign, causing transfusion reactions and transmission of infectious diseases, although this is now rare. Despite all the progress, mortality after hemorrhagic shock is still 31% within 2 hours of arrival in the emergency department.[75]

REFERENCES

1. Hess JR, Schmidt PJ. The first blood banker: Oswald Hope Robertson. Transfusion 2000;40:110–3.
2. Murray CJ, Lopez AD. Alternative projections of mortality and disability by cause 1990-2020: Global Burden of Disease Study. Lancet 1997;349:1498–504.
3. Brohi K, Cohen MJ, Davenport RA. Acute coagulopathy of trauma: mechanism, identification and effect. Curr Opin Crit Care 2007;13:680–5.
4. Dzik WH. Predicting hemorrhage using preoperative coagulation screening assays. Curr Hematol Rep 2004;3(5):324–30.
5. Hunt H, Hyde C, Stanworth S, et al. Thromboelastography (TEG) and thromboelastometry (ROTEM) for trauma induced coagulopathy in adult trauma patients with bleeding. Cochrane Database Syst Rev 2013;(3):CD010438. http://dx.doi.org/10.1002/14651858.CD010438.
6. Schochl H, Voelckl W, Grassetto A, et al. Practical application of point of care coagulation testing to guide treatment decisions in trauma. J Trauma Acute Care Surg 2013;74(6):1587–98.
7. Tapia NM, Chang A, Norman M, et al. TEG-guided resuscitation is superior to standardized MTP resuscitation in massively transfused penetrating trauma patients. J Trauma Acute Care Surg 2013;74:378–85 [discussion: 385–6].

8. Berger S, Salhanick SD, Chase M, et al. Hemorrhagic complications in emergency department patients who are receiving dabigatran compared with warfarin. Ann Emerg Med 2013;61(4):475–9.
9. Brohi K, Singh J, Heron M, et al. Acute traumatic coagulopathy. J Trauma 2003; 54(6):1127–30.
10. Holcomb JB, McMullin NR, Pearse L, et al. Causes of death in U.S. Special Operations forces in the global war on terrorism. Ann Surg 2007;245(6):968–91.
11. Napolitano LM, Kurek S, Luchette FA, et al. Clinical practice guidelines: red blood cell transfusion in adult trauma and critical care. Crit Care Med 2009; 37(12):3124–57.
12. Elmer J, Wilcox SR, Raja AS. Massive transfusion in hemorrhagic shock. J Emerg Med 2012;44(4):829–38.
13. Brohi K, Cohen MJ, Ganter MT, et al. Acute traumatic coagulopathy: initiated by hypoperfusion; modulated through protein C pathway? Ann Surg 2007;245: 812–8.
14. Mitra B, Cameron PA, Gruen RL, et al. The definition of massive transfusion in trauma: a critical variable in examining evidence for resuscitation. Eur J Emerg Med 2011;18(3):137–42.
15. Savage SA, Zarzaur BL, Croce MA, et al. Redefining massive transfusion when every second counts. J Trauma Acute Care Surg 2013;74(2):396–400 [discussion: 400–2].
16. Levy JH, Dutton RP, Hemphill JC, et al. Multidisciplinary approach to the challenge of hemostasis. Anesth Analg 2010;110:354–64.
17. Holcomb JB, Hess JR. Early massive transfusion for trauma: state of the art: editor's introduction. J Trauma 2006;60(6 Suppl):S1–2.
18. Malone DL, Hess JR, Fingerhut A. Massive transfusion practices around the globe and a suggestion for a common massive transfusion protocol. J Trauma 2006;60(6 Suppl):S91–6.
19. Holcomb JB, Jenkins D, Rhee P, et al. Damage control resuscitation: directly addressing the early coagulopathy of trauma. J Trauma 2007;62(2):307–10.
20. Davenport R, Manson J, De'Ath H, et al. Functional definition and characterization of acute trauma coagulopathy. Crit Care Med 2011;39:2652–8.
21. Murthi SB, Stansbury LG, Dutton RP, et al. Transfusion medicine in trauma patients: an update. Expert Rev Hematol 2011;4(5):527–37.
22. Holcomb JB, del Junco DJ, Fox EE, et al. The prospective, observational, multicenter, major trauma transfusion (PROMMTT) study. Comparative effectiveness of a time-varying treatment with competing risks. JAMA Surg 2013;148(2): 127–36.
23. Inaba K, Branco BC, Rhee P, et al. Impact of plasma transfusion in trauma patients who do not require massive transfusion. J Am Coll Surg 2010;210:957–65.
24. Sambasivan CN, Kunio NR, Nair PV, et al. High ratios of plasma and platelets to packed red blood cells do not affect mortality in nonmassively transfused patients. J Trauma 2011;71:S329–36.
25. Goodnough LT, Levy JH, Murphy MF. Blood transfusion 1. Concepts of blood transfusion in adults. Lancet 2013;381:1845–54.
26. Lefant C. Transfusion practice should be audited for both undertransfusion and overtransfusion. Transfusion 1992;32:873–4.
27. Hebert PC, Wells G, Blajchman MA, et al. A multicenter, randomized, controlled clinical trial of transfusion requirements in critical care. Transfusion Requirements in Critical Care Investigators, Canadian Critical Care Trials Group. N Engl J Med 1999;340:409–17.

28. Wu WC, Rathore SS, Wang Y, et al. Blood transfusions in elderly with acute myocardial infarction. N Engl J Med 2001;345:1230–6.
29. Carson JL, Terrin ML, Noveck H, et al, FOCUS Investigators. Liberal or restrictive transfusion in high-risk patients after hip surgery. N Engl J Med 2011;365(26): 2453–62.
30. Fatalities reported to FDA following blood collection and transfusion: annual summary for fiscal year 2012. US Food and Drug Administration Center for Biologics Evaluation and Research; 2013. Available at: http://www.fda.gov/BiologicsBloodVaccines/SafetyAvailability/ReportaProblem/TransfusionDonationFatalities/ucm346639.htm.
31. Triulzi DJ. Transfusion-related acute lung injury: current concepts for the clinician. Anesth Analg 2009;108:770–6.
32. Palfi M, Berg S, Berlin G. A randomized controlled trial of transfusion-related acute lung injury; is plasma from multiparous blood donors dangerous? Transfusion 2001;41:317–22.
33. Dzik WH, Blajchman MA, Fergusson D, et al. Clinical review: Canadian National Advisory Committee on blood and blood products-massive transfusion consensus conference 2011: report of the panel. Crit Care 2011;15:242.
34. Eder AF, Dy BA, Perez JM, et al. The residual risk of transfusion-related acute lung injury at the American Red Cross (2008-2011): limitations of a predominantly male-donor plasma mitigation strategy. Transfusion 2013. http://dx.doi.org/10.1111/j.1537-2995.2012.03935.x.
35. Vlaar AP, Binnekade JM, Prins D, et al. Risk factors and outcome of transfusion related acute lung injury in the critically ill: a nested case–control study. Crit Care Med 2010;38(3):771–7.
36. Murphy EL, Kwaan N, Looney MR, et al. Risk factors and outcomes in transfusion-associated circulatory overload. Am J Med 2013;126:357.e29–38.
37. Yazer M, Eder AF, Land KJ. How we manage AB plasma inventory in the blood center and transfusion service. Transfusion 2013;23(8):1627–33.
38. Inaba K, Branco BC, Rhee P, et al. Impact of ABO-identical vs ABO-compatible nonidentical plasma transfusion in trauma patients. Arch Surg 2010;145(9): 899–906.
39. Silliman CC, Moore EE, Johnson JL, et al. Transfusion of the injured patient: proceed with caution. Shock 2004;21:291–9.
40. Vamvakas EC, Blajchman MA. Transfusion-related mortality: the ongoing risks of allogenic blood transfusion and the available strategies for their prevention. Blood 2009;113(15):3406–17.
41. Alam HB, Bice LM, Butt MU, et al. Testing of blood products in a polytrauma model: results of a Multi-Institutional Randomized Preclinical Trial. J Trauma 2009;67:856–64.
42. Alam HB, Velmahos GC. Trends in resuscitation. Curr Probl Surg 2011;48(8): 531–64.
43. Uniformed Services University of the Health Sciences. Combat fluid resuscitation. Sponsored by US Office of Naval Research; US Army Medical Research and Material Command; Department of Surgery. Bethesda (MD): Department of Military and Emergency Medicine; 2001.
44. Koch CG, Li L, Sessler DI, et al. Duration of red-cell storage and complications after cardiac surgery. N Engl J Med 2008;358(12):1229–39.
45. Connolly SJ, Ezekowitz MD, Yusuf S, et al. Dabigatraban versus warfarin in patients with atrial fibrillation. N Engl J Med 2009;361(12):1139–51.

46. Patel MR, Mahaffey KW, Garg J, et al. Rivaroxaban verses warfarin in nonvalvular atrial fibrillation. N Engl J Med 2013;365(10):883–91.
47. Granger CB, Alexander JH, McMurray JJ, et al. Apixaban verses warfarin in patients with atrial fibrillation. N Engl J Med 2011;365(11):981–92.
48. Raja AS, Geyer B. Emergency department management of patients on novel oral anticoagulant agents. Emerg Med Pract 2013;15(10):1–19.
49. Yang L, Stanworth S, Hopewell S, et al. Is fresh-frozen plasma clinically effective? An update of a systematic review of randomized controlled trials. Transfusion 2012;52:1673–86.
50. Etemadrezaie H, Baharvahdat H, Shariati Z, et al. The effect of fresh frozen plasma in severe closed head injury. Clin Neurol Neurosurg 2007;109:166–71.
51. Society of Thoracic Surgeons Blood Conservation Guideline Task Force, Ferraris VA, Brown JR, et al. 2011 update to the Society of Thoracic Surgeons and the Society of Cardiovascular Anesthesiologists blood conservation clinical practice guidelines. Ann Thorac Surg 2011;91:944–82.
52. Zhou W, Schwarting S, Illanes S, et al. Hemostatic therapy in experimental intracerebral hemorrhage associated with direct thrombin inhibitor dabigatraban. Stroke 2011;42(12):3594–9.
53. Meehan R, Tavares M, Sweeney J. Clinical experience with oral versus intravenous vitamin K for warfarin reversal. Transfusion 2013;53(3):491–8.
54. Guyatt GH, Akl EA, Crowther M, et al, American College of Chest Physicians. Antithrombotic therapy and prevention of thrombosis, 9th ed: American College of Chest Physicians evidence-based clinical practice guidelines. Chest 2012; 141:10s.
55. Kenet G, Walden R, Eldad A, et al. Treatment of traumatic bleeding with recombinant factor VIIa. Surgical intervention failed to stop life-threatening bleeding caused by injury complicated by severe coagulopathy. Administration of recombinant factor VIIa immediately corrected the coagulopathy and bleeding stopped. Lancet 1999;354:1879.
56. Warkentin TE, Margetts P, Connolly SJ, et al. Recombinant factor VIIa (rFVIIa) and hemodialysis to manage massive dabigatran-associated postcardiac surgery bleeding. Blood 2012;119(9):2172–4.
57. Boffard KD, Riou B, Warren B, et al. Recombinant factor VIIa as adjunctive therapy for bleeding control in severely injured trauma patients: two parallel randomized placebo-controlled, double-blind clinical trials. J Trauma 2006;59: 8–15.
58. Hauser CJ, Boffard K, Dutton R, et al, CONTROL Study Group. Results of the CONTROL trial: efficacy and safety of recombinant activated Factor VII in the management of refractory traumatic hemorrhage. J Trauma 2010;69(3):489–500.
59. Dutton RP, Hess JR, Scalea TM. Recombinant factor VIIa for control of hemorrhage: early experience in critically ill trauma patients. J Clin Anesth 2003; 15(3):184–8.
60. Stein DM, Dutton RP, Kramer ME, et al. Recombinant factor VIIa: Decreasing time to intervention in coagulopathic patients with severe traumatic brain injury. J Trauma 2008;64(3):620–8.
61. Stein DM, Dutton RP, Kramer ME, et al. Reversal of coagulopathy in critically ill patients with traumatic brain injury: recombinant factor VIIa is more cost-effective than plasma. J Trauma 2009;66(1):63–72.
62. Stein DM, Dutton RP, Hess JR, et al. Low dose recombinant factor VIIa for trauma patients with coagulopathy. Injury 2008;39:1054–61.

63. Thomas GO, Dutton RP, Hemlock B, et al. Thromboembolic complications associated with factor VIIa administration. J Trauma 2007;62(3):564–9.
64. Quick JA, Bartels AN, Coughenour JP, et al. Experience with prothrombin complex for the emergent reversal of anticoagulation in rural geriatric trauma patients. Surgery 2012;152:722–8.
65. Sarode R, Milling TJ Jr, Refaai MA, et al. Efficacy and safety of a 4-factor prothrombin complex concentrate in patients on vitamin K antagonists presenting with major bleeding. A randomized, plasma-controlled, phase IIIb study. Circulation 2013;128:1234–43.
66. Sorenson B, Spahn DR, Innerhofer P, et al. Clinical review: prothrombin complex concentrates-evaluation of safety and thrombogenicity. Crit Care 2011;15:201.
67. Dager WE, Gosselin RC, Roberts AJ. Reversing dabigatraban in life-threatening bleeding during cardiac ablation with factor eight inhibitor bypassing activity. Crit Care Med 2013;41(5):e42–6.
68. Pernod G, Albaladejo P, Godier A, et al. Management of major bleeding complications and emergency surgery in patients on long-term treatment with direct oral anticoagulants, thrombin or factor-Xa inhibitors: proposals of the working group on perioperative hameostasis (GIHP). Arch Cardiovasc Dis 2013; 106(6–7):382–93.
69. Kaatz S, Kouides PA, Garcia DA, et al. Guidance on the emergent reversal of oral thrombin and factor Xa inhibitors. Am J Hematol 2012;87:S141–5.
70. Shakur H, Roberts I, Bautista R, et al. Effects of tranexamic acid on death, vascular occlusive events, and blood transfusion in trauma patients with significant hemorrhage (CRASH-2): a randomized, placebo-controlled trial. Lancet 2010;376(9734):23–32.
71. Roberts I, Shakur H, Afolabi A, et al. The importance of early treatment with tranexamic acid in bleeding trauma patients: an exploratory analysis of the CRASH-2 randomized controlled trial. Lancet 2011;377(9771):1096–101.
72. Kashuk JL, Moore EE, Johnson JL, et al. Postinjury life threatening coagulopathy: is 1:1 fresh frozen plasma:packed red blood cells the answer? J Trauma 2008;65:261–70.
73. Morrison JJ, Dubose JJ, Rasmussen TE, et al. Military application of tranexamic acid in trauma emergency resuscitation (MATTERs) study. Arch Surg 2012; 147:113.
74. Schwinn DA, Mackensen GB, Brown EN. Understanding the TXA seizure connection. J Clin Invest 2012;122(12):4339–41. http://dx.doi.org/10.1172/JCI66724.
75. Heckbert SR, Vedder NB, Hoffman W, et al. Outcome after hemorrhagic shock in trauma patients. J Trauma 1998;45(3):545–9.

Assessing Volume Status

Michael C. Scott, MD[a], Haney Mallemat, MD[b,*]

KEYWORDS

• Shock • Fluid resuscitation • Cardiac output • Stroke volume • Hemorrhage
• Hemodynamic monitoring • Noninvasive monitoring • Critical care

KEY POINTS

- Shock is a physiologic state associated with high morbidity and mortality rates.
- Fluid resuscitation has long been a part of the acute resuscitation armamentarium.
- Emergency physicians have a major impact on patient survival. The clinician has several tools available to evaluate volume status.
- Each modality has its benefits and limitations, but, to date, no one test can indicate with 100% accuracy which patients will be truly volume responsive.

INTRODUCTION

Shock, by definition, is a condition of inadequate tissue perfusion; during resuscitation, the clinician's goal is to restore the patient's perfusion of organs and tissues. The importance of early goal-directed therapy and early intervention by emergency physicians for hypotensive patients has been shown in multiple studies,[1,2] most classically by Rivers and colleagues[3] for patients presenting in septic shock. One of the most important principles of Rivers' study was the use of targeted and aggressive fluid resuscitation to improve tissue perfusion.

Fluid resuscitation has long been a part of the acute resuscitation armamentarium. Its goal is to increase cardiac filling and stroke volume (ie, cardiac output). What is often less clear, however, is accurately determining whether the patient who is currently hypotensive will actually respond to a fluid bolus (**Fig. 1**); that is, before administering a fluid bolus, it is very difficult to determine if the patient will respond.

Disclosures: None.
The article was copyedited by L.J. Kesselring, MS, ELS, the technical editor/writer in the Department of Emergency Medicine at the University of Maryland School of Medicine.
[a] Emergency Medicine/Internal Medicine/Critical Care Program, University of Maryland Medical Center, 110 South Paca Street, 6th floor, Suite 200, Baltimore, MD 21201, USA; [b] Emergency Medicine, University of Maryland School of Medicine, 110 South Paca Street, 6th Floor, Suite 200, Baltimore, MD 21201, USA
* Corresponding author.
E-mail address: haney.mallemat@gmail.com

Emerg Med Clin N Am 32 (2014) 811–822
http://dx.doi.org/10.1016/j.emc.2014.07.007 **emed.theclinics.com**
0733-8627/14/$ – see front matter

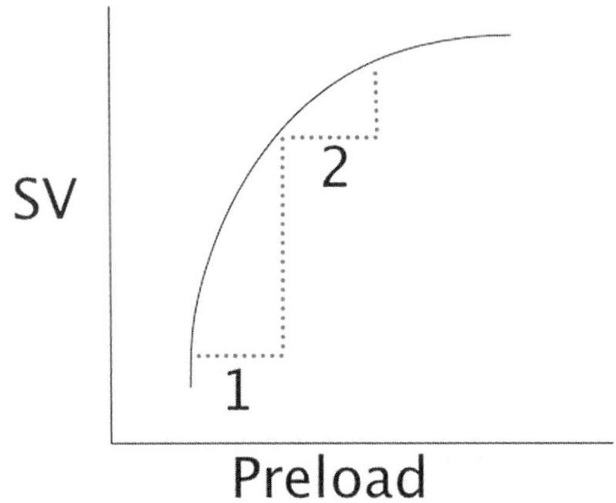

Fig. 1. Frank-Starling relationship of the heart. When the left ventricle is underfilled (1), an increase in preload brings on a large increase in stroke volume, and the patient is said to be volume responsive. When the left ventricle is closer to maximum end-diastolic volume (2), the increase in stroke volume is minimal for the same increase in preload.

This goal has proved to be perpetually elusive. In most studies, more than 40% of intensive care unit patients receiving a fluid bolus did not show the desired increase in cardiac output.[4] The harm of unnecessary and excessive fluid administration was shown in multiple studies, which suggest that the deleterious effects of fluid overload likely go far beyond simple pulmonary edema.[5–9] The endpoint of a goal-directed fluid strategy has placed increasing emphasis on finding a true "Goldilocks" state of fluid balance (ie, to not administer too much fluid or withhold too much).

This article describes the various tools available to the emergency physician to help answer an often perplexing question at the bedside: "Does this hemodynamically unstable patient need intravenous fluids?"

PHYSICAL EXAMINATION

Classic medical school teaching tells us to rely on the physical examination and vital signs to guide our resuscitation strategy, and this instruction extends into our clinical practice.[10] However, when the objective findings are evaluated for their correlation with actual changes in perfusion and cardiac output, few of them perform well.[11,12]

One example is estimation of jugular venous pressure during the physical examination, which is used to evaluate abnormalities of the left-sided circulation. Not only is jugular venous pressure difficult to measure under some circumstances (eg, when assessing an obese patient), but its true value can be confounded by numerous coexisting pathologies (eg, valvular disease, pulmonary hypertension). Another commonly used marker, urine output, can fail to accurately indicate the success of resuscitative efforts because it can be difficult to distinguish oliguria secondary to circulatory dysfunction (prerenal azotemia) from intrinsic kidney injury (eg, acute tubular necrosis) in the acute care setting. Even our most common and fundamental goal in resuscitation—improvement in the arterial pressure—does not necessarily correlate with improved cardiac output and, therefore, does not necessarily reflect improved perfusion.[13]

Once the limitations of the physical examination were realized, advanced resuscitation techniques for patients in shock shifted to using cardiac filling pressures as a guide to fluid therapy. The use of filling pressures makes theoretic sense because, as indicated by physiology and the Frank-Starling curve (see **Fig. 1**), ventricular pressures are directly proportional to ventricular volume until they reach a certain point at which this relationship is lost. Therefore, the goal during resuscitation is to administer intravenous fluids to optimally fill the left ventricle, which will increase the stroke volume, but not overfill it, which could result in deleterious side effects such as pulmonary edema.

When these filling pressures are interpreted randomly, they are known as *static measurements* and are thought to be a direct reflection of the ventricular pressure and hence the volume of the cardiac chambers. Central venous pressure (CVP) is the most popular of the static pressures and continues to be recommended in resuscitative protocols and guidelines.[3,10] Despite these recommendations, the reliability of CVP for guiding fluid resuscitation is controversial because of variations in patients' physiologies (eg, valvular pathology, right ventricular dysfunction)[14] as well as persistent inaccuracy when it is used as a predictor of response to a volume bolus.[15] An additional limitation to use of the CVP is that it requires insertion of a central venous catheter, which is invasive, and its placement is not readily possible in all emergency departments.

Another example of a static measurement of volume status is the estimation of right atrial pressure, based on an ultrasound image of the absolute size of the inferior vena cava (IVC) and its measured respiratory variation.[16] The IVC can be used to estimate right atrial pressures and, by indirect correlation, the CVP, which is the specified target in early goal-directed therapy. Ultrasound scan is an attractive hemodynamic monitor because it is noninvasive, rapid, and reproducible. Although there is debate as to its accuracy when predicting fluid responsiveness, it can be a useful measure when used as part of a comprehensive resuscitative protocol.[17,18]

The counterpart to static measurement of volume status is dynamic measurement. Dynamic measurements differ from static measurements because they involve the monitoring of hemodynamics followed by an intervention (eg, fluid bolus). Although dynamic measurements are better than static markers in predicting volume responsiveness,[4,19,20] their routine use in the emergency department has 2 major limitations. First, dynamic measurements require the concurrent use of monitoring devices that can detect increases in stroke volume (eg, ultrasound scan) during the assessment (such devices are explained in further detail later in this article). Second, most dynamic assessments require that patients be intubated and mechanically ventilated. This method is chosen because mechanical ventilation increases intrathoracic pressure, producing a significant respirophasic variation in preload, which mimics a fluid bolus, with venous return being at a minimum at end-inspiration (highest intrathoracic pressure) and a maximum at end-expiration (lowest intrathoracic pressure).

PULSE PRESSURE VARIATION AND STROKE VOLUME VARIATION

Pulse pressure variation (PPV), a well-studied dynamic marker of cardiac output, measures the change in pulse pressure (PP) throughout a respiratory cycle on a mechanical ventilator (**Fig. 2**). An arterial line is required to measure PPV, because systolic and diastolic measurements must be taken at specific points in the respiratory cycle. Once these measurements are recorded, the PPV can be calculated. Specialized monitors automatically perform both the measurements and the calculations in real time. Systolic pressure variation uses the same principal as PPV, except only the systolic pressures are measured at specific times in the respiratory cycle; therefore, it is not as reliable as PPV.

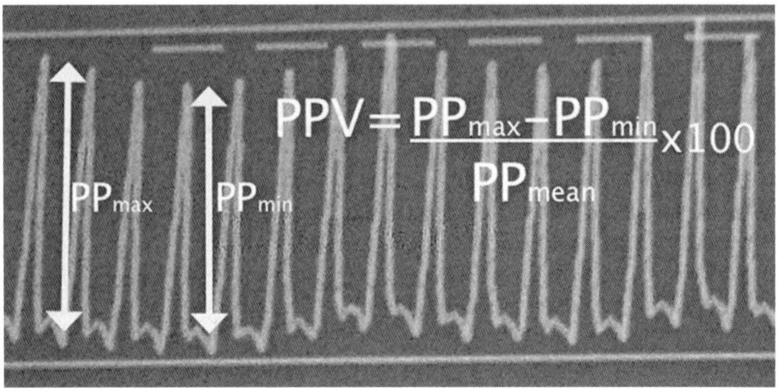

Fig. 2. Calculation of PPV using the tracing from an arterial catheter monitor. PPmax, maximum pulse pressure; PPmean, mean pulse pressure; PPmin, minimum pulse pressure (calculated by device).

PPV is a well-validated predictor of fluid responsiveness and can be applied in variety of clinical settings (emergency department, intensive care unit, operating room).[21–23] A PPV greater than 12.5% suggests that a patient's cardiac output would increase when given a fluid bolus. Conversely, a PPV less than 12.5% suggests that giving a fluid bolus would neither increase cardiac output nor improve hemodynamic status.[24]

The use of PPV for volume responsiveness in the emergency department has several limitations (**Box 1**). One limitation is that this measurement reflects a patient's hemodynamic status at only one point in time, so PPV must be calculated several times during resuscitation, especially before administering a fluid bolus.

IVC DISTENSIBILITY INDEX

The IVC distensibility index (IVCdI) is another commonly used dynamic assessment to determine fluid responsiveness. Ultrasound scan is used to assess the change in size of the IVC during a respiratory cycle in a mechanically ventilated patient. As was the case for PPV, positive intrathoracic pressure is essential to use this technique accurately. The benefit of IVCdI is that it is noninvasive (no arterial line is required) and is reproducible multiple times at the bedside.

During the delivery of a mechanical breath, a patient's intrathoracic pressure increases, and venous return decreases, resulting in IVC dilation (an increase in the diameter of the vessel). When the mechanical breath is released, the intrathoracic pressure decreases, and the IVC returns to its normal diameter. The degree of IVC diameter change is measured with ultrasound scan and then the IVCdI is calculated (**Fig. 3**).

Box 1
Limitations of dynamic indices

For IVCdI, PPV, or SVV to accurately predict volume responsiveness, the following criteria must be met:

- Mechanical ventilation
- Tidal volume of at least 8 mL/kg of ideal body weight
- Initiating no spontaneous breaths
- No cardiac arrhythmias

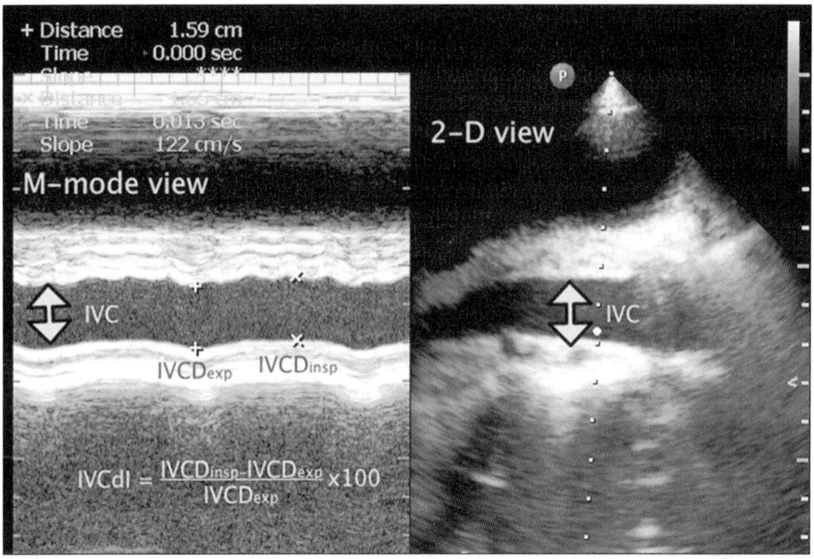

Fig. 3. IVC distensibility index. Calculation of IVCdI using M-mode ultrasound scan. IVCDexp, IVC diameter at end-expiration; IVCDinsp, IVC diameter at end-inspiration.

Many findings suggest that IVCdI is a useful bedside tool for assessing the status of the intravascular volume for patients undergoing fluid resuscitation. There has been, however, variation in the agreed cutoff values of the IVCdI across studies. Some studies found a cutoff of 12%, but others proposed values as high as 36%.[25–27]

Limitations of measuring the IVCdI are similar to those described for PPV (see **Box 1**). There is also debate in the literature on what level of the IVC is the best site for measurement. The location of measurement (eg, at the level of the hepatic or renal vein) can affect the recorded value of the IVC diameter.[28]

END-EXPIRATORY OCCLUSION TEST

The end-expiratory occlusion (EEO) test is a relatively new technique for dynamic assessment of fluid responsiveness in mechanically ventilated patients. The EEO test is executed by placing a 15-second expiratory hold on the ventilator (at the end of expiration). A prolonged state of increased preload is created by holding the positive pressure ventilation at it its lowest pressure, mimicking a fluid challenge. This test has the advantage of being able to assess fluid responsiveness even in the presence of arrhythmias, a notable difference from the techniques previously discussed.[29–31]

This technique requires concurrent measurement of stroke volume or cardiac output. Although this is a notable limitation, several monitoring approaches have been reported, such as measuring cardiac output by thermodilution or waveform analysis. When such monitoring is available, if the stroke volume or cardiac output during the final 5 seconds of the expiratory hold is 5% higher than the premaneuver value, the patient will likely respond to the administration of a fluid bolus.[29,31]

PASSIVE LEG RAISE

The dynamic techniques described above have one thing in common: the patient must be mechanically ventilated. Although these dynamic indices are fairly well validated, it would be helpful to have a test that is valid for spontaneously breathing patients. The passive leg raise (PLR) is the only dynamic index to date that has the ability to predict the response to fluids in a spontaneously breathing patient (**Fig. 4**).[32,33]

The PLR technique mobilizes pooled venous blood in the lower extremities (approximately 150–300 mL[34]) to the central circulation as an autologous and reversible fluid bolus. In this way, extrinsic fluids are not necessary, and patients do not receive an unnecessary fluid bolus if they are not volume responsive. The PLR is performed by first measuring the baseline stroke volume or cardiac output, followed by remeasuring it 30 to 90 seconds after lifting the patient's lower extremities.[35] A 10% to 15% change in stroke volume or cardiac output is an indicator that the patient will respond to exogenous fluid administration. Another benefit to this test is that it has been validated for patients with cardiac arrhythmias (eg, atrial fibrillation).[36] Similar to the EEO test, studies have used several monitoring systems, including bedside echocardiography, arterial waveform analysis, and bioreactance, to determine change in cardiac output or stroke volume.[37]

DEVICES FOR HEMODYNAMIC MONITORING

The methods described in this article permit the clinician to deliver fluid boluses in a goal-directed manner. Unfortunately, many of these methods are labor intensive and require the clinician to return to the bedside repeatedly to assess the patient's volume status. This requirement can be challenging and impractical in a busy emergency department.

Devices that automatically monitor and display a patient's hemodynamic information are desirable because they allow the use of nurse-directed resuscitation protocols while the clinician leaves the bedside temporarily. Another benefit of such monitors is as an early warning system that alerts clinicians to changes in a patient's hemodynamic status. These devices display hemodynamic information such as stroke volume, cardiac output, and stroke volume variation (SVV).

SVV is the amount of variation that occurs over a respiratory cycle in mechanically ventilated patients. It is similar in concept to PPV, except that a device is used to estimate the actual stroke volume rather than using the pulse pressure as a surrogate. Similar to PPV, SVV has been validated across multiple situations as a predictor of fluid responsiveness.[38,39] An SVV measurement greater than 11.5% suggests that giving a fluid bolus would be beneficial.[24] Conversely, an SVV less than 11.5% suggests that a fluid bolus would not improve the patient's hemodynamics and might cause harm (eg, pulmonary edema). Although PPV and SVV are very similar, PPV seems to slightly outperform SVV[23,24,38] and requires the same conditions for validity as do PPV and IVCdI (see **Box 1**).

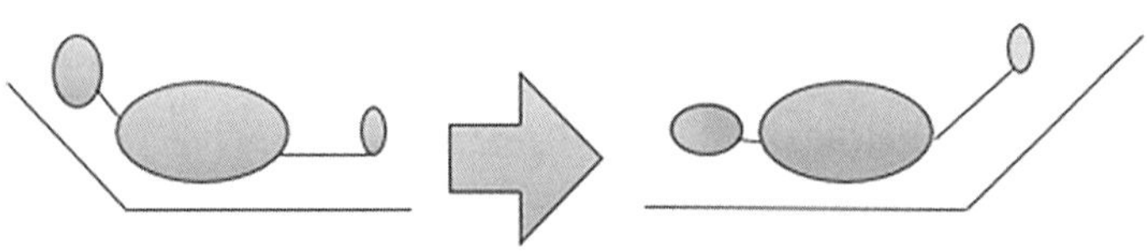

Fig. 4. Passive leg raising maneuver. The process begins with the head of the bed and the patient's trunk elevated to approximately 45°, at which time baseline parameters are recorded. The patient is then quickly laid back, with head and trunk flat and legs raised to 45°, allowing the venous blood pooled in the legs to return to the heart quickly, creating an autologous transfusion. Parameters should be rerecorded 30 to 90 seconds after raising the legs to evaluate for volume responsiveness.

Two main categories of devices provide hemodynamic data: invasive and noninvasive monitors. Each type has benefits and disadvantages, and neither is perfect. The choice of device depends on several factors, a full discussion of which can be found elsewhere.[40]

INVASIVE HEMODYNAMIC MONITORS

The pulmonary artery catheter (PAC) measures stroke volume and cardiac output by measuring the amount of time it takes for a known quantity of fluid to traverse the right side of the heart. The longer it takes, the worse the stroke volume. One of the major criticisms of the PAC is its invasive nature, given that it must be inserted through the superior vena cava, into the right side of the heart, across the tricuspid and pulmonary valves, and into the pulmonary artery. Major complications associated with the PAC include pneumothorax, arterial puncture, and hematoma—complications associated with the placement of any central line. Complications specific to PAC include ventricular arrhythmias, ventricular rupture, and pulmonary artery rupture.[41]

Two commercially available devices have monitoring principles similar to the PAC but are less invasive: the PiCCO and LidCO systems. These devices use an arterial catheter to perform pulse-contour analysis, which is a technique to determine hemodynamic parameters from an arterial waveform.

Both devices are periodically calibrated to improve accuracy. Calibration is performed by injecting a fluid into a venous line (ice-cold saline for the PiCCO and lithium for LidCO) and measuring the fluid in the arterial circulation after it traverses the heart.[42,43] The PiCCO system measures the degree of temperature elevation of the saline injected, and the LidCO system measures the dilution of the lithium that was injected; these measurements are made via a sensor in an arterial line.

Monitoring stroke volume and cardiac output with these monitors helps the clinician determine whether a hemodynamically unstable patient would benefit from a fluid bolus, because the response to fluid bolus can be measured. For example, an increase in either parameter by 10% to 15% after a fluid bolus suggests the patient was volume responsive as part of the hemodynamic resuscitation.[44] However, failure to increase the stroke volume or cardiac output by 10% to 15% after a fluid bolus suggests that the hemodynamically unstable patient would not improve with fluid administration and should perhaps receive vasopressors or an inotrope.

The PiCCO device is considered a minimally invasive device because it requires the placement of a central venous catheter (the tip of which resides at the junction of the superior vena cava and the right atrium) and a femoral arterial line that will detect changes in saline temperature distally. The limitations of the PiCCO device include decreased accuracy in patients with low-flow states (eg, severe heart failure), valvular regurgitation, intracardiac shunts, and aortic aneurysms.[43]

The LidCO device is somewhat less invasive than the PiCCO in that it requires placement of only a peripheral intravenous line and a radial arterial line (a central venous catheter can be used if it is already available). The major limitations to the accuracy of the LidCO device are similar to those associated with the PiCCO device, including low flow states, valvular regurgitation, and intracardiac shunts. A limitation specific to the LidCO device is its use of lithium dye. Although this dye is safe for most patients, it should be avoided in certain situations, including patients who weigh less than 40 kg, pregnant patients, and those taking lithium as a medication.[45]

A third minimally invasive system is the Flo Trac/Vigileo system. This system differs from the monitors discussed above in that it requires placement of only an arterial catheter. The monitor displays hemodynamic data such as stroke volume, cardiac output, and stroke volume variation by analyzing arterial waveforms and pressures and integrating this information into a complex algorithm based on the patient's demographics (height, sex, weight). This device does not require external calibration, and its manufacturer claims that the system is continuously fine tuning and auto calibrating each minute. Auto calibration is based on cadaveric studies, and its accuracy has been questioned.[46] The device has also been found to be inaccurate in certain clinical conditions (eg, in patients with rapidly changing cardiac output or high cardiac output states).[47]

Several studies found these minimally invasive monitors to be accurate. No single device, however, has gained widespread acceptance in emergency medicine; one of the major reasons for this is their invasiveness, requiring at least an arterial line (and a central line in the case of the PiCCO). Despite their limitations, these devices provide clinicians with hemodynamic monitoring that is otherwise difficult to achieve with traditional methods.

NONINVASIVE HEMODYNAMIC MONITORS

Invasive catheters have the potential to create complications, such as discomfort during placement, infection, and bleeding, so a noninvasive hemodynamic monitor is an appealing concept in the emergency department. Two examples of completely noninvasive monitors are the ultrasonic cardiac output monitor (USCOM) and the noninvasive cardiac output monitor (NICOM).

USCOM

The USCOM is a small probe that can be applied intermittently to a patient's chest or suprasternal notch whenever hemodynamic information is needed. The device works by providing a continuous Doppler signal, which measures the velocity of blood flow in the aorta (parasternal view) or the pulmonary blood flow (suprasternal notch).[43,48,49] This information is used in conjunction with the patient's height to calculate several hemodynamic parameters, including stroke volume and cardiac output. Beyond the noninvasive nature of this device, another advantage is that bedside nurses can obtain the information for use in resuscitative algorithms.

The USCOM seems to be a promising addition to the emergency department armamentarium, although there are several limitations to its general use. The device can easily be applied to a patient, but obtaining an adequate and accurate Doppler signal can be a challenge for novice users and altogether impossible in a percentage of certain populations (eg, the elderly).[50] Another limitation is that hemodynamic information is not obtained continuously but rather only when the device is applied; this means that crucial information might be missed in patients with a rapidly changing hemodynamic state. Another criticism of the USCOM is the assumption that 2 patients with the same height will have the same hemodynamic changes when faced with a similar stressor, which might not actually be true. A detailed discussion of this concept is beyond the scope of this article, but it is a valid limitation that should be considered.[51]

NiCOM: Bioreactance

The NiCOM requires the placement of 4 adhesive electrodes on the patient's anterior thorax. These electrodes measure changes in the frequency of electrical currents as they cross the thorax, converting this information into relevant hemodynamic information, including stroke volume, cardiac output, and stroke volume variation.[52–54] Newer versions of this device incorporate the use of a passive leg raise maneuver to determine volume responsiveness.[55,56] This device has been found to correlate well with more invasive means of hemodynamic monitoring, such as the pulmonary artery catheter.

The greatest clinical benefit of this device is that it provides continuous hemodynamic monitoring noninvasively for critically ill patients. Rapidly changing hemodynamics are more likely to be detected with this monitor compared with monitors that use intermittent measurements.[54] Additionally, little training is required to set up and use the device because the sensors are applied to the thorax and do not require constant manipulation, minimizing sampling errors between readings. More clinical trials are needed to determine whether this device improves patient outcomes, but it is a promising technology for continuous hemodynamic monitoring in the emergency department.

SUMMARY

Shock is a physiologic state associated with high morbidity and mortality rates. Emergency physicians have a major impact on patient survival. The clinician has several tools available to evaluate volume status. Each modality has its benefits and limitations but, to date, no one test can indicate with 100% accuracy which patients will be truly volume responsive. Although the search for the Holy Grail of a perfect intravascular monitor continues, we must remember the importance of early, aggressive, and goal-directed interventions for patients in shock. We, therefore, must be astute clinicians and integrate the multitude of variables available at the bedside to assist in our decision making; this is truly the art of medicine. Finally, there is no substitute for the most important intervention—the frequent presence of the physician at the patient's bedside.

REFERENCES

1. Kumar A, Roberts D, Wood KE, et al. Duration of hypotension before initiation of effective antimicrobial therapy is the critical determinant of survival in human septic shock. Crit Care Med 2006;34:1589–96.
2. Marchick MR, Kline JA, Jones AE. The significance of non-sustained hypotension in emergency department patients with sepsis. Intensive Care Med 2009;35:1261–4.
3. Rivers E, Nguyen B, Havstad S, et al. Early goal-directed therapy in the treatment of severe sepsis and septic shock. N Engl J Med 2001;345:1368–77.
4. Michard F, Teboul J. Predicting fluid responsiveness in ICU patients: a critical analysis of the evidence. Chest 2002;121:2000–8.
5. Vincent JL, Sakr Y, Ranieri VM, et al. Sepsis in European intensive care units: results of the SOAP study. Crit Care Med 2006;34:344–53.
6. Rosenberg AL, Dechert RE, Park PK, et al. Association of cumulative fluid balance on outcome in acute lung injury: a retrospective review of the ARDSnet tidal volume study cohort. J Intensive Care Med 2009;24:35–46.
7. Boyd JH, Forbes J, Nakada TA, et al. Fluid resuscitation in septic shock: a positive fluid balance and elevated central venous pressure are associated with increased mortality. Crit Care Med 2011;39:259–65.
8. Sadaka F, Juarez M, Naydenov S, et al. Fluid resuscitation in septic shock: the effect of increasing fluid balance on mortality. J Intensive Care Med 2013;29:213–7.
9. Micek ST, McEvoy C, McKenzie M, et al. Fluid balance and cardiac function in septic shock as predictors of hospital mortality. Crit Care 2013;17:R246.

10. Dellinger RP, Levy MM, Rhodes A, et al. Surviving sepsis campaign: international guidelines for management of severe sepsis and septic shock, 2012. Intensive Care Med 2013;39:165–228.
11. Rady MY, Rivers EP, Martin GB, et al. Continuous central venous oximetry and shock index in the emergency department: use in the evaluation of clinical shock. Am J Emerg Med 1992;10:538–41.
12. Rady MY, Rivers EP, Nowak RM. Resuscitation of the critically ill in the ED: responses of blood pressure, heart rate, shock index, central venous oxygen saturation, and lactate. Am J Emerg Med 1996;14:218–25.
13. Pierrakos C, Velissaris D, Scolletta S, et al. Can changes in arterial pressure be used to detect changes in cardiac index during fluid challenge in patients with septic shock? Intensive Care Med 2012;38:422–8.
14. Nahouraii RA, Rowell SE. Static measures of preload assessment. Crit Care Clin 2010;26:295–305.
15. Marik P, Baram M, Vahid B. Does central venous pressure predict fluid responsiveness? A systematic review of the literature and the tale of seven mares. Chest 2008;134:172–8.
16. Otto C. Textbook of clinical echocardiography. 2nd edition. Philadelphia: WB Saunders; 2000.
17. Perera P, Mailhot T, Riley D, et al. The RUSH exam: rapid ultrasound in shock in the evaluation of the critically ill. Emerg Med Clin North Am 2010;28:29–56.
18. Ferrada P, Anand RJ, Whelan J, et al. Qualitative assessment of the inferior vena cava: useful tool for the evaluation of fluid status in critically ill patients. Am Surg 2012;78:468–70.
19. Michard F, Boussat S, Chemla D, et al. Relationship between respiratory changes in arterial pulse pressure and fluid responsiveness in septic patients with acute circulatory failure. Am J Repir Crit Care Med 2000;162:134–8.
20. Osman D, Ridel C, Ray P, et al. Cardiac filling pressures are not appropriate to predict hemodynamic response to volume challenge. Crit Care Med 2007;35:64–8.
21. Solus-Biguenet H, Fleyfel M, Tavernier B, et al. Non-invasive prediction of fluid responsiveness during major hepatic surgery. Br J Anaesth 2006;97:808–16.
22. Zhang Z, Lu B, Sheng X, et al. Accuracy of stroke volume variation in predicting fluid responsiveness: a systematic review and meta-analysis. J Anesth 2011;25: 904–16.
23. Biais M, Cottenceau V, Stecken L, et al. Evaluation of stroke volume variations obtained with the pressure recording analytic method. Crit Care Med 2012;40: 1186–91.
24. Marik PE, Cavallazzi R, Vasu T, et al. Dynamic changes in arterial waveform derived variables and fluid responsiveness in mechanically ventilated patients: a systematic review of the literature. Crit Care Med 2009;37:2642–7.
25. Feissel M, Michard F, Faller J, et al. The respiratory variation in inferior vena cava diameter as a guide to fluid therapy. Intensive Care Med 2004;30:1834–7.
26. Barbier C, Loubieres Y, Schmit C, et al. Respiratory changes in inferior vena cava diameter are helpful in predicting fluid responsiveness in ventilated septic patients. Intensive Care Med 2004;30:1740–6.
27. Vieillard-Baron A, Chergui K, Rabiller A, et al. Superior vena caval collapsibility as a gauge of volume status in ventilated septic patients. Intensive Care Med 2004;30:1734–9.
28. Machare-Delgado E, Decaro M, Marik PE. Inferior vena cava variation compared to pulse contour analysis as predictors of fluid responsiveness: a prospective cohort study. J Intensive Care Med 2011;26:116–24.

29. Wallace DJ, Allison M, Stone MB. Inferior vena cava collapse during respiration is affected by the sampling location: an ultrasound study in healthy volunteers. Acad Emerg Med 2010;17:96–9.
30. Monnet X, Osman D, Ridel C, et al. Predicting volume responsiveness by using the end-expiratory occlusion in mechanically ventilated intensive care unit patients. Crit Care Med 2009;37:951–6.
31. Monnet X, Bleibtreu A, Ferre A, et al. Passive leg-raising and end-expiratory occlusion tests perform better than pulse pressure variation in patients with low respiratory system compliance. Crit Care Med 2012;40:152–7.
32. Monnet X, Dres M, Ferre A, et al. Prediction of fluid responsiveness by a continuous non-invasive assessment of arterial pressure in critically ill patients: comparison with four other dynamic indices. Br J Anaesth 2012;109:330–8.
33. Teboul J, Monnet X. Prediction of volume responsiveness in critically ill patients with spontaneous breathing activity. Curr Opin Crit Care 2008;14:334–9.
34. Biais M, Vidil L, Sarrabay P, et al. Changes in stroke volume induced by passive leg raising in spontaneously breathing patients: comparison between echocardiography and Vigileo/FloTrac device. Crit Care 2009;13:R195.
35. Rutlen DL, Wackers FJ, Zaret BL. Radionuclide assessment of peripheral intravascular capacity: a technique to measure intravascular volume changes in the capacitance circulation in man. Circulation 1981;64:146–52.
36. Monnet X, Teboul J. Passive leg raising. Intensive Care Med 2008;34:659–63.
37. Cavallaro F, Sandroni C, Marano C, et al. Diagnostic accuracy of passive leg raising for prediction of fluid responsiveness in adults: systematic review and meta-analysis of clinical studies. Intensive Care Med 2010;36:1475–83.
38. Marik PE, Levitov A, Young A, et al. The use of bioreactance and carotid Doppler to determine volume responsiveness and blood flow redistribution following passive leg raising in hemodynamically unstable patients. Chest 2013;143: 364–70.
39. Cecconi M, Monti G, Hamilton MA, et al. Efficacy of functional hemodynamic parameters in predicting fluid responsiveness with pulse power analysis in surgical patients. Minerva Anestesiol 2012;78:527–33.
40. Reuter DA, Kirchner A, Felbinger TW, et al. Usefulness of left ventricular stroke volume variation to assess fluid responsiveness in patients with reduced cardiac function. Crit Care Med 2003;31:1399–404.
41. Vincent JL, Rhodes A, Perel A, et al. Clinical review: update on hemodynamic monitoring - a consensus of 16. Crit Care 2011;15:229.
42. Marik PE. Obituary: pulmonary artery catheter 1970 to 2013. Ann Intensive Care 2013;3:38.
43. Ramsingh D, Alexander B, Cannesson M. Clinical review: does it matter which hemodynamic monitoring system is used? Crit Care 2013;17(2):208.
44. Mohammed I, Phillips C. Techniques for determining cardiac output in the intensive care unit. Crit Care Clin 2010;26:355–64.
45. Napoli A. Physiologic and clinical principles behind noninvasive resuscitation techniques and cardiac output monitoring. Cardiol Res Pract 2012;2012: 531908.
46. Reuter DA, Huang C, Edrich T, et al. Cardiac output monitoring using indicator-dilution techniques: basics, limits, and perspectives. Anesth Analg 2010;110: 799–811.
47. Benington S, Ferris P, Nirmalan M. Emerging trends in minimally invasive haemodynamic monitoring and optimization of fluid therapy. Eur J Anaesthesiol 2009;26:893–905.

48. Mayer J, Boldt J, Poland R, et al. Continuous arterial pressure waveform-based cardiac output using the Flo Trac/Vigileo: a review and meta-analysis. J Cardiothorac Vasc Anesth 2009;23:401–6.
49. Boyle M, Steel L, Flynn GM, et al. Assessment of the clinical utility of an ultrasonic monitor of cardiac output (the USCOM) and agreement with thermodilution measurement. Crit Care Resusc 2009;11:198–203.
50. Tan HL, Pinder M, Parsons R, et al. Clinical evaluation of USCOM ultrasonic cardiac output monitor in cardiac surgical patients in intensive care unit. Br J Anaesth 2005;94:287–91.
51. Chong SW, Peyton PJ. A meta-analysis of the accuracy and precision of the ultrasonic cardiac output monitor (USCOM). Anaesthesia 2012;67:1266–71.
52. Huang L, Critchley LA. Accuracy and precision of the USCOM: does a meta-analysis provide the answer? Anaesthesia 2013;68:431–2.
53. Keren H, Burkhoff D, Squara P. Evaluation of a noninvasive continuous cardiac output monitoring system based on thoracic bioreactance. Am J Physiol Heart Circ Physiol 2007;293:H583–9.
54. Raval NY, Squara P, Cleman M, et al. Multicenter evaluation of noninvasive cardiac output measurement by bioreactance technique. J Clin Monit Comput 2008;22:113–9.
55. Squara P, Denjean D, Estagnasie P, et al. Noninvasive cardiac output monitoring (NICOM): a clinical validation. Intensive Care Med 2007;33:1191–4.
56. Benomar B, Ouattara A, Estagnasie P, et al. Fluid responsiveness predicted by noninvasive bioreactance-based passive leg raise test. Intensive Care Med 2010;36:1875–81.

Pressors and Inotropes

Joe Kanter, MD, MPH*, Peter DeBlieux, MD

KEYWORDS

- Vasopressors • Inotropes • Chronotropes • Hemodynamic effect

KEY POINTS

- Although disease-specific guidelines provide a framework for vasopressor, inotrope, and chronotrope selection and usage, real-world applications demand therapy be tailored to the individual patient.
- Physiologic parameters, such as fluid status or cardiovascular reserve, may alter an individual patient's response to a particular agent.
- Patients with preexisting, poorly controlled hypertension may require higher than normal goal blood pressures to achieve treatment goals.

INTRODUCTION

To effectively treat an aging and increasingly complex patient population, emergency physicians and other acute-care providers must be comfortable with the use of vasopressors, inotropes, and chronotropes. These medicines are used to augment the cardiovascular function of critically ill patients.

Each class of medication produces a different hemodynamic effect. Vasopressors induce peripheral vasoconstriction, increasing systemic vascular resistance (SVR) and mean arterial pressure (MAP). Inotropes increase the force of cardiac contractility, increasing cardiac output and MAP. Chronotropes increase heart rate. Some agents produce only one of these actions, whereas others have multiple effects. For the emergency physician, these agents are used with the explicit goal of preserving vital organ perfusion during acute and severe illness. This article reviews the physiologic receptors targeted by such drugs, common agents used, and specific clinical indications for their use.

PHYSIOLOGY

Vasopressors, inotropes, and chronotropes act on various adrenergic receptors (**Table 1**). Ubiquitous within the smooth muscle of arterial walls, α_1 receptors induce

Disclosure: None.
Section of Emergency Medicine, LSU Health Sciences Center, 5th Floor Rm 548W, New Orleans, LA 70112, USA
* Corresponding author.
E-mail address: joekanter@gmail.com

Emerg Med Clin N Am 32 (2014) 823–834
http://dx.doi.org/10.1016/j.emc.2014.07.006 **emed.theclinics.com**

Table 1
Commonly used vasopressors, inotropes, and chronotropes

Drug	Action	Common Doses	Adverse Effects
Norepinephrine	$\alpha_1 > \beta_1$	0.01–0.5 μg/kg/min	Tachyarrhythmias, increased myocardial oxygen consumption, myocardial banding necrosis with prolonged infusions
Vasopressin	α_1, V_1, V_2, V_3	0.04 U/min	Possible gastrointestinal hypoperfusion
Dopamine	α_1, β_1, dopa 1	0.5–25 μg/kg/min	Tachyarrhythmias, increased myocardial oxygen consumption
Epinephrine	α_1, β_1, β_2	0.01–0.75 μg/kg/min	Tachyarrhythmias, leukocytosis, increased myocardial oxygen consumption
Phenylephrine	α_1	0.15–0.75 μg/kg/min	Reflex bradycardia
Isoproterenol	$\beta_1 > \beta_2$	0.01–0.02 μg/kg/min	Tachyarrhythmias, flushing, increased myocardial oxygen consumption
Dobutamine	$\beta_1 > \beta_2$	2.0–20 μg/kg/min	Tachyarrhythmias, increased myocardial oxygen consumption, pharmacologic tolerance in prolonged infusions
Milrinone	Phosphodiesterase inhibition	0.3–0.8 μg/kg/min	Headache, hypotension, tachycardia
Levosimendan	Increased calcium-dependent binding of troponin C	0.05–0.2 μg/kg/min	Headache, hypotension, prolonged half-life of active metabolites

arterial vasoconstriction, increasing SVR. They are also present to a lesser extent in the heart and can increase systolic contraction without affecting chronotropy, although the clinical significance of this action is unclear.[1] β_1 receptors predominate in cardiac smooth muscle. They act on the sinoatrial node to produce positive chronotropy and on atrial and ventricular muscle to produce inotropy. Located throughout the body but notably in bronchial smooth muscle, β_2 receptors increase calcium uptake by the sarcoplasmic reticulum, resulting in mild vasodilation and, of particular importance, pulmonary bronchodilation.[2] They are also located in uterine muscle, and are targeted during tocolysis treatment. Dopamine receptors are located in renal, splanchnic, and coronary vasculature and the central nervous system; their actions are complicated and diverse. Vasopressin receptors are located in vascular smooth muscle, the anterior pituitary gland, and the renal collecting duct. Their activation results in vasoconstriction, adrenocorticotropic hormone and prolactin release, and renal water reabsorption.[3]

Although each drug carries its own side effect profile, some adverse effects can be seen with multiple agents. All catecholamines may cause myocardial contraction band necrosis, mostly by protein kinase A activation and increased cytosolic calcium influx,[4] which can result in ventricular aneurysm, rupture, or irreversible impairment of cardiac function. The risk of this increases with prolonged infusions. Also, any vasopressor usage carries the risk of tissue necrosis if intravenous (IV) extravasation occurs. Vasopressors are traditionally delivered by central venous access for this reason, although evidence-based trials supporting the long-followed practice are lacking.

COMMON PHARMACOLOGIC AGENTS

Norepinephrine (Levophed) is an endogenous catecholamine with strong α_1 agonist activity and modest β_1 activity, resulting in potent vasoconstriction and less potent inotropy. The net clinical effect is an increase in systolic blood pressure (SBP), diastolic blood pressure, and pulse pressure, with minimal effect on cardiac output. Chronotropic effects are also minimal.

Vasopressin, or antidiuretic hormone, is an endogenous hormone stored in the posterior pituitary gland and released in response to increased plasma osmolality, hypotension, pain, nausea, and hypoxia. It is also synthesized by the heart in response to cardiac wall stress,[5] and by the adrenal glands in response to increased catecholamine secretion.[6] It acts on V_1 receptors in vascular smooth muscle to induce vasoconstriction, and V_2 receptors in the renal collecting tubules to increase collecting duct permeability and renal water reabsorption. Vasopressin increases SVR but reflexive increases in systemic vagal tone result in a minimal net effect on cardiac output. Vascular sensitivity to norepinephrine is increased when vasopressin is coadministered, thus creating a synergistic effect and decreasing the needed dose (and side effects) of norepinephrine. Some have suggested it is particularly useful in sepsis because its vasoconstrictive effects are preserved in hypoxic and acidotic conditions.[7–9]

Dopamine is a central neurotransmitter and the immediate precursor to norepinephrine in the endogenous catecholamine synthesis pathway. Traditionally, systemic effects are considered dose-dependent. At low infusion rates (0.5–3 μg/kg/min), stimulation of D_1 postsynaptic receptors in coronary, renal, mesenteric, and cerebral vascular beds, and D_2 presynaptic receptors in renal tissue, result in mild vasodilation and diuresis.[10] The clinical significance of this "renal dose" of dopamine is unclear. In critically ill patients, low-dose dopamine infusions have been shown not to increase glomerular filtration rate and to confer no protection against increases in serum creatinine, progression toward oliguria, or eventual need of hemodialysis.[11] Similarly, the increase in splanchnic blood flow is of questionable clinical significance and does not alter other key metrics of mesenteric perfusion.[12] Intermediate doses of dopamine (3–10 μg/kg/min) activate β_1 receptors and increase endogenous norepinephrine release, increasing cardiac inotropy and SVR.[13] At high doses (10–20 μg/kg/min), α_1 activity predominates resulting in vasoconstriction and increased SVR.[14] It should be noted that these distinctions are derived generally and in clinical practice the response is patient-specific.

Epinephrine is an endogenous catecholamine with high affinity for α_1, β_1, and β_2 receptors resulting in vasoconstriction, positive inotropy, and bronchodilation. At high infusion rates the duration of diastole is increased and myocytes are stimulated to release local vasodilators leading to increased coronary blood flow.[15] When compared with norepinephrine, dopamine, and vasopressin, a higher risk exists for dysrhythmia and splanchnic vasoconstriction.[16]

Phenylephrine is a synthetic α agonist that rapidly increases SVR. In addition to standard infusions, it can be bolused to correct sudden, severe hypotension. It has no direct chronotropic effects but rapid increases in MAP can induce baroreceptor-mediated reflex bradycardia.

Isoproterenol is a synthetic nonselective β agonist and acts as a strong chronotrope and inotrope. Increased systemic vasodilation and mild pulmonary vasodilation are also seen. Stroke volume is increased, but because of its β_2-mediated decrease in SVR, the net effect on cardiac output is neutral. It may be safely administered by peripheral IV access but caution must be taken in patients at-risk for cardiac ischemia.

Dobutamine is a synthetic catecholamine that binds β_1 and, to a lesser extent, α_1 and β_2 receptors. This results in strong inotropic and weaker chronotropic activity. A mild reduction in SVR can be seen and is a reflexive response to increased inotropy. Dobutamine's activation of α_1 and β_2 receptors is of questionable clinical significance. Similar to isoproterenol, it increases myocardial oxygen consumption (useful in pharmacologic cardiac stress testing) and is potentially harmful to patients at-risk for cardiac ischemia. Significant pharmacologic tolerance can develop after only 72 hours of continued infusion.[17] It is safe to administer by peripheral IV but can induce ventricular arrhythmias at any dose.[18]

Milrinone is a second-generation phosphodiesterase inhibitor that improves cardiac output and reduces SVR. Through inhibition of type 3 phosphodiesterase, conversion of cAMP to AMP is blocked, increasing available cAMP and resulting in increased myocardial contractility and mild peripheral vasodilation. Pulmonary vascular resistance is decreased and diastolic relaxation is improved. Milrinone may be preferable in patients with significant pulmonary venous hypertension.[19] It does not induce pharmacologic tolerance, has a relatively longer half-life (2–4 hours) than most other inotropes, and is safe for peripheral infusion.[20] It has largely replaced its predecessor inamrinone (Amrinone) because of fewer associated side effects, particularly the risk of thrombocytopenia.

Levosimendan, a newer "calcium sensitizer" that increases calcium-dependent binding of troponin C, enhances ventricular contractility without increasing intracellular calcium concentration or affecting diastolic relaxation. It improves cardiac output and also opens vascular smooth muscle potassium channels, which provide arteriolar and venous vasodilation.[21,22] It may increase glomerular filtration rate in acute decompensated heart failure (ADHF)[23] and is potentially cardioprotective during periods of ischemia.[24,25] Levosimendan is an unproved but promising treatment of heart failure.[26,27]

SEPTIC SHOCK

In the patient with sepsis, functional intravascular hypovolemia caused by decreased oral intake, insensible losses, increased venous capacitance, reduced myocardial contractility, vascular damage, and increased peripheral vasodilation lead to hypotension and impaired end-organ perfusion. Management begins with infectious source control, timely and appropriate antimicrobials, volume assessment, and initial correction of hypovolemia. Concurrent vasopressors are often needed to maintain organ perfusion. In a noted change from previous recommendations, norepinephrine is now the pressor-of-choice in septic shock. Compared with dopamine, it is less arrhythmogenic[28,29] and, in meta-analysis, seems to confer a mortality benefit.[30] The Surviving Sepsis Campaign now recommends it as the first-line agent.[31] Infusions should be initially titrated to an MAP of 65. This target has been shown to provide adequate perfusion as measured by systemic oxygen metabolism, skin microcirculatory blood flow, urine output, and splanchnic perfusion, and no benefit has been seen with higher MAP targets.[32] Importantly, MAP goals must always be individualized and based on clinically relevant perfusion markers, such as urine output, mental status, skin perfusion, and serum lactate clearance. Initial vasopressor treatment should be concomitant with volume repletion; one should not wait for euvolemia before initiating pressors.

Fixed, low-dose vasopressin should be added to norepinephrine as the "first-line additional agent" if resuscitation goals are not met. Lower levels of endogenous anti-diuretic hormone are common in shock and contribute to systemic hypotension.[33] Low doses of vasopressin (0.04 U/min) are safe and effective,[34,35] and are particularly beneficial when coadministered with norepinephrine.[36] Vasopressin is not recommended as an agent that should be titrated.

Considered less safe but still acceptable, epinephrine may be substituted as the "first-line alternative" in patients intolerant of norepinephrine. Its use may be accompanied by metabolic side effects, such as tachycardia, increased lactic acidosis, and increased insulin requirements. These side effects have been shown to be reversible on discontinuation of epinephrine infusions and of questionable effect on mortality.[37] Phenylephrine should be used only if tachycardia or arrhythmias make norepinephrine and epinephrine intolerable, if cardiac output is known to be high with a persistently low blood pressure, or as salvage therapy. Previous studies have shown it may decrease stroke volume and impair hepatosplanchnic perfusion,[38,39] but more recent studies suggest it may be safer than previously thought.[40] Dopamine should only be used in patients with a low risk of tachyarrhythmia. A trial of dobutamine, in addition to a vasopressor, may be considered if myocardial dysfunction is present as inferred from elevated cardiac filling pressures and low cardiac output, or signs of ongoing hypoperfusion despite fluid repletion and vasopressor therapy. The use of inotropes to increase tissue oxygen delivery beyond physiologic levels confers no additional benefit.[41,42]

CARDIOGENIC SHOCK FOLLOWING ACUTE MYOCARDIAL INFARCTION

Definitive treatment of shock following acute myocardial infarction is revascularization. Mechanical augmentation of cardiac function with intra-aortic balloon pumps or left ventricular assist devices is a temporizing option. The use of vasopressors and inotropes carries the risk of increasing myocardial oxygen consumption, inducing ventricular arrhythmias, contraction-band necrosis, and infarct expansion. However, hypotension also compromises myocardial perfusion. When used as a bridge to definitive treatment, the hemodynamic benefits of vasopressors and/or inotropes usually outweigh the systemic risks of severe hypotension. Agents should be kept to the lowest efficacious dose and close attention paid toward the risk of arrhythmia and infarct expansion.

There exists no clear evidence-based recommendation for choice of agents in the setting of cardiogenic shock. The best strategy seems to be norepinephrine if hypotension is severe (SBP <70), or dopamine or dobutamine (or perhaps both, coadministered at lower doses of each) if hypotension is moderate (SBP 70–100).[13] Dopamine has traditionally been recommended over norepinephrine, but newer all-type shock studies have challenged this practice.[28] The 2004 American College of Cardiology/American Heart Association Guidelines recommend dobutamine if SBP is 70 to 100 without shock, dopamine if shock is present, and norepinephrine if a second agent is needed.[43] These recommendations are not evidence-based, and the group's 2013 update makes no comment, except noting that dopamine can be associated with "excess hazard."[44] Some evidence suggests dopamine and dobutamine may be coadministered in doses of 7.5 μg/kg/min each to increase MAP, maintain normal pulmonary capillary wedge pressure, and prevent hypoxemia more effectively than either single agent dosed alone at 15 μg/kg/min.[45] Other studies suggest vasopressin may be effective at increasing MAP without decreasing cardiac index or increasing pulmonary capillary wedge pressure.[46] Regardless, patients with postinfarct shock demand prompt specialty consultation, and treatment generally should be chosen in collaboration with the cardiologist who will inherit care of the patient.

Considerable expertise in treating cardiogenic shock has been gained through the perioperative management of patients undergoing cardiac surgery. Despite the widespread use of inotropes in this setting, particularly dobutamine, there remains considerable variation in practice between surgeons and centers,[47] no clear evidence-based guidelines,[48,49] and a growing discussion regarding the side effects of inotrope use.[50–52]

ACUTE DECOMPENSATED HEART FAILURE (ADHF)

Treatment of ADHF often involves inotropic support to lower end-diastolic pressure; improve diuresis; and allow typical regimens of angiotensin-converting enzyme inhibitors, diuretics, and β-blockers to be reinstated gradually. Despite the presence of hypotension, patients may have elevated SVR because of renal-angiotensin-aldosterone stimulation and the release of endogenous catecholamines and vasopressin. Inotropes with peripheral vasodilatory properties are therapeutic.[13]

Dobutamine or milrinone are recommended for consideration in patients with hypotensive ADHF and signs of decreased peripheral perfusion or end-organ dysfunction, or in patients unresponsive to or intolerant of IV vasodilation. Inotropes are not recommended unless left heart filling pressures are elevated, or cardiac index is severely impaired as noted on direct measurement or inferred from clinical signs. Inotropic support should be immediately discontinued if the patient experiences worsening hypotension or tachyarrhythmia.[18] Evidence-based guidelines in this area are scarce. The European Society of Cardiology gives tenuous recommendations for a trial of dopamine in ADHF without shock, or dobutamine if there exists peripheral hypoperfusion with or without pulmonary edema, in patients unresponsive to standard diuretic and vasodilator therapy. For ADHF patients in shock, the Society advises proceeding with extreme caution because vasopressors can further increase SVR to the point of threatening end-organ perfusion.[53] Any use of dobutamine in a patient with ADHF should be done under close watch for signs of ischemia or arrhythmia, and serum potassium should particularly be monitored.

In clinical trials, dobutamine and milrinone have shown similar outcomes. Dobutamine increases contractility with only minimal systemic vasodilation, but β receptors can become blunted in patients with ADHF. Milrinone provides pulmonary vasodilatation, right ventricular afterload reduction, and causes less of an increase in cardiac oxygen consumption, but has been noted at times to worsen systemic hypotension.[54,55] Despite earlier enthusiasm for the newer "calcium sensitizer" levosimendan, it has been shown to confer no mortality benefit over dobutamine.[56]

POSTCARDIOPULMONARY ARREST CARE

In the postarrest patient, MAP goals are typically 70 to 90. Without clear evidence-based support, professional consensus statements[57,58] and expert opinion[59] offer this recommendation based mostly on small observational reports noting that postarrest patients treated accordingly have enjoyed favorable outcomes.[60,61] These case series are confounded by other notable interventions, such as therapeutic hypothermia and percutaneous coronary intervention. The presumption is the postischemic brain loses much of its autoregulatory ability, and MAP goals of 65 may not be adequate to maintain cerebral perfusion.[58,62–64] No clear recommendations on choice of pressor are offered. Given the risk for arrhythmia in postarrest patients, norepinephrine, as opposed to dopamine, is a reasonable first-line selection. Future areas of study include the role of vasopressin and steroids during arrest, and a short course of stress-dose steroids in the week following return of circulation.[65]

NEUROGENIC SHOCK

In neurogenic shock, vasopressor support is frequently indicated to counter the vasodilation, hypotension, and bradycardia resulting from spinal cord injury and the disruption of autonomic pathways and sympathetic tone. Hypotension impairs spinal cord perfusion and leads to propagation of secondary injury.[66] MAP should be kept at 85 or above immediately postinjury and in the week following. This recommendation is based on consensus statements from The American Association of Neurologic Surgeons[67] and The Consortium for Spinal Cord Medicine,[68] expert opinion,[69–71] and small case reports.[72] There are no official recommendations for choice of vasopressor. Dopamine and norepinephrine are reasonable choices to augment α_1 and β_1 activity in cervical injuries, and phenylephrine may be adequate for lower thoracic injuries.[73]

One must balance these higher MAP goals against suspected traumatic brain injury. Impaired cerebral autoregulation often accompanies traumatic brain injury and increased intracranial pressure may exacerbate cerebral edema.[74] Additionally, cerebral perfusion pressures greater than 70 have been associated with pulmonary edema and acute respiratory distress syndrome. In the setting of traumatic brain injury, one must heed these concerns and use higher MAP goals judiciously.

Excessive IV fluids can be dangerous. Impaired respiratory mechanics and loss of mobility in a bed-bound patient can lead to pulmonary edema. Also, cardiac pacing may be indicated in patients who remain bradycardic despite pharmacologic support.[75,76] Autonomic deregulation is common and patients must be monitored closely for abrupt changes in heart rate and blood pressure.

ANAPHYLAXIS

Anaphylaxis is a difficult clinical entity to define and there exists a general consensus that health care providers are slow to recognize and treat the disease.[77–79] To satisfy the World Allergy Organization's definition, one of three criteria must be fulfilled: (1) acute-onset involvement of skin or mucosal tissue with either respiratory compromise or clinically significant hypotension; (2) two or more of the following conditions arising after exposure to a likely allergen: skin or mucosal involvement, respiratory compromise, hypotension, or persistent gastrointestinal symptoms, such as abdominal pain or vomiting; or (3) hypotension after exposure to a known allergen with SBP less than 90, or greater than 30% decrease from a patient's baseline.[79]

Epinephrine is first-line treatment. It should be given immediately on suspicion of anaphylaxis as 0.01 mg/kg of 1:1000 solution, up to a maximum of 0.5 mg in adults and 0.3 mg in children, intramuscular to the lateral thigh.[79] Intramuscular injections in this location achieve therapeutic plasma concentrations rapidly and reliably. The dose may be repeated every 5 to 15 minutes if clinical response is inadequate, but providers should not delay initiation of a titratable IV infusion of 1:10,000 concentration epinephrine. This is usually dosed at 0.5 to 5 μg/min and is titrated to clinical response and tolerated tachycardia.[78–80] Feared side effects, such as tachyarrhythmia, hypertensive crisis, and pulmonary edema, are rare following intramuscular dosing and, when seen with IV infusions, are frequently caused by erroneous administration of 1:1000 concentration.[80] Patients on β-blocking medications and unresponsive to epinephrine infusions may respond to glucagon, dosed 1 to 5 mg (0.02–0.03 mg/kg to maximum of 1 mg in children) of slow IV push over 5 minutes, then infused at 5 to 15 mg/min and titrated to clinical response.[81,82] Adjunctive therapy, such as antihistamines and corticosteroids, may be of use but should not replace or delay first-line treatment with epinephrine. Any patient treated for anaphylaxis must undergo a period of close and meaningful observation because symptoms can recur after an initial resolution.

SUMMARY

Although disease-specific guidelines provide a framework for vasopressor, inotrope, and chronotrope selection and usage, real-world applications demand therapy be tailored to the individual patient. Physiologic parameters, such as fluid status or cardiovascular reserve, may alter an individual patient's response to a particular agent. Patients with preexisting, poorly controlled hypertension may require higher than normal goal blood pressures to achieve treatment goals. Medications should be titrated to meaningful indicators of clinical response, such as urine output, skin perfusion, and mental status. If side effects render a patient intolerant of a particular medication, an alternative agent should be tried. Treatment of the critically ill patient with vasoactive medications must always be closely monitored and individualized.

REFERENCES

1. Williamson AP, Seifen E, Lindemann JP, et al. WB4101- and CEC-sensitive positive inotropic actions of phenylephrine in rat cardiac muscle. Am J Physiol 1994; 266:H2462.
2. Purves D, Augustine GJ, Fitzpatrick D, et al, editors. Neuroscience. 2nd edition. Sunderland (MA): Sinauer Associates; 2001. Catecholamine receptors. Available at: http://www.ncbi.nlm.nih.gov/books/NBK11062/.
3. Russell JA. Bench-to-bedside review: vasopressin in the management of septic shock. Crit Care 2011;15(4):226.
4. Communal C, Singh K, Pimentel DR, et al. Norepinephrine stimulates apoptosis in adult rat ventricular myocytes by activation of the β-adrenergic pathway. Circulation 1998;98:1329–34.
5. Hupf H, Grimm D, Riegger GAJ, et al. Evidence for a vasopressin system in the rat heart. Circ Res 1999;84:365–70.
6. Guillon G, Grazzini E, Andrez M, et al. Vasopressin: a potent autocrine/paracrine regulator of mammal adrenal functions. Endocr Res 1998;24:703–10.
7. Salzman AL, Vromen A, Denenberg A, et al. K(ATP)-channel inhibition improves hemodynamics and cellular energetics in hemorrhagic shock. Am J Physiol 1997;272:H688–94.
8. Kusano E, Tian S, Umino T, et al. Arginine vasopressin inhibits interleukin-1 beta-stimulated nitric oxide and cyclic guanosine monophosphate production via the V1 receptor in cultured rat vascular smooth muscle cells. J Hypertens 1997;15:627–32.
9. Hamu Y, Kanmura Y, Tsuneyoshi I, et al. The effects of vasopressin on endotoxin-induced attenuation of contractile responses in human gastroepiploic arteries in vitro. Anesth Analg 1999;88(3):542–8.
10. Denton MD, Chertow GM, Brady HR. "Renal-dose" dopamine for the treatment of acute renal failure: scientific rationale, experimental studies and clinical trials. Kidney Int 1996;50:4–14.

11. Bellomo R, Chapman M, Finfer S, et al. Low-dose dopamine in patients with early renal dysfunction: a placebo-controlled randomized trial. Australian and New Zealand Intensive Care Society (ANZICS) Clinical Trials Group. Lancet 2000;356:2139–43.
12. Meier-Hellmann A, Bredle DL, Specht M, et al. The effects of low-dose dopamine on splanchnic blood flow and oxygen update in patients with septic shock. Intensive Care Med 1997;23:31.
13. Overgaard CB, Džavík V. Inotropes and vasopressors: review of physiology and clinical use in cardiovascular disease. Circulation 2008;118(10):1047–56.
14. MacGregor DA, Smith TE, Prielipp RC, et al. Pharmacokinetics of dopamine in healthy male subjects. Anesthesiology 2000;92:338.
15. Jones CJ, DeFily DV, Patterson JL, et al. Endothelium-dependent relaxation competes with α1- and α2-adrenergic constriction in the canine epicardial coronary microcirculation. Circulation 1993;87:1264–74.
16. De Backer D, Creteur J, Silva E, et al. Effects of dopamine, norepinephrine, and epinephrine on the splanchnic circulation in septic shock: which is best? Crit Care Med 2003;31:1659.
17. Unverferth DA, Blanford M, Kates RE, et al. Tolerance to dobutamine after a 72 hour continuous infusion. Am J Med 1980;69:262–6.
18. Givertz MM, Teerlink JR, Albert NM, et al. Acute decompensated heart failure: update on new and emerging evidence and directions for future research. J Card Fail 2013;19(6):371–89.
19. Majure DT, Teerlink JR. Update on the management of acute decompensated heart failure. Curr Treat Options Cardiovasc Med 2011. [Epub ahead of print].
20. Shipley JB, Tolman D, Hastillo A, et al. Milrinone: basic and clinical pharmacology and acute and chronic management. Am J Med Sci 1996;311(6): 286–91.
21. Yildiz O. Vasodilation mechanisms of levosimendan: involvement of K+ channels. J Pharmacol Sci 2007;104(1):1–5.
22. Ng TM, Akhter MW. Levosimendan: dual mechanisms for acute heart failure-...and beyond? Minerva Cardioangiol 2005;53(6):565–84.
23. Yilmaz MB. Levosimendan improves renal function in patients with acute decompensated heart failure: comparison with dobutamine. Cardiovasc Drugs Ther 2007;21(6):431–5.
24. Lehtonen L, Poder P. The utility of levosimendan in the treatment of heart failure. Ann Med 2007;39:2–17.
25. Pollesello P, Papp Z. The cardioprotective effects of levosimendan: preclinical and clinical evidence. J Cardiovasc Pharmacol 2007;50(3):257–63.
26. Follath F, Yilmaz MB, Delgado JF, et al. Clinical presentation, management and outcomes in the acute heart failure global survey of standard treatment. Intensive Care Med 2011;37(4):619–26. http://dx.doi.org/10.1007/s00134-010-2113-0.
27. Archan S, Toller W. Levosimendan: current status and future prospects. Curr Opin Anaesthesiol 2008;21(1):78–84.
28. De Backer D, Biston P, Devriendt J, et al. SOPA II investigators: comparison of dopamine and norepinephrine in the treatment of shock. N Engl J Med 2010; 362:779–89.
29. Patel GP, Grahe JS, Sperry M, et al. Efficacy and safety of dopamine versus norepinephrine in the management of septic shock. Shock 2010;33:375–80.
30. De Backer D, Aldecoa C, Njimi H, et al. Dopamine versus norepinephrine in the treatment of septic shock: a meta-analysis. Crit Care Med 2012;40:725–30.

31. Dellinger RP, Levy MM, Rhodes A, et al. Surviving sepsis campaign: international guidelines for management of severe sepsis and septic shock: 2012. Crit Care Med 2013;41:580–637.
32. LeDoux D, Astiz ME, Carpati CM, et al. Effects of perfusion pressure on tissue perfusion in septic shock. Crit Care Med 2000;28:2729–32.
33. Landry DW, Levin HR, Gallant EM, et al. Vasopressin deficiency contributes to the vasodilation of septic shock. Circulation 1997;95:1122–5.
34. Malay MB. Low-dose vasopressin in the treatment of vasodilatory septic shock. J Trauma 1999;47:699–703.
35. Patel BM, Chittock DR, Russell JA, et al. Beneficial effects of short-term vasopressin infusion during severe septic shock. Anesthesiology 2002;96:576–82.
36. Dunser MW, Mayr AJ, Ulmer H, et al. Arginine vasopressin in advanced vasodilatory shock: a prospective, randomized, controlled study. Circulation 2003;107(18):2313–9.
37. Myburgh JA, Higgins A, Jovanovska A, et al. CAT Study investigators: a comparison of epinephrine and norepinephrine in critically ill patients. Intensive Care Med 2008;34:2226–34.
38. Gregory JS, Bonfiglio MF, Dasta JF, et al. Experience with phenylephrine as a component of the pharmacologic support of septic shock. Crit Care Med 1991;19:1395–400.
39. Flancbaum L, Dick M, Dasta J, et al. A dose-response study of phenylephrine in critically ill, septic surgical patients. Eur J Clin Pharmacol 1997;51:461–5.
40. Morelli A, Ertmer C, Rehberg S, et al. Phenylephrine versus norepinephrine fir initial hemodynamic support of patients with septic shock: a randomized, controlled trial. Crit Care 2008;12:R143.
41. Hayes MA, Timmins AC, Yau EH, et al. Elevation of systemic oxygen delivery in the treatment of critically ill patients. N Engl J Med 1994;330:1717–22.
42. Gattinoni L, Brazzi L, Pelosi P, et al. A trial of goal-oriented hemodynamic therapy in critically ill patients. N Engl J Med 1995;333:1025–32.
43. Antman EM, Anbe DT, Armstrong PW, et al. ACC/AHA guidelines for the management of patients with ST-elevation myocardial infarction: a report of the American College of Cardiology/American Heart Association Task Force on practice guidelines (Committee to revise the 1999 guidelines for the management of patients with acute myocardial infarction). J Am Coll Cardiol 2004;44(3):E1–211.
44. O'Gara PT, Kushner FG, Ascheim DD, et al. 2013 ACCF/AHA guideline for the management of ST-elevation myocardial infarction: a report of the American College of Cardiology Foundation/American Heart Association Task Force on Practice Guidelines. Circulation 2013;127(4):e362–425.
45. Richard C, Ricome JL, Rimailho A, et al. Combined hemodynamic effects of dopamine and dobutamine in cardiogenic shock. Circulation 1983;67:620–6.
46. Jolly S, Newton G, Horlick E, et al. Effect of vasopressin on hemodynamics in patients with refractory cardiogenic shock complicating acute myocardial infarction. Am J Cardiol 2005;96:1617–20.
47. Hernandez AF, Li S, Dokholyan RS, et al. Variation in perioperative vasoactive therapy in cardiovascular surgical care: data from the Society of Thoracic Surgeons. Am Heart J 2009;158:47–52.
48. Gillies M, Bellomo R, Doolan L, et al. Bench-to-bedside review: inotropic drug therapy after adult cardiac surgery: a systematic literature review. Crit Care 2005;9:266–79.

49. Mebazaa A, Pitsis AA, Rudiger A, et al. Clinical review: practical recommendations on the management of perioperative heart failure in cardiac surgery. Crit Care 2010;14(2):201.
50. Singer M, Brealey D. Another nail in the hammer's coffin? Crit Care 2011; 15(4):179.
51. Fellahi JL, Parienti JJ, Hanouz JL, et al. Perioperative use of dobutamine in cardiac surgery and adverse cardiac outcome: propensity-adjusted analyses. Anesthesiology 2008;108:979–87.
52. Shahin J, deVarennes B, Wing Tse C, et al. The relationship between inotrope exposure, six-hour physiological variables, and hospital mortality and renal dysfunction in patients undergoing cardiac surgery. Crit Care 2011;15:R162.
53. Nieminen MS, Böhm M, Cowie MR, et al. Executive summary of the guidelines on the diagnosis and treatment of acute heart failure: the Task Force on Acute Heart Failure of the European Society of Cardiology. Eur Heart J 2005;26:384–416.
54. Karlsberg RP, DeWood MA, DeMaria AN, et al. Comparative efficacy of short-term intravenous infusions of milrinone and dobutamine in acute congestive heart failure following acute myocardial infarction. Clin Cardiol 1996;19:21–30.
55. Aranda JM Jr, Schofield RS, Pauly DF, et al. Comparison of dobutamine versus milrinone therapy in hospitalized patients awaiting cardiac transplantation: a prospective, randomized trial. Am Heart J 2003;145(2):324–9.
56. Mebazaa A, Nieminen MS, Packer M, et al. Levosimendan vs dobutamine for patients with acute decompensated heart failure: the SURVIVE randomized trial. JAMA 2007;297(17):1883–91.
57. Bell DD, Brindley PG, Forrest D, et al. Management following resuscitation from cardiac arrest: recommendations from the 2003 Rocky Mountain Critical Care Conference. Can J Anaesth 2005;52:309–22.
58. Neumar RW. Post-cardiac arrest syndrome: epidemiology, pathophysiology, treatment, and prognostication: a consensus statement from the International Liaison Committee on Resuscitation. Circulation 2008;118:2452–83.
59. Stub D, Bernard S, Duffy SJ, et al. Contemporary reviews in cardiovascular medicine: post cardiac arrest syndrome: a review of therapeutic strategies. Circulation 2011;123:1428–35.
60. Gaieski DF. Early goal-directed hemodynamic optimization combined with therapeutic hypothermia in comatose survivors of out-of-hospital cardiac arrest. Resuscitation 2009;80:418–24.
61. Sunde K, Pytte M, Jacobsen D, et al. Implementation of a standardized treatment protocol for post resuscitation care after out-of-hospital cardiac arrest. Resuscitation 2007;73:29–39.
62. Nishizawa H, Kudoh I. Cerebral autoregulation is impaired in patients resuscitated after cardiac arrest. Acta Anaesthesiol Scand 1996;40:1149.
63. Sundgreen C, Larsen FS, Herzog TM, et al. Autoregulation of cerebral blood flow in patients resuscitated from cardiac arrest. Stroke 2001;32:128–32.
64. Shaffner DH, Eleff SM, Brambrink AM, et al. Effect of arrest time and cerebral perfusion pressure during cardiopulmonary resuscitation on cerebral blood flow, metabolism, adenosine triphosphate recovery, and pH in dogs. Crit Care Med 1999;27:1335–42.
65. Mentzelopoulos SD. Vasopressin, steroids, and epinephrine and neurologically favorable survival after in-hospital cardiac arrest: a randomized clinical trial. JAMA 2013;310(3):270–9.
66. Dumont RJ, Okonkwo DO, Verma S, et al. Acute spinal cord injury, part I: pathophysiologic mechanisms. Clin Neuropharmacol 2001;24(5):254–64.

67. Blood pressure management after acute spinal cord injury. Neurosurgery 2002; 50(3 Suppl):S58–62.
68. Consortium for Spinal Cord Medicine. Early acute management in adults with spinal cord injury: a clinical practice guideline for health-care professionals. J Spinal Cord Med 2008;31(4):1–69.
69. Jia X, Kowalski RG, Sciubba DM, et al. Critical care of traumatic spinal cord injury. J Intensive Care Med 2013;28:12.
70. Furlan JC, Fehlings MG. Cardiovascular complications after acute spinal cord injury: pathophysiology, diagnosis, and management. Neurosurg Focus 2008; 25(5):E13.
71. Ryken TC, Hurlbert RJ, Hadley MN, et al. The acute cardiopulmonary management of patients with cervical spinal cord injuries. Neurosurgery 2013;72(Suppl. 2):84–92.
72. Vale FL, Burns J, Jackson AB, et al. Combined medical and surgical treatment after acute spinal cord injury: results of a prospective pilot study to assess the merits of aggressive medical resuscitation and blood pressure management. J Neurosurg 1997;87(2):239–46.
73. Ploumis A, Yadlapalli N, Fehlings MG, et al. A systematic review of the evidence supporting a role for vasopressor support in acute SCI. Spinal Cord 2010;48(5): 356–62.
74. Muzevich KM, Voils SA. Role of vasopressor administration in patients with acute neurologic injury. Neurocrit Care 2009;11(1):112–9.
75. Lehmann KG, Lane JG, Piepmeier JM, et al. Cardiovascular abnormalities accompanying acute spinal cord injury in humans: incidence, time course and severity. J Am Coll Cardiol 1987;10:46.
76. Bilello JF, Davis JW, Cunningham MA, et al. Cervical spinal cord injury and the need for cardiovascular intervention. Arch Surg 2003;138(10):1127–9.
77. Simons FER, Clark S, Camargo CA. Anaphylaxis in the community: learning from the survivors. J Allergy Clin Immunol 2009;124:301–6.
78. Pumphrey RS. Lessons for management of anaphylaxis from a study of fatal reactions. Clin Exp Allergy 2000;30:1144–50.
79. Simons FE, Ardusso LRF, Bilò B, et al. World Allergy Organization guidelines for the assessment and management of anaphylaxis. World Allergy Organ J 2011; 4:13–37.
80. Kanwar M, Irvin CB, Frank JJ, et al. Confusion about epinephrine dosing leading to iatrogenic overdose: a life-threatening problem with a potential solution. Ann Emerg Med 2010;55:341–4.
81. Thomas M, Crawford I. Best evidence topic report. Glucagon infusion in refractory anaphylactic shock in patients on beta-blockers. Emerg Med J 2005;22: 272–3.
82. Lieberman P, Nicklas RA, Oppenheimer J, et al. The diagnosis and management of anaphylaxis practice parameter: 2010 update. J Allergy Clin Immunol 2010;126:477–80.

Emergency Department Antimicrobial Considerations in Severe Sepsis

Robert S. Green, MD, FRCPC, FRCP(Edin)[a,b,*],
Sean K. Gorman, BSc(Pharm), PharmD[c]

KEYWORDS

- Severe sepsis • Emergency medicine • Timing of antimicrobials
- Antimicrobial pharmacodynamics and pharmacokinetics • Procalcitonin
- Antimicrobial shortages

KEY POINTS

- The administration of antimicrobials in the emergency department (ED) is of paramount importance for optimal patient outcomes.
- Various factors need to be considered when choosing antimicrobials in the ED, including patient factors, infective microbe factors, and drug-related factors.
- Prompt administration of antimicrobials is a key management strategy.
- Clinicians should use a basic understanding of pharmacokinetic and pharmacodynamic properties when empirically selecting antimicrobials in septic ED patients.
- Antimicrobial shortages are a recurrent threat to the optimal treatment of septic patients, and clinicians should understand how a systems approach can ensure adequate antimicrobial options during these periods.

INTRODUCTION

There were more than 3.5 million emergency department (ED) visits in the United States in 2010 associated with a primary diagnosis of infectious and parasitic diseases.[1]

Disclosures: The authors have no actual or perceived conflicts of interest to disclose.
[a] Division of Critical Care Medicine, Department of Anesthesia, Faculty of Medicine, Trauma Nova Scotia, Dalhousie University, 1276 South Park Street, Halifax, Nova Scotia B3H 2Y9, Canada; [b] Department of Emergency Medicine, Faculty of Medicine, Trauma Nova Scotia, Dalhousie University, Room 377 Bethune Building, 1276 South Park Street, Halifax, Nova Scotia B3H 2Y9, Canada; [c] Clinical Quality & Research, Critical Care, Pharmacy Services, Interior Health Authority, Faculty of Pharmaceutical Sciences, The University of British Columbia, #200-1835 Gordon Drive, Kelowna, British Columbia V1Y3H5, Canada
* Corresponding author. Department of Emergency Medicine, Faculty of Medicine, Trauma Nova Scotia, Dalhousie University, Room 377 Bethune Building, 1276 South Park Street, Halifax, Nova Scotia B3H 2Y9, Canada.
E-mail address: Dr.robert.green@dal.ca

Emerg Med Clin N Am 32 (2014) 835–849
http://dx.doi.org/10.1016/j.emc.2014.07.014 **emed.theclinics.com**
0733-8627/14/$ – see front matter

Sepsis, which is defined as the systemic inflammatory response syndrome (SIRS) accompanied by the probable or documented presence of infection, is an advanced manifestation of infectious diseases and can lead to severe sepsis, septic shock, and multiple organ dysfunction syndrome.[2] Between 1992 and 2001, approximately 2.8 million visits to EDs in the United States were related to sepsis, and more than 10% of these patients required admission to an intensive care unit (ICU).[3] The most prevalent sources of infection leading to sepsis were the lower respiratory tract and the genitourinary tract.[3] Despite recent advances in the understanding and treatment of severe sepsis and septic shock, this syndrome remains a leading cause of death.[4]

Clinical practice guidelines have been developed to aid clinicians in the identification and treatment of patients with severe sepsis and septic shock. Recommended treatment strategies include early goal-directed therapy, obtaining appropriate microbiological specimens before antimicrobial administration (if feasible), identifying and controlling the source of infection in a timely fashion, and administering timely, appropriate empiric intravenous antimicrobial therapy.[2]

Appropriate initial antimicrobial therapy has been defined in numerous ways, and a recent systematic review identified that most studies incorporated in vitro antimicrobial susceptibility test results in the definition of appropriateness; however, timeliness and dosage were rarely included in the definition.[5] Therefore, it is suggested that antimicrobial appropriateness be defined based on the spectrum of activity, route of administration, dosage, and timing.[6–9]

The published literature concerning appropriate antimicrobial utilization in severe infections is rapidly expanding. Accordingly, the aim of this article was to provide a comprehensive, up-to-date review of the key antimicrobial-related considerations in the critically ill patient presenting to the ED.

General Approach to Antimicrobial Selection in ED Patients with Sepsis

Emergency medicine (EM) physicians have a critical role in the management of patients with severe sepsis and septic shock. In many cases, the EM physician is the initial point of contact for a patient's medical care. The identification and timely intervention of septic patients in the ED may be the most important phase of care, because delays in therapy are associated with increased morbidity and mortality.[10]

Although guidelines have been published to assist clinicians in the identification and management of patients with severe sepsis/septic shock, optimal antimicrobial administration principles have received relatively little attention.[2,11] Elements that should be considered when administrating antimicrobials include the following: (1) patient-related factors, (2) microorganism-related factors, (3) the importance of the timing of antimicrobial administration, and (4) source control.[12]

EM physicians should primarily consider their patient's age, weight, allergy status, and comorbidities when choosing antimicrobial medication.[13] Renal and hepatic dysfunction may impact the pharmacokinetic properties of antimicrobials, with some medications eliminated primarily by one system or the other.[14] Patients who are pregnant or lactating require special consideration to minimize any potential negative impact on the fetus or newborn. In addition, any recent exposure to antimicrobials is very important to consider, as previous exposure to an antimicrobial may increase the incidence of resistance, therefore leading to treatment failure and increased morbidity and mortality.[15]

Important microorganism factors include the site of infection, intrinsic microbial susceptibility to anti-infectives, and local resistance patterns.[13] Often the site of infection is suspected in EM patients with severe sepsis/septic shock, which provides the clinician valuable information for antimicrobial selection. For instance, infections of the lower respiratory tract are often caused by predictable organisms and therefore clinicians should administer antimicrobials that cover these bacteria. Similarly, microbes that are unlikely to cause an infection in the presumed site of infection need not be covered, therefore limiting broad-spectrum antimicrobial use. Although the susceptibility of a microbe in ED patients is usually unknown, knowledge of local antimicrobial resistance patterns is extremely important to protect against inadequate antimicrobial coverage. Resistance patterns vary from hospital to hospital and, in some cases, ward to ward, and every effort should be made to ensure that accurate patterns of resistance are available and reviewed regularly because antimicrobial administration with insufficient activity against a microbe can result in treatment failure and progression of the sepsis syndrome.[13] Bacteria of particular concern in the ED include drug-resistant *Streptococcus pneumoniae*, methicillin-resistant *Staphylococcus aureus* (MRSA), and multi-drug-resistant gram-negative infections caused by extended spectrum β-lactamases (ESBL). Valid screening tools to help identify patients at risk for antibiotic-resistant organisms (ARO) do not exist. However, there are several ARO risk factors that should be considered, in addition to local susceptibility patterns, when choosing empiric antibiotic therapy.

Risk factors for infection with β-lactam-resistant *S pneumoniae* in adults include age greater than 65 years, previous β-lactam therapy within 90 days, alcoholism, medical comorbidities, immunosuppression, and exposure to a child in a daycare center.[16] The risk of *S pneumoniae* resistance to β-lactams, macrolides, or fluoroquinolones appears highest if the patient has been exposed to the respective antibiotic within 90 days.[16] Therefore, administration of a different class of antibiotics with activity against the most likely organisms is a recommended strategy in this situation.[16]

Risk factors for MRSA in patients presenting to the ED include past colonization or infection with MRSA, history of previous antibiotic use in the past 90 days, hospitalization in the past 3 months, a history of hospitalization for an acute illness, residence in a long-term care facility, chronic dialysis, home wound care or infusion therapy, immunosuppression, and contact with family members with MRSA.[17,18] Patients with these risk factors who present to the ED with severe sepsis should be provided a regimen that includes vancomycin or linezolid.

The rate of ESBL production among the most common Enterobacteriaceae (*Klebsiella pneumoniae* and *Escherichia coli*) approaches 8% in North America.[19] Urinary tract infections (UTI) due to *E coli* represent the most frequent community-acquired infection because of ESBL and important risk factors include advanced age, diabetes mellitus, recurrent UTI, and previous receipt of aminopenicillins (eg, amoxicillin, ampicillin), cephalosporins, or fluoroquinolones.[19] Patients suspected to be infected with ESBL-producing bacteria should be treated with a carbapenem or a fluoroquinolone; however, co-resistance to fluoroquinolones is frequent in these organisms.[19]

The timing of appropriate antimicrobial medication administration is of paramount importance for patient outcomes in severe sepsis/septic shock.[8,20,21] Kumar and colleagues[8] demonstrated an increase in mortality of 7.6% for every hour delay in administration of appropriate antimicrobials after onset of hypotension in septic shock patients. Therefore, after the recognition and diagnosis of a septic patient in the ED, every effort should be made to administer appropriate empiric antimicrobials as soon as possible. Guidelines have called for antimicrobial administration within 30 to 60 minutes.[2,11]

An often-overlooked aspect in the management of septic patients is the importance of source control of infected tissue.[22,23] Tissue infected with a significant burden of microbes, such as a soft tissue abscess, obstructive pyelonephritis, or pleural empyema, is best managed with both antimicrobial administration and surgical drainage.

Similar to antimicrobial administration, source control should be performed as soon as possible. In some instances, this will require consultation and transfer to a surgical theater and therefore emergency physicians should ensure that the appropriate specialties are rapidly notified. Perhaps the best example of the importance of these principles comes from the management of patients with necrotizing fasciitis. In these patients, immediate surgical debridement of infected tissue in addition to appropriate antimicrobial is necessary for patient survival. Any delay in source control is associated with poor patient outcomes. Although necrotizing fasciitis is an extreme example, surgical drainage of any potential source should be a time-sensitive management objective in the ED.

In addition to inappropriate antimicrobial selection and delayed administration, low initial dosing may also lead to suboptimal outcomes. Consequences of suboptimal dosing in sepsis include treatment failure, higher mortality rates, increased costs and adverse effects, and emergence of antimicrobial-resistant organisms.[24–26] Suboptimal low initial dosing is primarily driven by pharmacokinetic changes associated with severe sepsis and septic shock and the fear of toxicity in the setting of organ dysfunction.[27,28] Both of these factors can be mitigated by considering the key pharmacologic characteristics of antimicrobial agents when determining dosing.[27] Patients with severe sepsis and septic shock are often transferred to the ICU within 6 hours; therefore, ED clinicians should aim to provide delivery of an appropriate initial antimicrobial dose to maximize the chances for a positive outcome.[29,30]

Important Pharmacokinetic and Pharmacodynamic Principles for the EM Physician

Antimicrobial selection should also be guided by its pharmacokinetic and pharmacodynamic profile.[31] Pharmacokinetics is the study of the time course of the primary pharmacokinetic processes of absorption, distribution, metabolism, and elimination and the overall disposition of the drug. In basic terms, it describes the relationship between the dose administered and the changes in drug concentration with time.[28,32]

When selecting an antimicrobial and its respective initial dose in severe sepsis and septic shock, the primary pharmacokinetic consideration is the degree of distribution of the antimicrobial to the site of infection. Absorption, metabolism, and elimination are important factors to consider when considering subsequent maintenance dosing regimens.

The pharmacokinetic parameter that reflects the relationship between initial dose and initial intravascular concentration is the apparent volume of distribution (V_d). In general, the initial antimicrobial concentration (mg/L) achieved in the vascular compartment is equal to the dose (mg) administered divided by the V_d (L).

Fluid shifts lead to an increase in V_d for many hydrophilic antimicrobials, such as aminoglycosides, β-lactams, vancomycin, and linezolid in severe sepsis and shock, whereas lipophilic agents, such as ciprofloxacin, are largely unaffected.[28] For antimicrobials that are highly bound to serum albumin, hypoalbuminemia results in higher than usual unbound fractions and therefore a higher tissue distribution and V_d. Increased tissue distribution of antimicrobials should be advantageous because the unbound antimicrobial is free to distribute to the interstitial space that is most often the site of infection; however, this is usually offset by the antimicrobial dilutional effect caused by third spacing during early goal-directed therapy.[28] Because of the higher V_d for many antimicrobials administered in severe sepsis and septic shock, a higher initial dose is often required to achieve the same desired intravascular concentrations as in nonseptic patients with a normal V_d.[28]

Pharmacodynamics is the study of the relationship between serum drug concentration and the clinical (and microbiological) response observed.[32] **Table 1** provides

Table 1
Antimicrobial pharmacodynamic properties

Pharmacodynamic Parameter	Definition	Relevance to EM
Bacteriostatic	Antibacterial inhibits bacterial growth (but does not "kill" at usual concentrations)	Avoid if possible for treatment of endocarditis, meningitis, and infections in the neutropenic host
Bactericidal	Antibacterial kills bacteria at similar concentrations needed to inhibit growth	Proven or hypothesized to produce improved cure rates in patients with endocarditis, meningitis, and neutropenia
Concentration-dependent killing	Demonstrates a greater rate and extent of activity when the microorganism is exposed to higher concentrations of drug	Dosing regimens that result in higher concentration at some point during the dosing interval are desired. In general, give higher doses less often
Time-dependent killing	Demonstrates a greater rate and extent of activity by maintaining drug concentrations above a threshold for a greater proportion of time	Dosing regimens that result in maintaining drug concentrations at a threshold higher than the MIC (usually 4–5 times higher than MIC) are desired. In general, give lower doses more often

antimicrobial pharmacodynamic properties of relevance when considering initial antimicrobial dosing in patients with sepsis.

Antimicrobials that require significantly higher concentrations to kill a microorganism than are required to inhibit microorganism growth are considered bacteriostatic agents. Antimicrobials that kill at concentrations similar to those required to inhibit in vitro growth are considered bactericidal. This method of classifying antimicrobials is based on lethality and is useful to guide antimicrobial selection and dosing in patient subpopulations with sepsis, such as those with neutropenia. These patients should receive bactericidal agents because of a relatively poor host immune response.[33]

Antimicrobials can also be classified based on the rate and extent of bacterial killing. Antimicrobials can be considered concentration-dependent bacterial killers or time-dependent bacterial killers. Aminoglycosides are considered concentration-dependent bactericidal agents because they demonstrate a greater rate and extent of bacterial killing when the microorganism is exposed to higher concentrations of drug. A clinically relevant example of exploitation of this effect is the administration of single daily dosing of aminoglycosides. Rather than administering smaller doses more frequently, one large dose is given once daily to achieve high postdose concentrations. The aminoglycosides also possess another pharmacodynamic characteristic that allows for single daily dosing and that is the postantibiotic effect (PAE). The PAE is defined as the time required for an organism to demonstrate viable regrowth after the removal of an antimicrobial.[34,35]

Penicillins, cephalosporins, and carbapenems are examples of time-dependent bactericidal antimicrobials because the rate and extent of bacterial killing activity becomes saturated at a particular drug concentration. For example, desired activity for time-dependent bactericidal antimicrobials is usually achieved by maintaining drug concentrations at various thresholds above the minimum inhibitory concentration (MIC), most commonly 4 to 5 times higher than the MIC.[32]

Using traditional intermittent infusion dosing strategies, patients with severe sepsis and septic shock may experience insufficient β-lactam concentrations.[36] A potential strategy to optimize the efficacy of time-dependent bactericidal antimicrobials is to extend the duration of intermittent infusion or administer via continuous infusion. These strategies have been investigated for the carbapenems and piperacillin/tazobactam and have been shown to improve pharmacokinetic/pharmacodynamic endpoints such as the frequency of plasma antimicrobial concentrations above the MIC in patients with severe sepsis.[37] However, it is not clear whether these strategies improve clinical outcomes compared with standard intermittent infusion administration and it has not been adequately evaluated in the ED setting.[38] Larger randomized controlled studies are required to determine whether this strategy improves clinical cure and survival in severe sepsis.

It is also important to note that certain antimicrobials, such as fluoroquinolones and vancomycin, demonstrate both concentration-dependent and time-dependent activity.[28] **Table 2** outlines the integrated antimicrobial pharmacokinetic/pharmacodynamic targets with dose recommendations from the manufacturer as compared with the best available evidence.[39–48]

A good example of the importance of these principles applies to the initial dosing of antibiotics in severe sepsis and septic shock. These patients will often have multiple organ dysfunction, including acute kidney injury. Tertiary references provide drug-dosing recommendations for varying degrees of renal function; if these recommendations are implemented for certain antibiotics in these situations, the patient

Table 2
Pharmacokinetics/pharmacodynamic parameters and initial dosing recommendations for bactericidal antibiotics in severe sepsis and septic shock[a]

Antibiotic	PK:PD Parameter	Recommended Initial Dose[b]	Literature-Based Initial Dose
Aminoglycosides			
Amikacin	C_{max}: MIC	15 mg/kg	25 mg/kg[39,40]
Gentamicin/Tobramycin	C_{max}: MIC	4.5–7 mg/kg[c]	7 mg/kg[41]
β-Lactams			
Ceftriaxone	T > MIC	1–2 g	1–2 g[42]
Meropenem		1–2 g	1–2 g[43]
Piperacillin	T > MIC	3–4 g	4 g[44]
Fluoroquinolones			
Ciprofloxacin	AUC_{0-24}/MIC	400 mg	400 mg[45]
Levofloxacin	AUC_{0-24}/MIC	500–750 mg	500–750 mg[46]
Glycopeptides			
Vancomycin	AUC_{0-24}/MIC	15 mg/kg	25–30 mg/kg[47]
Macrolides			
Azithromycin	AUC_{0-24}/MIC	500 mg	500 mg[48]

Abbreviations: AUC 0-24, area under the concentration-time curve from 0 to 24 hours; Cmax, peak serum concentration; PD, pharmacodynamic; PK, pharmacokinetic; T, time.

[a] Intermittent infusion administration.

[b] Derived from tertiary drug information references/manufacturer.

[c] Once daily dosing.

may receive subtherapeutic doses. For example, a patient with septic shock caused by *Pseudomonas aeruginosa* pneumonia has an estimated creatinine clearance (CrCL) of 25 mL/min. After incorporating the aforementioned considerations for selection of antimicrobial therapy, it is decided to initiate piperacillin/tazobactam plus ciprofloxacin as initial therapy because of the relatively high incidence of multidrug-resistant *P aeruginosa* in the location. This antibiotic choice provides double-bactericidal coverage in a time-dependent (piperacillin/tazobactam) and concentration-dependent (ciprofloxacin) fashion. Many tertiary drug information references will recommend reducing the dose of piperacillin/tazobactam when CrCL decreases to less than 40 mL/min to 2.25 to 3.375 G per dose. Piperacillin/tazobactam is a hydrophilic antibiotic whose V_d significantly increases in severe sepsis and septic shock; therefore, concentrations achieved with the aforementioned dose may be significantly lower than required to ensure cure. To mitigate this, an initial loading dose of 4.5 G of piperacillin/tazobactam is recommended in this situation. The initial 400 mg intravenous loading dose of ciprofloxacin does not change because fluid shifts observed early in severe sepsis and shock do not significantly alter the V_d of this lipophilic antibiotic. The maintenance dosing regimen should be selected after considering the potential safety implications of antibiotic accumulation in end-organ dysfunction, such as renal failure.

SEPSIS BIOMARKERS IN THE ED

A biological laboratory marker, otherwise known as biomarker, "refers to a broad subcategory of medical signs which can be measured accurately and reproducibly".[49] More than 150 biomarkers have been evaluated in the context of sepsis, and they reflect several pathophysiological mechanisms.[50]

Biomarkers can potentially indicate the presence, absence, or severity of sepsis, differentiate bacterial from viral and fungal infection, assist with prognostication, guide initial antimicrobial therapy decisions, and help evaluate the response to therapy to guide antimicrobial de-escalation decision-making.[50] The various types of biomarkers include cytokines, receptors, coagulation system markers, acute phase proteins, cell surface markers, apoptosis markers, and markers of endothelial function.[51] Although there are numerous biomarkers of sepsis, procalcitonin (PCT) has recently been the focus of much investigation in patients with sepsis.

PCT is a prohormone of calcitonin and is synthesized in the C cells of the thyroid.[52] Bacterial toxins and bacterial-specific proinflammatory cytokines trigger an increased PCT release from parenchymal organs.[52,53] One of the most attractive properties of PCT supporting its investigation as a clinically useful biomarker in sepsis is its attenuated release in response to viral infection-triggered cytokine release, therefore potentially allowing a degree of discrimination between bacterial and viral infections.[53]

Within 2 to 12 hours of bacterial infection onset, serum PCT demonstrates a measurable increase.[53] Serum PCT concentrations rapidly drop by approximately 50% each day when the infection is well under control by a combination of host response and antimicrobial therapy.[52,53] It is also noteworthy that the serum dynamic profile of PCT is not affected by neutropenia or the administration of systemic corticosteroids.[53] There are several PCT assays available; however, the most commonly investigated assays in sepsis are quantitative.

The most relevant application of PCT in the context of sepsis in the ED is as a diagnostic marker. The specific aim of using PCT is to help guide timely diagnosis and treatment of sepsis. Three meta-analyses have been published since 2006 that have evaluated the diagnostic accuracy of PCT in sepsis.[54–56] The results of the first

2 meta-analyses were conflicting in terms of the diagnostic accuracy of PCT in critically ill patients.[54,55] However, because of methodological limitations of these analyses, an additional meta-analysis was performed with the aim to determine the ability of PCT to differentiate between sepsis and SIRS of noninfectious origin in a heterogeneous mix of critically ill patients.[56]

This meta-analysis included 30 studies accounting for 3244 patients. Four studies included only critically ill pediatric patients representing 177 patients, and 4 studies were conducted in the ED. Most studies used quantitative manual PCT assays; however, the sepsis diagnostic cutoff for PCT concentration differed substantially between studies with a median cutoff of 1.1 ng/mL and interquartile range of 0.5 ng/mL to 2 ng/mL. The mean sensitivity and specificity of PCT as a diagnostic marker were 0.77 (95% CI 0.72–0.81) and 0.79 (95% CI 0.74–0.84), respectively, and the area under the receiver operating characteristic curve was 0.85 (95% CI 0.81–0.88).

The results of this meta-analysis were limited by the presence of significant statistical heterogeneity between the included studies and the presence of publication bias. Therefore, PCT should not be used as the single definitive test for sepsis diagnosis, but can be a helpful marker when used in the context of information provided from medical history, physical examination, and microbiological assessment.[56] When used as a tool in assisting with diagnosis, a PCT diagnostic cutoff of 1 to 2 ng/mL could be useful to discriminate sepsis from other inflammatory conditions.[56] Further investigation in this population of patients presenting to the ED is warranted.

Clinical Practice Guidelines Review

The surviving sepsis guidelines

Clinical practice guidelines are "systematically developed statements to assist practitioners and patients in making decisions about appropriate health care for specific clinical circumstances."[57] Adherence to high-quality clinical practice guidelines in clinical practice can reduce variations in care and ultimately improve the quality of care.[58]

Since the launch of the Surviving Sepsis Campaign in 2002, there have been 3 published versions of international guidelines focusing on the management of severe sepsis and septic shock.[2,59,60] The initial version of these guidelines was of variable quality; however, the most recent versions are of high quality and their recommendations should be incorporated into clinical decision-making.[61]

The most recently published severe sepsis and septic shock guidelines make 18 recommendations related to infection diagnosis, antimicrobial therapy, source control, and infection prevention. However, not all of these recommendations are applicable to the initial management of a patient with severe sepsis or shock in the ED.

Diagnostic recommendations in the latest iteration of these guidelines are very similar to the 2008 version. The recommendation is to obtain clinically appropriate cultures that include at least 2 sets of blood cultures before antimicrobial initiation provided that there will be no significant delay in the start of antimicrobials.[2] Two sets of blood cultures remains a strong recommendation based on low-quality evidence. However, the latest guidelines now define a significant antimicrobial delay as greater than 45 minutes, whereas the older version of the guidelines did not define delay.[2,60] The recommendation to promptly perform imaging studies to confirm a potential source of infection remains; however, it has changed from a strong recommendation to an ungraded recommendation because the guideline development committee did not think that topic was conducive to the GRADE (Grading of Recommendations Assessment, Development and Evaluation) process.

Antimicrobial-related recommendations that are most applicable to the ED patient with severe sepsis and shock remain largely unchanged. Strong recommendations remain for administration of effective intravenous antimicrobials within 1 hour of onset of severe sepsis and shock and for administration of an initial intravenous antimicrobial regimen that consists of at least one drug with activity against likely pathogens and that adequately penetrate into infected tissues. There also remains the strong recommendation that antimicrobial regimens should be reassessed daily for potential de-escalation to prevent resistance development, reduce toxicity, and reduce costs, although this is likely outside the ED phase of care.

A new weak recommendation has been made for using PCT or other biomarkers to assist clinicians in discontinuation of antimicrobials in patients who initially appeared septic but no subsequent evidence of infection was found. However, there is no recommendation addressing whether biomarkers should assist with the decision whether to initiate empiric therapy or guide initial antimicrobial choice.

Consistent with the previous version of the guidelines, combination empiric antimicrobial therapy is weakly recommended in neutropenic patients with severe sepsis and patients with difficult-to-treat multidrug-resistant pathogens such as *Acinetobacter* and *Pseudomonas* species. A new weak recommendation is made to combine a β-lactam and macrolide for patients with septic shock due to bacteremic *S pneumoniae* infections. If empiric combination therapy is initiated, the latest guidelines continue to weakly recommend that combination empiric therapy should not exceed 3 to 5 days and should be de-escalated to monotherapy once the microbial susceptibility profile is known.

Another new weak recommendation is to initiate antiviral therapy if severe sepsis or shock is of viral origin. This recommendation is focused on early antiviral therapy with a neuraminidase inhibitor (oseltamivir or zanamivir) for patients with suspected or confirmed influenza.

The recommendations related to source control are not dramatically different in the new guidelines; however, it is now strongly recommended that a target time window of no more than 12 hours elapse before achieving source control, if applicable, after diagnosis.

For those patients who are intubated and ventilated for a prolonged period in the ED, there are 2 new weak recommendations suggesting the use of selective oral and digestive tract decontamination to reduce the risk for ventilator-associated pneumonia in settings where this strategy has been found to be effective. Specifically, it is suggested that oral chlorhexidine gluconate topical antiseptic be used with oral care in the intubated patient as a form of oropharyngeal decontamination. Clinical equipoise exists around the effectiveness of selective decontamination of the digestive tract in these critically ill patients; future research that involves longer follow-up to assess antimicrobial resistance is required.[62] A broader review of the latest sepsis guidelines for ED clinicians has been published elsewhere.[63]

Other sepsis-related guidelines

Lower respiratory and genitourinary infections are the most common reasons patients present to the ED with severe sepsis in the United States.[29] However, a recent search for North American adult community-acquired pneumonia clinical practice guidelines revealed that the latest version was published in 2007, although an update is currently in progress.[16]

The latest clinical practice guidelines for the treatment of acute uncomplicated cystitis and pyelonephritis in women were last updated in 2010 and are considered current by the Infectious Disease Society of America (IDSA). However, because uncomplicated cystitis rarely progresses to sepsis in otherwise healthy, nonpregnant women, the authors have reviewed only the section addressing the management of pyelonephritis.[64] It is recommended that a urine culture and susceptibility test be performed followed by timely administration of empiric antimicrobial therapy. Initial antimicrobials for women with pyelonephritis requiring hospitalization should provide coverage for the most common uropathogens, which primarily consist of *E coli*. Other species may occasionally cause uncomplicated pyelonephritis, and these include other species of Enterobacteriaceae and *Staphylococcus saprophyticus*.

Recommended initial therapy should be dictated by local resistance data. For example, expert opinion drives the recommendation that a local fluoroquinolone resistance prevalence threshold of 10% should prompt using alternative empiric antimicrobial agents.[64] Depending on local resistance patterns, initial options include intravenous ciprofloxacin, an aminoglycoside with or without intravenous ampicillin, an extended-spectrum penicillin such as piperacillin/tazobactam with or without an aminoglycoside, or a carbapenem, which subsequently should be tailored based on the culture and susceptibility results.

ANTIMICROBIAL SELECTION IN THE ERA OF ANTIMICROBIAL SHORTAGES

A drug shortage is defined as "a supply issue that affects how the pharmacy prepares or dispenses a drug product or influences patient care when prescribers must use an alternative agent."[65] Several factors affecting the supply chain contribute to drug shortages and can be attributed to reduced supply or increased demand.

Common reasons for drug shortages include disruptions in the supply of raw or bulk materials, manufacturing disruptions due to regulatory issues such as noncompliance with current good manufacturing practices and voluntary recalls related to manufacturing problems, changes in a product's formulation or manufacturer, and manufacturer business decisions to reduce production. In addition, manufacturer mergers that result in decisions to narrow the product-line focus or move production to another facility, restricted distribution methods that are the result of market approval requirements or postmarketing surveillance, "just-in-time" inventory management practices, unexpected increases in demand and shifts in clinical practice, and natural disasters have also been cited as potential reasons for drug shortages.[65]

Patient-specific consequences of antimicrobial shortages include delays in treatment, use of antimicrobials that are not considered first-line therapy, and increased potential for worsened patient outcomes.[66,67] These shortages also impact health systems by increasing time-expenditures and labor costs associated with managing the shortages.[68]

As of November 2013, antimicrobials represented approximately 12% of the 235 currently unavailable drugs in the United States.[69] These shortages are further exacerbated by the reality that there are significantly fewer new antimicrobials coming down the pipeline and increasing antimicrobial resistance.[66]

American guidelines for the management of drug shortages have been published, but these guidelines are broad in scope and do not discuss managing the specific challenges associated with antimicrobial shortages.[65] To lessen the impact of antimicrobial shortages on patient care, a prospective management strategy has been proposed.[70] This approach recommends institutional prospective tracking of shortages and maximizing inventory through antimicrobial usage management, preferably by an interprofessional team that specializes in antimicrobial stewardship. The institutional antimicrobial stewardship team can play a large role in spearheading these efforts to achieve the best possible outcomes in the era of antimicrobial drug shortages.[71]

Identification of potential foreign suppliers of first-line antimicrobials is a recommended early step. Other tactics necessary for successful management include the selection of appropriate alternative agents before the inventory of a first-line antimicrobial has been completely depleted. This inventory can be accomplished using a multidisciplinary approach to assessing clinical practice guidelines, such as those from the IDSA, and by incorporating local antimicrobial resistance patterns into the decision to use alternative agents.

Ongoing shortages should be regularly communicated to clinical leadership and creation of temporary guidelines for alternatives should be created that are supported by ongoing educational support for clinicians. Other strategies for managing ongoing shortages include rationing the inventory of first-line agents, which should be supported by ethical considerations.[70]

The ultimate role of the EM physician caring for critically ill patients with infections is to understand the current state in terms of which antimicrobials are currently on shortage and which antimicrobials have zero inventories. EM physicians should work with the stakeholders, such as the pharmacy department inventory managers, the antimicrobial stewardship team if available, infectious disease specialist physicians and pharmacists, EM clinical pharmacists, and other colleagues in emergency and critical care medicine to proactively manage this challenge.

SUMMARY

The recognition and rapid institution of appropriate management strategies in septic ED patients are paramount in optimizing good outcomes. Although available guidelines address most strategies, evidence-based antimicrobial administration methods for EM physicians are required. These factors include patient illness, microorganism, timing of antimicrobial administration, and source control. EM physicians should also use a basic understanding of pharmacokinetic and pharmacodynamic principles when choosing appropriate antimicrobials and their method of delivery. Finally, because of the recent problem of antimicrobial deficiencies that limit the availability of medications, EM physicians should also proactively address issues relating to the administration of antimicrobials during shortages.

REFERENCES

1. Centers for Disease Control and Prevention. National Hospital Ambulatory Medical Care Survey: 2010 Emergency Department summary tables. Available at: http://www.cdc.gov/nchs/data/ahcd/nhamcs_emergency/2010_ed_web_tables.pdf. Accessed October 15, 2013.
2. Dellinger RP, Levy MM, Rhodes A, et al. Surviving sepsis campaign: international guidelines for management of severe sepsis and septic shock: 2012. Crit Care Med 2013;41:580–637.
3. Strehlow MC, Emond SD, Shapiro NI, et al. National study of emergency department visits for sepsis, 1992 to 2001. Ann Emerg Med 2006;48:326–31.
4. Levy MM, Dellinger RP, Townsend SR, et al. The surviving sepsis campaign: results of an international guideline-based performance improvement program targeting severe sepsis. Crit Care Med 2010;38:367–74.
5. McGregor JC, Rich SE, Harris AD, et al. A systematic review of the methods used to assess the association between appropriate antibiotic therapy and mortality in bacteremic patients. Clin Infect Dis 2007;45:329–37.
6. Kollef MH, Sherman G, Ward S, et al. Inadequate antimicrobial treatment of infections: a risk factor for hospital mortality among critically ill patients. Chest 1999;115:462–74.

7. Taccone FS, Hites M, Beumier M, et al. Appropriate antibiotic dosage levels in the treatment of severe sepsis and septic shock. Curr Infect Dis Rep 2011;13: 406–15.
8. Kumar A, Roberts D, Wood KE, et al. Duration of hypotension before initiation of effective antimicrobial therapy is the critical determinant of survival in human septic shock. Crit Care Med 2006;34:1589–96.
9. Kumar A, Ellis P, Arabi Y, et al. Initiation of inappropriate antimicrobial therapy results in a fivefold reduction of survival in human septic shock. Chest 2009; 136:1237–48.
10. Capp R, Chang Y, Brown DF. Effective antibiotic treatment prescribed by emergency physicians in patients admitted to the intensive care unit with severe sepsis or septic shock: where is the gap? J Emerg Med 2011;41:573–80.
11. Green RS, Djogovic D, Gray S, et al. Canadian Association of Emergency Physicians sepsis guidelines: the optimal management of severe sepsis in Canadian emergency departments. CJEM 2008;10:443–59.
12. Green RS, Gorman SK. Optimizing initial antibiotic delivery for adult patients with severe sepsis and septic shock in the emergency department. EM Critical Care 2012;(Suppl):1–16.
13. Leekha S, Terrell CL, Edson RS. General principles of antimicrobial therapy. Mayo Clin Proc 2011;86:156–67.
14. Brun-Buisson C, Doyon F, Carlet J, et al. Incidence, risk factors, and outcome of severe sepsis and septic shock in adults. A multicenter prospective study in intensive care units. JAMA 1995;274:968–74.
15. Johnson MT, Reichley R, Hoppe-Bauer J, et al. Impact of previous antibiotic therapy on outcome of Gram-negative severe sepsis. Crit Care Med 2011;39: 1859–65.
16. Mandell LA, Wunderink RG, Anzueto A, et al. Infectious Diseases Society of America/American Thoracic Society consensus guidelines on the management of community-acquired pneumonia in adults. Clin Infect Dis 2007;44: S27–72.
17. Wakatake H, Fujitani S, Kodama T, et al. Positive clinical risk factors predict a high rate of methicillin-resistant Staphylococcus aureus colonization in emergency department patients. Am J Infect Control 2012;40:988–91.
18. Niederman MS, Craven DE, Bonten MJ, et al. Guidelines for the management of adults with hospital-acquired, ventilator-associated, and healthcare-associated pneumonia. Am J Respir Crit Care Med 2005;171:388–416.
19. Falagas ME, Karageorgopoulos DE. Extended-spectrum β-lactamase-producing organisms. J Hosp Infect 2009;73:345–54.
20. Cullen M, Fogg T, Delaney A. Timing of appropriate antibiotics in patients with septic shock: a retrospective cohort study. Emerg Med Australas 2013;25: 308–15.
21. Puskarich MA, Trzeciak S, Shapiro NI, et al. Association between timing of antibiotic administration and mortality from septic shock in patients treated with a quantitative resuscitation protocol. Crit Care Med 2011;39:2066–71.
22. Marshall JC, Maier RV, Jimenez M, et al. Source control in the management of severe sepsis and septic shock: an evidence-based review. Crit Care Med 2004;32(Suppl 11):S513–26.
23. Tabah A, Koulenti D, Laupland K, et al. Characteristics and determinants of outcome of hospital-acquired bloodstream infections in intensive care units: the EUROBACT international cohort study. Intensive Care Med 2012;38: 1930–45.

24. Scaglione F, Paraboni L. Pharmacokinetics/pharmacodynamics of antibacterials in the intensive care unit: setting appropriate dosing regimens. Int J Antimicrob Agents 2008;32:294–301.
25. Roberts JA, Kruger P, Paterson DL, et al. Antibiotic resistance – what's dosing got to do with it? Crit Care Med 2008;36:2433–40.
26. Sanchez Garcia M. Early antibiotic treatment failure. Int J Antimicrob Agents 2009;34(S3):S14–9.
27. Eyler RF, Mueller BA. Antibiotic dosing in critically ill patients with acute kidney injury. Nat Rev Nephrol 2011;7:226–35.
28. Varghese JM, Roberts JA, Lipman J. Pharmacokinetic and pharmacodynamic issues in the critically ill with severe sepsis and septic shock. Crit Care Clin 2011;27:19–34.
29. Wang HE, Shapiro NI, Angus D, et al. National estimates of severe sepsis in United Stated emergency departments. Crit Care Med 2007;35:1928–36.
30. Patel GW, Roderman N, Gehring H, et al. Assessing the effect of the Surviving Sepsis Campaign treatment guidelines on clinical outcomes in a community hospital. Ann Pharmacother 2010;44:1733–8.
31. Nicolau DP. Optimizing antimicrobial therapy and emerging pathogens. Am J Manag Care 1998;4(10 Suppl 2):S525–30.
32. Slavik RS, Jewesson PJ. Selecting antibacterials for outpatient parenteral antimicrobial therapy: pharmacokinetic-pharmacodynamic considerations. Clin Pharmacokinet 2003;42:793–817.
33. Pankey GA, Sabath LD. Clinical relevance of bacteriostatic versus bactericidal mechanisms of action in the treatment of Gram-positive bacterial infections. Clin Infect Dis 2004;38:864–70.
34. Levison ME. Pharmacodynamics of antimicrobial drugs. Infect Dis Clin North Am 2004;18:451–65.
35. Gonzalez US, Spencer JP. Aminoglycosides: a practical review. Am Fam Physician 1998;15:1811–20.
36. Taccone FS, Laterre PF, Dugernier T, et al. Insufficient β-lactam concentrations in the early phase of severe sepsis and septic shock. Crit Care 2010; 14:R126.
37. Dulhunty JM, Roberts JA, Davis JS, et al. Continuous infusion of beta-lactam antibiotics in severe sepsis: a multicenter double-blind, randomized controlled trial. Clin Infect Dis 2013;56:236–44.
38. Falagas ME, Tansarli GS, Ikawa K, et al. Clinical outcomes with extended or continuous versus short-term intravenous infusion of carbapenems and piperacillin/tazobactam: a systematic review and meta-analysis. Clin Infect Dis 2013; 56:272–82.
39. Taccone FS, Laterre PF, Spapen H, et al. Revisiting the loading dose of amikacin for patients with severe sepsis and septic shock. Crit Care 2010;14:R53.
40. Galvez R, Luengo C, Cornejo R, et al. Higher than recommended amikacin loading doses achieve pharmacokinetic targets without associated toxicity. Int J Antimicrob Agents 2011;38:146–51.
41. Kashuba AD, Bertino JS, Nafziger AN. Dosing of aminoglycosides to rapidly attain pharmacodynamic goals and hasten therapeutic response by using individualized pharmacokinetic monitoring of patients with pneumonia caused by Gram-negative organisms. Antimicrob Agents Chemother 1998;42:1842–4.
42. Garot D, Respaud R, Lanotte P, et al. Population pharmacokinetics of ceftriaxone in critically ill septic patients: a reappraisal. Br J Clin Pharmacol 2011;72: 758–67.

43. Roberts JA, Kirkpatrick CM, Roberts MS, et al. Meropenem dosing in critically ill patients with sepsis and without renal dysfunction: intermittent bolus versus continuous administration? Monte Carlo dosing simulations and subcutaneous tissue distribution. J Antimicrob Chemother 2009;64:142–50.
44. Roberts JA, Kirkpatrick CM, Roberts MS, et al. First-dose and steady-state population pharmacokinetics and pharmacodynamics of piperacillin by continuous or intermittent dosing in critically ill patients with sepsis. Int J Antimicrob Agents 2010;35:156–63.
45. Gous A, Lipman J, Scribante J, et al. Fluid shifts have no influence on ciprofloxacin pharmacokinetics in intensive care patients with intra-abdominal sepsis. Int J Antimicrob Agents 2005;26:50–5.
46. Tayab ZR, Hochhaus G, Kaufmann S, et al. Do intensive care patients need an individualized dosing regimen for levofloxacin? Int J Clin Pharmacol Ther 2006; 44:262–9.
47. Rybak M, Lomaestro B, Rotschafer JC, et al. Therapeutic monitoring of vancomycin in adult patients: a consensus review of the American Society of Health-System Pharmacists, the Infectious Diseases Society of America, and the Society of Infectious Diseases Pharmacists. Am J Health Syst Pharm 2009; 66:82–98.
48. Ulldemonlins M, Roberts JA, Lipman J, et al. Antibiotic dosing in multiple organ dysfunction syndrome. Chest 2011;139:1210–20.
49. Strimbu K, Tavel JA. What are biomarkers? Curr Opin HIV AIDS 2010;5:463–6.
50. Pierrakos C, Vincent JL. Sepsis biomarkers: a review. Crit Care 2010;14:R15.
51. Vincent JL, Beumier M. Diagnostic and prognostic markers in sepsis. Expert Rev Anti Infect Ther 2013;11:265–75.
52. Kruger S, Welte T. Biomarkers in community-acquired pneumonia. Expert Rev Respir Med 2012;6:203–14.
53. Haubitz S, Mueller B, Schuetz P. Streamlining antibiotic therapy with procalcitonin protocols: consensus and controversies. Expert Rev Respir Med 2013;7: 145–57.
54. Uzzan B, Cohen R, Nicolas P, et al. Procalcitonin as a diagnostic test for sepsis in critically ill adults and after surgery or trauma: a systematic review and meta-analysis. Crit Care Med 2006;34:1996–2003.
55. Tang BM, Eslick GD, Craig JC, et al. Accuracy of procalcitonin for sepsis diagnosis in critically ill patients: systematic review and meta-analysis. Lancet Infect Dis 2007;7:210–7.
56. Wacker C, Prkno A, Brunkhorst FM, et al. Procalcitonin as a diagnostic marker for sepsis: a systematic review and meta-analysis. Lancet Infect Dis 2013;13: 426–35.
57. Field MJ, Lohr KN, editors. Institute of Medicine Committee to Advise the Public Health Service on Clinical Practice Guidelines. Clinical practice guidelines: direction for a new program. Washington, DC: National Academy Press; 1990. p. 55–77.
58. Gundersen L. The effect of clinical practice guidelines on variations in care. Ann Intern Med 2000;133:317–8.
59. Dellinger RP, Carlet JM, Masur H, et al. Surviving Sepsis Campaign guidelines for the management of severe sepsis and septic shock. Crit Care Med 2004;32: 858–73.
60. Dellinger RP, Levy MM, Carlet JM, et al. Surviving Sepsis Campaign: international guidelines for management of severe sepsis and septic shock: 2008. Crit Care Med 2008;36:296–327.

61. Gorman SK, Chung MH, Slavik RS, et al. A critical appraisal of the quality of critical care clinical practice guidelines and their strength of recommendations. Intensive Care Med 2010;36:1636–43.
62. Cuthbertson BH, Campbell MK, MacLennan G, et al. Clinical stakeholders' opinions on the use of selective decontamination of the digestive tract in critically ill patients in intensive care units: an international Delphi study. Crit Care 2013;17:R266.
63. Jones AE, Puskarich MA. The surviving sepsis campaign guidelines 2012: update for emergency physicians. Ann Emerg Med 2014;63:35–47.
64. Gupta K, Hooton TM, Naber KG, et al. International clinical practice guidelines for the treatment of acute uncomplicated cystitis and pyelonephritis in women: a 2010 update by the Infectious Diseases Society of America and the European Society for Microbiology and Infectious Diseases. Clin Infect Dis 2011;52:e103–20.
65. Fox ER, Birt A, James KB, et al. ASHP guidelines on managing drug product shortages in hospitals and health systems. Am J Health Syst Pharm 2009;66:1399–406.
66. Griffith MM, Gross AE, Sutton SH, et al. The impact of anti-infective drug shortages on hospitals in the United States: trends and causes. Clin Infect Dis 2012;54:684–91.
67. Hall R, Bryson GL, Flowerdew G, et al. Drug shortages in Canadian anesthesia: a national survey. Can J Anaesth 2013;60:539–51.
68. Kaakeh R, Sweet BV, Reilly C, et al. Impact of drug shortages on U.S. health systems. Am J Health Syst Pharm 2011;68:e13–21.
69. American Society of Health-System Pharmacists (ASHP). Drug Shortages Resource Center. Available at: http://www.ashp.org/drugshortages/current. Accessed November 24, 2013.
70. Griffith MM, Patel JA, Sutton SH, et al. Prospective approach to managing antimicrobial drug shortages. Infect Control Hosp Epidemiol 2012;33:745–52.
71. Griffith MM, Pentoney Z, Scheetz MH. Antimicrobial drug shortages: a crisis amidst the epidemic and the need for antimicrobial stewardship efforts to lessen the effects. Pharmacotherapy 2012;32:665–7.

Mechanical Circulatory Support

John C. Greenwood, MD[a,*], Daniel L. Herr, MD[b]

KEYWORDS

- Mechanical circulatory support • Intra-aortic balloon pump
- Ventricular assist device • Extracorporeal membrane oxygenation (ECMO)
- Cardiogenic shock

KEY POINTS

- The routine use of an intra-aortic balloon pump is no longer recommended for patients with refractory cardiogenic shock.
- Common ventricular assist device (VAD) complications include thrombosis, bleeding, right-sided heart failure, infection, cerebral vascular accidents, arrhythmias, and device failure.
- Driveline infection is the most common infectious complication for the patient with a VAD.
- Ventricular arrhythmias are most common within the first 3 months after VAD placement and should be cardioverted in a timely fashion.
- Venoarterial ECMO is a treatment modality that can be considered in the patient with refractory cardiogenic shock or cardiac arrest from a reversible cause.

INTRODUCTION

Mechanical circulatory support, a term that most emergency physicians did not concern themselves with 10 years ago, is now an area of patient care that emergency physicians must understand. The role of mechanical support for both acute and chronic heart failure is rapidly growing. For example, as of April 2012 more than 10,000 HeartMate (Pleasanton, CA, USA) left ventricular assist devices (LVADs) had been implanted, yet only a handful of the patients who received these devices will go on to receive a heart transplant.[1] Most of these patients will never receive a transplant and will spend most of their time receiving outpatient care. The use of extracorporeal membrane oxygenation (ECMO) for refractory cardiogenic shock and cardiac

Funding Sources: Nothing to disclose.
Conflict of Interest: Nothing to disclose.
[a] Division of Pulmonary & Critical Care Medicine, University of Maryland School of Medicine, 110 South Paca Street, 2nd Floor, Baltimore, MD 21201, USA; [b] Critical Care Service, Cardiac Surgery ICU, Shock Trauma Center, University of Maryland School of Medicine, 22 South Greene Street, Baltimore, MD 21201, USA
* Corresponding author.
E-mail address: johncgreenwood@gmail.com

Emerg Med Clin N Am 32 (2014) 851–869
http://dx.doi.org/10.1016/j.emc.2014.07.009 **emed.theclinics.com**

arrest is also rapidly growing. As of January 2013, more than 200 centers provide some type of extracorporeal support and more than 4200 cardiac patients have been treated by extracorporeal cardiopulmonary resuscitation (CPR).[2]

This review has several purposes: (1) to discuss the use of the intra-aortic balloon pump (IABP) in patients with cardiogenic shock, (2) to describe the complications and management strategies for the critically ill patient with an LVAD, and (3) to explore the emerging role of ECMO in the emergency department for patients presenting in cardiac arrest.

IABP

The IABP has classically been regarded as the mainstay of mechanical support for patients in cardiogenic shock (CS). This device provides hemodynamic support by augmenting diastolic arterial blood pressure during the normal cardiac cycle. By increasing diastolic blood pressure, IABP counterpulsation is believed to improve coronary perfusion, reduce myocardial oxygen demand, and reduce left ventricular afterload during systole.[3] IABP therapy is the most widely used form of mechanical hemodynamic support in patients with CS secondary to acute myocardial infarction.[4] Historically, American and European guidelines have recommended the use of IABP therapy, giving it a class IB and class IC recommendation, respectively.[5,6] However, an emerging body of literature questions the outcome and mortality benefits of IABP therapy for CS associated with acute myocardial infarction (AMI).[7–9] As a result, American and European guidelines have downgraded the use of IABP therapy to class IIa and IIb recommendations, respectively.[10–13]

Despite the recent controversy surrounding the routine use of IABP therapy, it is important for the emergency physician to be aware of the traditional indications for an IABP, the mechanisms of support, and the contraindications. The traditional indications for IABP insertion include refractory CS caused by AMI, refractory unstable angina, and mechanical causes, such as acute mitral regurgitation, papillary muscle rupture, and ventricular septal defect. Generally accepted contraindications to counterpulsation therapy are aortic insufficiency, aortic dissection, and chronic end-stage heart failure with no anticipation of recovery.

The device consists of a double-lumen 8.0-French to 9.5-French catheter with a 25-mL to 50-mL balloon at the distal end. The IABP catheter is inserted percutaneously using a Seldinger technique through the femoral artery. Traditionally, the IABP balloon is placed after measuring the distance from the insertion point to the manubrium, followed by confirmation with a chest radiograph, or alternatively it can be placed under direct fluoroscopic guidance. Ultrasound is also being used to guide tube placement at some centers.[14] The balloon itself is positioned 2 to 3 cm distal to the left subclavian artery and is inflated during the diastolic portion of the cardiac cycle.

Evidence behind the use of IABP therapy for refractory CS has historically been mixed, especially for CS secondary to myocardial infarction. There is some evidence that IABP therapy reduces preoperative mortality in a subset of patients, including those with CS secondary to acute mitral regurgitation or a ventricular septal defect after myocardial infarction.[15] The routine use of IABP therapy in refractory CS has fallen out of favor. A meta-analysis performed on the use of IABP in ST-elevation myocardial infarction (STEMI) found insufficient evidence to routinely recommend this therapy.[16] These findings were followed by the IABP Shock-II Trial, a multicenter, randomized, prospective study,[8,9] which found no significant reduction in short-term (30-day) or long-term (12-month) all-cause mortality for patients in CS related to AMI undergoing early revascularization. Despite these observations, a small subset of patients, specifically those with acute mitral regurgitation or ventricular septal defect, could benefit from this intervention. Therefore, it may be considered as a temporizing measure while the patient is being prepared for the operating room.

VENTRICULAR ASSIST DEVICE

Ventricular assist devices (VADs) are being used more commonly today as a durable form of mechanical circulatory support, especially for patients awaiting long-term recovery or transplantation. It is important that the emergency physician be able to recognize the type of device, and become aware of the indications and complications for this type of mechanical circulatory support, as well as how to promptly manage them.

There are 3 major indications for placement of a VAD. Similar to most other mechanical circulatory devices, VADs are used as either a bridge to transplantation, bridge to recovery, or destination therapy. Permanent LVAD implantation (destination therapy) can be performed in certain patients with advanced heart failure and a low chance of transplant.[17,18] In some patients, a VAD can be considered as a “bridge to decision” when more time is needed to determine if further definitive treatment would benefit the patient.[19] In the most recent American College of Cardiology Foundation/American Heart Association STEMI guidelines, VADs were given a IIa recommendation as an alternative treatment for refractory CS.[11]

There are 2 major types of VADs, which are classified by their mechanism of support. Older, first-generation VADs provide circulatory support through a pulsatile flow pump that is driven by a pneumatic motorized pump. Except for patients with right ventricular failure, these devices are less frequently used today. The older, external VAD pumps are large and bulky, which decreases the patient’s mobility. Pulsatile VADs require frequent pump exchanges, which makes them less desirable as well.

Newer-generation VADs provide circulatory support though continuous-flow pumps that work by axial or centrifugal flow. Continuous-flow pumps have a number of advantages over the older, pulsatile-flow devices. They are often smaller, more durable, and have higher energy efficiency and lower thrombogenicity. These devices are surgically implanted and have minimal external hardware.

VAD commercial brands include the Heart Assist 5 (Houston, TX, USA), HeartWare HVAD (Framingham, MA, USA), Jarvic 2000 (New York, NY, USA), and Thoratec HeartMate II (Pleasanton, CA, USA). The most common LVAD in use today is the axial flow HeartMate II; however, with recent advances in VAD technology, the HeartWare centrifugal flow device is now more commonly inserted. The centrifugal pumps are connected directly to the patient’s left ventricle and lie within the pericardium (above the diaphragm). Blood returns to the ascending aorta by way of a separate return cannula. Axial flow pumps have a left ventricular outflow cannula that is connected in series to an intracorporeal pump located either above or below the diaphragm (**Fig. 1**).

The evaluation and management of a patient with a VAD can be challenging. It is important that the emergency physician be aware of common complications that can occur with VAD patients, as well as the laboratory and diagnostic tests that should be considered. During the initial evaluation, it is important to ask the patient or the patient’s family how to contact their VAD coordinator and cardiothoracic surgeon. These contacts are often able to provide vital information about the patient and can help coordinate the patient’s care and disposition through the emergency department.

The initial evaluation of any VAD patient should begin with a thorough initial history, physical examination, and laboratory testing. When evaluating the device, the first step should be to auscultate the motor to listen for a characteristic “hum” to ensure the device is running.

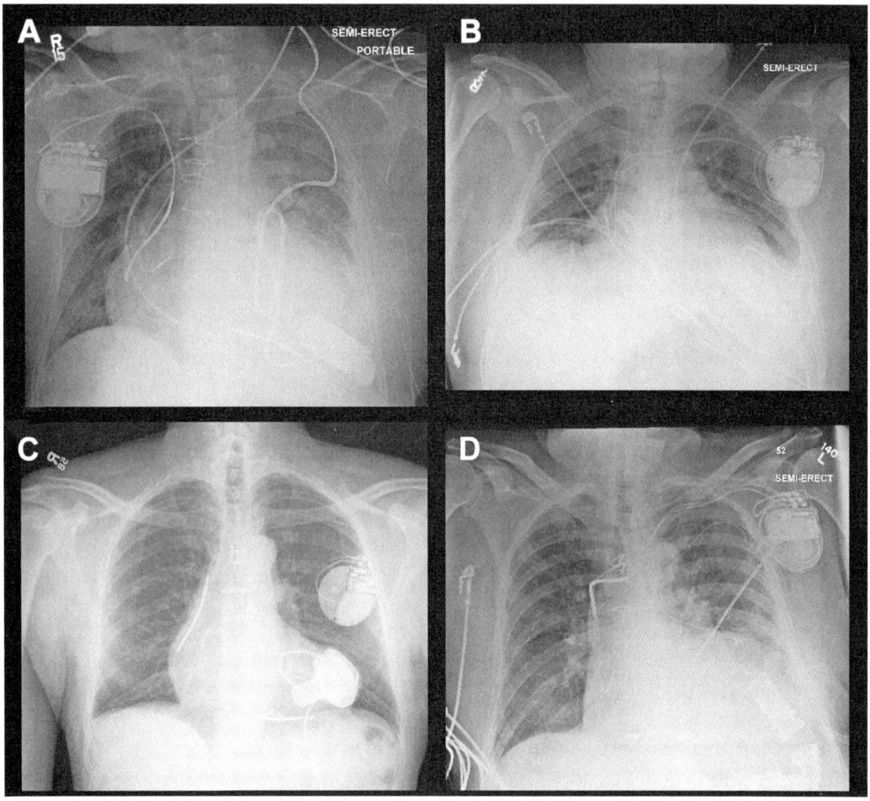

Fig. 1. The appearance of different LVAD pumps on chest radiograph. (*A*) Jarvic 2000 post-auricular driveline placement. (*B*) Jarvic-2000 abdominal placement. (*C*) HeartWare centrifugal flow device. (*D*) Thoratec HeartMate II.

Assessing vital signs can be challenging in the patient with a continuous-flow device. These patients often lack central or peripheral pulses if the patient's intrinsic cardiac contractility is poor. Therefore, their blood pressure should be measured with a manual blood pressure cuff and arterial Doppler. To obtain the mean arterial pressure (MAP), locate either the brachial or radial artery with your Doppler device. Inflate the cuff until you no longer hear auditory flow, then slowly release pressure from the manual cuff. The patient's MAP is determined at the pressure where arterial flow is heard. The goal MAP is between 70 and 80 mm Hg, with a maximum of 90 mm Hg. Excessive elevations in blood pressure can significantly increase the risk for stroke. Consider arterial line placement early, as this will provide continuous, accurate measurements of the patient's MAP. Closely examine the VAD driveline for signs of infection, damage, or bleeding (**Fig. 2**). Last, review the patient's control box for any alarms and ensure the VAD has adequate battery power (**Fig. 3**).

Pulse oximetry also can be difficult to obtain, and may be unreliable in patients with a subtle pulse or no pulse. It is important to confirm low values with a rapid arterial blood gas sample.

VADs are preload dependent. For a VAD to run efficiently, the patient's intravascular volume must be filled appropriately. Hypovolemia can lead to a reduction in VAD power secondary to reduced blood flow.

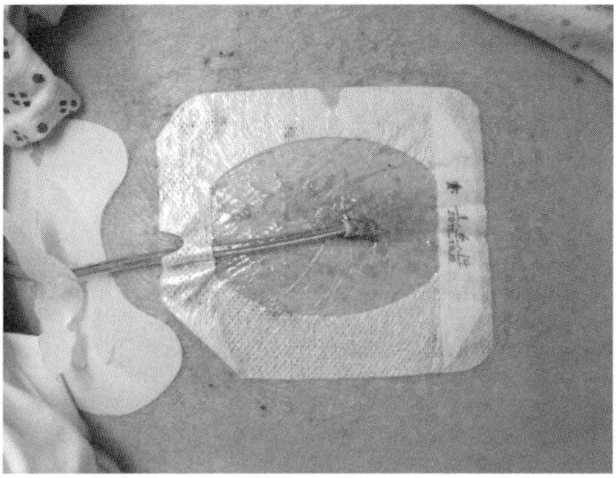

Fig. 2. Abdominal driveline location with surrounding erythema concerning for cellulitis.

These devices are also afterload sensitive. Uncontrolled increases in MAP higher than 90 mm Hg will often reduce LVAD power, flow, cardiac output, and distal perfusion. Patients with a MAP greater than 80 are at increased risk of cerebral vascular events (ie, hemorrhage, ischemia) and should be treated promptly with afterload-reducing medications.[20] A flow diagram for the differential diagnosis based on common VAD alarms is presented in **Fig. 4**.

Common VAD Complications

Common complications associated with VADs include thrombosis, bleeding, right-sided heart failure, infection, cerebral vascular accidents, arrhythmias, and device failure. Patients with VADs are at increased risk for bleeding complications, as they are usually on chronic systemic anticoagulation (ie, Coumadin [warfarin]) and antiplatelet therapy (ie, aspirin, dipyridamole). The most common international normalized ratio (INR) target for patients with LVADs is 2.0 to 3.0; however, patients with a HeartWare device target a slightly higher INR of 2.5 to 3.5. The most commonly reported types of bleeding that VAD patients encounter are epistaxis, gastrointestinal, mediastinal, and intracranial hemorrhage.[21] Hemorrhagic events are commonly caused by a supratherapeutic INR, intestinal arteriovenous malformations, or bleeding dyscrasias, such as acquired von Willebrand disease.[22,23]

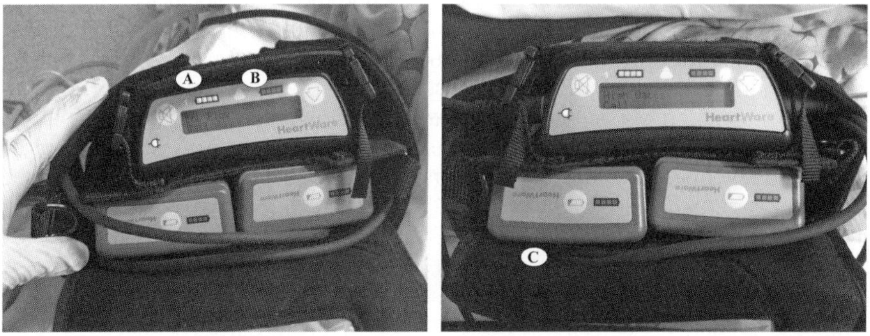

Fig. 3. HeatWare control box and battery packs. (*A*) Battery/power bar. (*B*) Alarm notification light. (*C*) Extra battery packs.

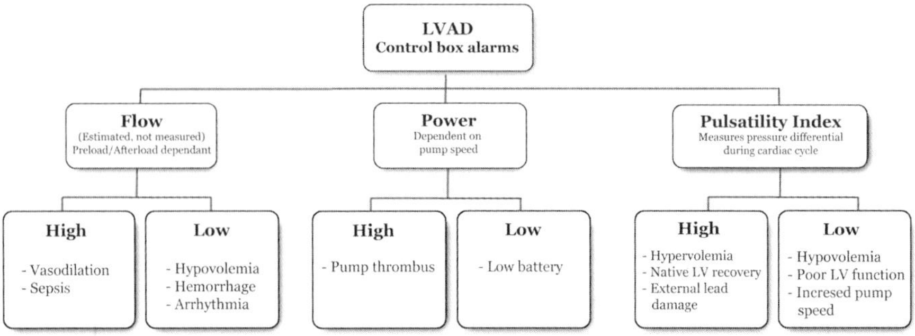

Fig. 4. Common VAD complications and their associated control box alarms. LV, left ventricular.

Treatment of the bleeding VAD patient should begin with standard therapy to reverse an elevated INR with fresh frozen plasma or prothrombin complex concentrate, if available. Platelet dysfunction due to acquired von Willebrand disease is common and is believed to be the result of platelet exposure to the mechanical sheer stress that occurs with continuous-flow devices.[22,24] Treatment with desmopressin or cryoprecipitate may be effective. Platelet transfusions may also be necessary if the patient is taking antiplatelet medications. Rapid thrombelastography may assist in targeted blood component therapy to reverse coagulopathy.[25]

VAD pump thrombosis should be considered in any patient presenting with cardiac arrest, decreased pump flow, pump power spikes, recurrent heart failure, or echocardiographic findings that raise concern for abnormal left ventricular unloading.[26] Thrombosis is a worrisome long-term complication, as it can result in stroke, peripheral embolism, heart failure, and death.[27,28] Thromboembolic events have been reported in 2.7% to 35.0% of all patients.[29] HeartMate devices were once thought to have a lower incidence of thrombosis of approximately 3%, because of their specific mechanical design.[30,31] However, a recent study detected a rapid increase in HeartMate II VAD thrombosis: up to 8.4% at 3 months for devices implanted after 2011.[32] The reason for this increase is unclear.

Pump thrombus should be suspected if hemolysis is detected by laboratory studies, if the lactate dehydrogenase is greater than 1500 mg/dL or 2.5 to 3.0 times the upper limit of normal, if the patient has hemoglobinuria, or if the plasma-free hemoglobin level is elevated.[21,26,33] Systemic anticoagulation with a continuous heparin infusion should be initiated if pump thrombosis is suspected. The VAD team should be consulted quickly to discuss emergent treatment options, including thrombolytic agents, antiplatelet therapy, and the potential need for emergent surgical pump replacement or explantation of the device.

Suction (or "suck-down") events can occur in patients with decreased left ventricular filling caused by right ventricular failure, restrictive or hypertrophic cardiomyopathies, arrhythmias, or hypovolemia.[20,34] These patients often present with hypotension. Suck-down events can be visualized under bedside echocardiography as the left ventricular chamber being equivalent in size to the VAD cannula (**Fig. 5**). Prompt recognition and treatment with an intravenous fluid bolus can reverse this problem rapidly.

Infectious Complications

Infectious complications are a major concern for patients with implanted hardware and can occur anywhere along the device circuit. Driveline, pump pocket, and device infections can be devastating and occur most frequently within the first 3 months after

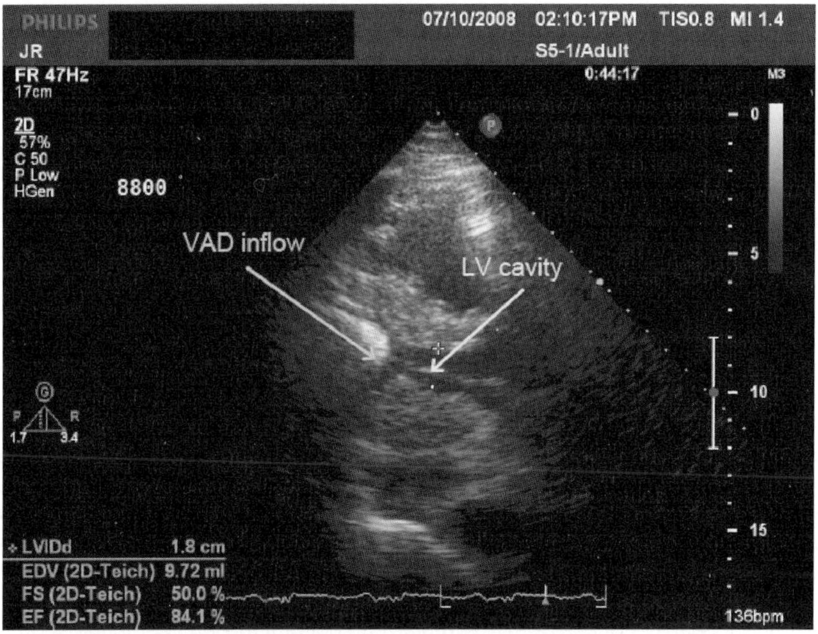

Fig. 5. A suck-down event visualized by bedside echocardiography.

placement, although they can occur at any time.[35,36] VAD infections are the most common cause of death among patients who require this device for long-term mechanical circulatory support.[35]

The most common location of infection is the driveline insertion site. Patients with infected hardware often present with symptoms of malaise, low-grade fever, and mild tenderness around the driveline. The most common infecting organisms are skin and gastrointestinal pathogens: *Staphylococcus aureus, Staphylococcus epidermidis, Enterococcus, Pseudomonas, Enterobacter,* and *Klebsiella* species.[37–40] Fungal infections have been reported and are estimated to occur in approximately 9% of VAD patients. *Candida* infections are less frequent than bacterial infections but are responsible for the highest mortality rates.[41–43]

During implantation, the VAD pump is commonly placed within the pericardium, in an anatomic "pocket" within the intra-abdominal cavity, or in the preperitoneal space below the lateral rectus muscle. The "pump pocket" is at risk for infection because it is contiguous with the driveline. Consider a pump pocket infection in VAD patients presenting with fever, leukocytosis, and abdominal pain, especially in the setting of a driveline infection.[36,44] An abdominal ultrasound or computed tomography scan is highly recommended to identify a VAD-related fluid collection or abscess.

Pump endocarditis can occur when the hardware itself becomes colonized with a bacterial pathogen. The presentation is similar to that of nonmechanical endocarditis. Symptoms include low-grade fever, signs of septic emboli on physical examination, and even pump obstruction. Sources include the driveline infection, transient bacteremia or fungemia, and other health care–associated infections from urinary or pulmonary sources.[45] Pump endocarditis carries a particularly high mortality, estimated to be as high as 50% in several case series.[46,47]

Treatment of any suspected VAD infection should begin with aggressive fluid resuscitation to maintain adequate preload. Early broad-spectrum antibiotic administration should include treatment for both methicillin-resistant *S aureus* (MRSA) and gram-negative bacterial infections. Empiric antifungal therapy should probably be given as well. Definitive source control with surgical drainage of the localized fluid collection, device exchange, or explantation for transplant is often required.

Arrhythmias

Patients with a VAD may present to the emergency department with cardiac arrhythmia, classified as either primary or secondary, based on the underlying cause.

Primary arrhythmias are intrinsic to the electrical conduction pathways of the heart and occur independently of the VAD itself. Ventricular arrhythmias are common and can be caused by cannula migration, malposition over time, electrical remodeling, secondary scaring, or fibrosis.[48,49] Because the patient's cardiac output is supported by the VAD, primary arrhythmias, such as a supraventricular tachycardia or ventricular tachycardia, are often tolerated without clinical signs or symptoms.[50]

A persistent primary arrhythmia can eventually cause right ventricular failure and reduced left ventricular filling, ultimately leading to reduced cardiac output. As a result, primary arrhythmias should be managed in a timely fashion with cardioversion or antiarrhythmic medications. There is limited evidence to guide the choice of antiarrhythmic medication in patients with a primary arrhythmia. Amiodarone is often used as a first-line agent, although the use of β-blockers can also be considered. Mexiletine can be given during in-patient management for refractory ventricular tachycardia.[48,49]

Secondary causes of cardiac arrhythmias can occur if the left ventricular septum or free wall is sucked into the VAD outflow tract. Hypovolemia and inadequate pulmonary venous return are the most common causes of a secondary arrhythmia.[51]

In the emergency department, it is often difficult to determine whether the patient's arrhythmia has a primary or secondary cause. The management of any VAD patient presenting with an abnormal rhythm should begin with a prompt fluid challenge followed by an emergent bedside echocardiogram to determine if the patient would benefit from more aggressive volume resuscitation or adjustments of the VAD settings.

Mechanical Failure

Pump failure is one of the most feared complications in VAD patients. Signs of pump failure include an absence of detectable blood pressure by Doppler, the absence of a running motor on auscultation, or the absence of power displayed on the VAD's control box. If pump failure is suspected, it is important to immediately contact the patient's cardiothoracic surgeon, VAD engineer, and on-call nurse to obtain vital information about the make and model of the hardware.

In any patient without evidence of perfusion (eg, MAP <40 with at least one other sign of hypoperfusion, such as loss of consciousness or cyanosis), it is important to promptly begin treatment with volume resuscitation and standard advanced cardiac life support (ACLS) interventions. Strongly consider initiation of a heparin infusion if there is any suspicion for pump thrombosis. An epinephrine infusion should be initiated to maximize intrinsic cardiac output. Rapid initiation of veno-arterial ECMO (VA ECMO) can also be considered in conjunction with the patient's cardiac surgeon.

First-generation VADs can be pumped manually to provide adequate blood flow. In general, it is recommended that the provider deliver 60 to 90 pumps per minute to provide adequate cardiac output if the VAD has failed. Newer-generation VADs generally do not have manual hand pumps. One of the biggest misperceptions about the patient with a VAD is that you should never perform CPR on a patient with mechanical pump failure. Although CPR may increase the risk of device dislodgement, it is not contraindicated. If the patient continues to have a MAP of zero after 1 minute, connect the patient's manual hand pump or initiate chest compressions.

ECMO

Overview

Over the years, major advances in technology have increased the availability and ability to use ECMO as a viable form of prolonged mechanical circulatory support. The historical roller pumps used for cardiopulmonary bypass were associated with higher rates of pump-induced hemolysis and lower flow rates compared with the newer centrifugal pump heads.[52,53] The transition from older bubble-type oxygenators to newer hollow-membrane silicone oxygenators has also reduced blood trauma significantly, allowing increased duration of extracorporeal support.[54]

Two major forms of ECMO circuits are used today. Venovenous ECMO (VV ECMO) is used primarily for patients in refractory respiratory failure. Currently there are no universally agreed on indications for the initiation of VV ECMO, but general indications include *refractory* hypoxemia, hypercapnia, and the failure of conventional mechanical ventilatory strategies.[55] In general, initiation of VV ECMO is rare in the emergency department, because this modality is chosen well after more advanced resuscitation measures have been attempted.

VV ECMO can be considered the "ultimate" form of lung rest therapy, as ventilator strategies can be used to minimize barotrauma, volutrauma, and biotrauma. In the patient with refractory respiratory failure on ECMO, it is generally acceptable to follow ARDSnet ventilation strategies (between 4 and 8 mL/kg of ideal body weight, with plateau pressures <30 cm H_2O), which can be readily used without worrying about alveolar gas exchange.[56]

The second major form of extracorporeal support is VA ECMO. VA ECMO not only provides assistance with gas exchange, but also provides hemodynamic support by way of venous and arterial cannulation. VA ECMO can be considered for any patient with CS that is refractory to standard medical management, especially if the cause of the patient's shock is believed to be reversible.

Cardiogenic shock can be defined as heart failure resulting in hypotension (systolic blood pressure <80–90 mm Hg, mean arterial pressure <30 from baseline), end-organ dysfunction, cardiac index less than 1.8 (without support) to 2.2 L/min/m^2 (with support), or evidence of pulmonary edema (objectively defined with a pulmonary capillary wedge pressure >18 mm Hg).[13,57] When a patient with CS has failed traditional medical management, VA ECMO can be a used as a potential salvage therapy; however, although a number of international organizations recognize the role of extracorporeal support, they have not agreed on strict inclusion criteria.[13,19] The ultimate goal of VA ECMO is to provide temporary support as a bridge to shock recovery, bridge to a more durable form of cardiovascular support (ie, LVAD or total artificial heart), heart or lung transplantation, or termination of further efforts (if futile).

ECMO Pump Set-Up and Cannulation

Current ECMO circuits are composed of heparin-coated polyvinylchloride tubing running to and from the patient, a centrifugal pump, a membrane oxygenator, a heat exchanger, and a bladder reservoir (**Fig. 6**). Blood is driven through the oxygenator by the centrifugal pump head, warmed to a prespecified temperature, then returned to the patient by way of continuous, nonpulsatile flow. Systemic anticoagulation with unfractionated heparin is used to prevent thrombosis of the ECMO circuit.

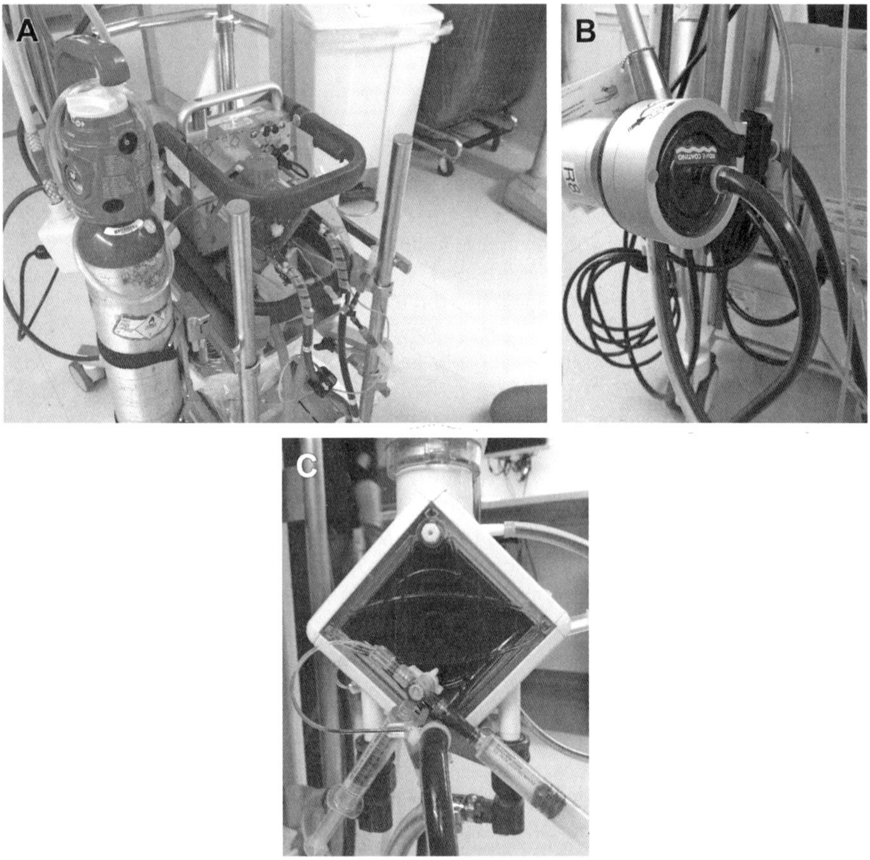

Fig. 6. (*A*) Maquet CARDIOHELP ECMO circuit. (*B*) Centrifugal pump. (*C*) Silicone membrane oxygenator.

VV ECMO cannulation can be performed by a number of methods under ultrasound or fluoroscopic guidance. Traditionally, two 21-French to 28-French cannulas are used. Deoxygenated blood is removed from the inferior vena cava by way of a multiport cannula inserted into the right femoral vein and advanced to the level of T11/T12. It is important to avoid advancing this catheter higher than approximately the level of T8, as this can lead to hepatic vein obstruction. Deoxygenated blood is then sent to the pump's oxygenator and finally returned to the right heart through a cannula inserted into the right internal jugular vein.

Access can also be obtained by placing a single, 23-French, dual-lumen catheter (eg, Avalon) in the right internal jugular vein. When using a single-cannula, bicaval approach, the internal jugular ECMO catheter is advanced through the right atrium so that the proximal drainage port rests in the superior vena cava and the distal port rests just beyond the cavoatrial junction in the inferior vena cava.[58] Oxygenated blood is returned through a separate cannula by way of a central port located in the right atrium to provide flow across the tricuspid valve.

VA ECMO cannulation can be performed centrally in the operating room under direct vascular visualization, but is more frequently being performed percutaneously at the patient's bedside. Using a Seldinger technique with serial dilations, a

21-French venous catheter is inserted into the common femoral vein and a 15-French or 17-French arterial catheter is inserted into the contralateral femoral artery. The arterial catheter is advanced to the distal aorta to deliver retrograde blood flow for perfusion.

The catheter can be directly visualized with fluoroscopy or ultrasound. A great deal of care must be taken when performing the serial dilations to avoid laceration of the femoral vessels. Complications such as acute embolism/thrombosis, common femoral artery dissection, perforation, and compartment syndrome can be devastating.[59] Once the femoral arterial cannula is in place, it is important to monitor for critical limb ischemia. A supplemental backflow cannula can be placed distal to the ascending arterial cannula in the superficial femoral artery to provide blood flow if there is concern for limb hypoperfusion.[60,61] After cannulation, initial cardiac output targets of 1.5 to 2.0 L/min are acceptable but should be titrated up gradually to 3.0 to 6.0 L/min. Because arterial flow will be continuous, a pulse pressure of approximately 10 mm Hg is considered acceptable.[62]

During VA ECMO, the retrograde aorta-to-left ventricular pressure gradient is very high, but the aortic valve should be able to function normally. A post cannulation transesophageal or transthoracic echocardiogram should be performed to check for proper opening of the aortic valve, aortic regurgitation, left ventricular distention, and tamponade.[63] Although usually unnecessary, vasopressor and inotropic agents are occasionally required to reach target blood pressure and cardiac output, respectively.

Unlike VV ECMO, which allows the left heart to provide pulsatile flow to the systemic vasculature, VA ECMO provides continuous blood flow through the arterial system. After initiation, VA ECMO usually rapidly reduces pulmonary arterial pressures, improves end-organ perfusion, and increases Pa_{O_2}. For the postarrest patient, the pump's heat exchanger can be used to facilitate targeted temperature management.

Clinical Uses for ECMO

Toxic overdoses

Medical management of most cardiotoxic ingestions remains largely supportive, as the effects of these toxic ingestions are often self-limited. A number of case series and reports have been published about the utility of VA ECMO in the overdose patient presenting with refractory CS. For patients presenting early to medical centers with personnel experienced with extracorporeal support, this technology can be used as a bridge to recovery.

Cardiovascular failure is a leading cause of death in patients with severe, acute drug intoxication.[64–66] In 2010 alone, cardiovascular medication overdoses accounted for 9.4% of all fatalities. According to the American Association of Poison Control Centers, calcium-channel and beta-blocking medications were involved in 30% of these overdoses and accounted for more than 45% of deaths related to cardiovascular medications.[64]

A growing body of literature supports the use of VA ECMO in the overdose patient, especially when the offending agent leads to refractory CS or arrhythmias. Case series describe overdoses with diltiazem, verapamil, flecainide, acebutolol, and other antidepressants agents.[67–72] In many of these reports, VA ECMO was instituted early to provide effective perfusion and avoid multiorgan dysfunction. After the initiation of extracorporeal support, the duration of therapy was generally less than 1 week.

Myocarditis

One well-described use of ECMO is in fulminant CS secondary to acute myocarditis. Infective myocarditis is an acquired inflammatory muscle disorder that is more common in the pediatric patient population.[73] It can be caused by a wide spectrum of infectious organisms, as well as toxic and hypersensitivity reactions. Viral pathogens are the most common offending agents, specifically parvovirus B19 and human herpes virus 6.[74,75]

Fulminant myocarditis is characterized by the presence of hypotension, respiratory failure, and signs of end-organ hypoperfusion. For patients presenting in shock, initial management often requires mechanical ventilation, inotropic agents, and vasopressors. If the patient is unresponsive to initial medical management, mechanical circulatory support might be required. Extracorporeal membrane oxygenation appears to be an effective therapy for these patients and can be used as a bridge to recovery.[76]

The decision to initiate mechanical circulatory support can be difficult, because there are no absolute indications. Most experts agree that the decision to initiate ECMO should be strongly considered in the patient presenting with acute end-organ dysfunction, a refractory ventricular arrhythmia, or cardiac arrest.[77]

ECMO for out-of-hospital cardiac arrest and ECMO-assisted CPR (eCPR)

The utility of ECMO in managing out-of-hospital cardiac arrest is perhaps one of the most exciting developments in the expanded role of extracorporeal support. Historically, out-of-hospital cardiac arrest outcomes remained poor despite advances in ACLS protocols and the use of conventional CPR. Return of spontaneous circulation (ROSC) rates are regularly reported to be less than 40%. Additionally, survival to hospital discharge rates range from 7% to 11%, and for those who do leave the hospital, favorable neurologic outcome is achieved in only 3% to 5%.[78,79] Outcomes have improved with post-ROSC therapeutic hypothermia,[80,81] rapid defibrillation,[82] cardiocerebral resuscitation,[83–85] and rapid revascularization.[86,87]

Initiating ECMO for a patient in cardiac arrest remains a heroic procedure, with a small body of growing literature to support its use. In general, there is a lack of large randomized trials evaluating the efficacy of eCPR. Most of the published reports supporting its use are case reports and small observational studies with heterogeneous patient populations.

Appropriate patient selection is critical, as the use of ECMO should be only a temporizing, not definitive, treatment strategy. Accepted indications include a brief arrest period, a condition believed to be reversible (such as coronary occlusion, refractory arrhythmia, or toxin-induced arrest), or a condition that is amenable to transplantation or rapid revascularization. There are a number of suggested contraindications to eCPR, which are listed in **Box 1**. With respect to the duration of CPR, most published reports have included only those who had not achieved ROSC within 10 to 30 minutes of conventional CPR.[88–91]

Box 1
Common exclusion criteria for initiation of ECMO-assisted CPR

- History of severe neurologic damage
- Intracranial hemorrhage
- Terminal malignancy
- Traumatic arrest with uncontrolled bleeding
- Unwitnessed arrest or prolonged arrest
- Aortic dissection
- Severe peripheral arterial disease

A number of studies have reported improved survival and neurologic outcomes with the use of eCPR for patients with in-hospital cardiac arrest.[89,92,93] When used as a bridge to revascularization in patients who experienced cardiac arrest due to ST-elevation myocardial infarction, a significant 30-day mortality benefit has been achieved.[92] More importantly, for those with a primary cardiac cause of arrest or shock, an improved 6-month survival with minimal neurologic impairment has been reported.[93]

The ability to initiate ECMO for patients presenting to the emergency department with out-of-hospital cardiac arrest (OHCA) has become possible with advances in ECMO technology. In 2012, Bellezzo and colleagues[94] published a staged approach for the initiation of ECMO for OHCA in the emergency department. This small study demonstrated that ECMO can be initiated in the emergency department and, if done carefully, can significantly improve neurologic recovery. Larger reports have shown a significant 30-day survival and improvement in neurologic outcomes as well.[95–97]

The use of ECMO is extremely resource intensive and the cost alone could prohibit its widespread adoption. The amount of data for the use of VA ECMO in patients with OHCA remains limited, and it is still unclear which patients will benefit most from ECMO therapy. But as the body of literature continues to grow, it appears that rapid initiation of ECMO in the emergency department for OHCA is possible. It is important for the emergency physician to keep in mind that ECMO can be used as a temporary bridge to a more definitive procedure, such as revascularization, the use of a VAD, or transplantation.

SUMMARY

Patients who require mechanical circulatory support are some of the most critically ill patients one can encounter in the emergency department. As the use of these technologies continues to grow, emergency physicians have increasing opportunities to participate in the advancement of these potentially life-saving technologies. It is imperative that emergency physicians not only understand the complexities of these patients, but also be well-prepared to handle the many complications that can occur with these emerging therapies.

ACKNOWLEDGMENTS

The authors thank and acknowledge Linda J. Kesselring, MS, ELS, for copyediting the article and incorporating revisions into the final article.

REFERENCES

1. HeartMate II® left ventricular assist device (LVAD) fact sheet. Available at: www.thoratec.com/downloads/heartmate-II-fact-sheet-b100-0812-final.pdf. Accessed January 21, 2014.
2. Extracorporeal Life Support Organization. ECLS Registry report. International summary. 2013. Available at: www.elso.org/index.php?option=com_content&;view=article&id=85&Itemid=653. Accessed January 21, 2014.
3. Scheidt S, Wilner G, Mueller H, et al. Intra-aortic balloon counterpulsation in cardiogenic shock: report of a co-operative clinical trial. N Engl J Med 1973;288:979–84.
4. Thiele H, Allam B, Chatellier G, et al. Shock in acute myocardial infarction: the Cape Horn for trials? Eur Heart J 2010;31:1828–35.
5. Antman EM, Anbe DT, Armstrong PW, et al. ACC/AHA guidelines for the management of patients with ST-elevation myocardial infarction–executive summary.

A report of the American College of Cardiology/American Heart Association Task Force on Practice Guidelines (Writing Committee to revise the 1999 guidelines for the management of patients with acute myocardial infarction). J Am Coll Cardiol 2004;44:671–719.

6. Van de Werf F, Bax J, Betriu A, et al. Management of acute myocardial infarction in patients presenting with persistent ST-segment elevation: the Task Force on the Management of ST-Segment Elevation Acute Myocardial Infarction of the European Society of Cardiology. Eur Heart J 2008;29:2909–45.
7. Zeymer U, Bauer T, Hamm C, et al. Use and impact of intra-aortic balloon pump on mortality in patients with acute myocardial infarction complicated by cardiogenic shock: results of the Euro Heart Survey on PCI. EuroIntervention 2011;7:437–41.
8. Thiele H, Zeymer U, Neumann FJ, et al. Intra-aortic balloon counterpulsation in acute myocardial infarction complicated by cardiogenic shock (IABP-SHOCK II): final 12 month results of a randomised, open-label trial. Lancet 2013;382:1638–45.
9. Thiele H, Zeymer U, Neumann FJ, et al. Intraaortic balloon support for myocardial infarction with cardiogenic shock. N Engl J Med 2012;367:1287–96.
10. O'Gara PT, Kushner FG, Ascheim DD, et al. 2013 ACCF/AHA guideline for the management of ST-elevation myocardial infarction: executive summary: a report of the American College of Cardiology Foundation/American Heart Association Task Force on Practice Guidelines. J Am Coll Cardiol 2013;61:485–510.
11. American College of Emergency Physicians, Society for Cardiovascular Angiography and Interventions, O'Gara PT, et al. 2013 ACCF/AHA guideline for the management of ST-elevation myocardial infarction: a report of the American College of Cardiology Foundation/American Heart Association Task Force on Practice Guidelines. J Am Coll Cardiol 2013;61:e78–140.
12. Steg PG, James SK, Atar D, et al. ESC guidelines for the management of acute myocardial infarction in patients presenting with ST-segment elevation. Eur Heart J 2012;33:2569–619.
13. Wijns W, Kolh P, Danchin N, et al. Guidelines on myocardial revascularization: the Task Force on Myocardial Revascularization of the European Society of Cardiology (ESC) and the European Association for Cardio-Thoracic Surgery (EACTS). Eur Heart J 2010;31:2501–55.
14. Sustiíc A, Medved I, Simić O. Ultrasound-guided placement of intra-aortic balloon pump. Eur J Anaesthesiol 2002;19:149–50.
15. Kettner J, Sramko M, Holek M, et al. Utility of intra-aortic balloon pump support for ventricular septal rupture and acute mitral regurgitation complicating acute myocardial infarction. Am J Cardiol 2013;112:1709–13.
16. Sjauw KD, Engström AE, Vis MM, et al. A systematic review and meta-analysis of intra-aortic balloon pump therapy in ST-elevation myocardial infarction: should we change the guidelines? Eur Heart J 2009;30:459–68.
17. Kirklin JK, Naftel DC, Kormos RL, et al. Third INTERMACS Annual Report: the evolution of destination therapy in the United States. J Heart Lung Transplant 2011;30:115–23.
18. Kirklin JK, Naftel DC, Pagani FD, et al. Long-term mechanical circulatory support (destination therapy): on track to compete with heart transplantation? J Thorac Cardiovasc Surg 2012;144:584–603.
19. Peura JL, Colvin-Adams M, Francis GS, et al. Recommendations for the use of mechanical circulatory support: device strategies and patient selection: a scientific statement from the American Heart Association. Circulation 2012;126:2648–67.

20. Slaughter MS, Pagani FD, Rogers JG, et al. Clinical management of continuous-flow left ventricular assist devices in advanced heart failure. J Heart Lung Transplant 2010;29(Suppl 4):S1–39.
21. Slaughter MS, Rogers JG, Milano CA, et al. Advanced heart failure treated with continuous-flow left ventricular assist device. N Engl J Med 2009;361:2241–51.
22. Geisen U, Heilmann C, Beyersdorf F, et al. Non-surgical bleeding in patients with ventricular assist devices could be explained by acquired von Willebrand disease. Eur J Cardiothorac Surg 2008;33:679–84.
23. Letsou GV, Shah N, Gregoric ID, et al. Gastrointestinal bleeding from arteriovenous malformations in patients supported by the Jarvik 2000 axial-flow left ventricular assist device. J Heart Lung Transplant 2005;24:105–9.
24. Klovaite J, Gustafsson F, Mortensen SA, et al. Severely impaired von Willebrand factor-dependent platelet aggregation in patients with a continuous-flow left ventricular assist device (HeartMate II). J Am Coll Cardiol 2009;53:2162–7.
25. Ashbrook M, Walenga JM, Schwartz J, et al. Left ventricular assist device-induced coagulation and platelet activation and effect of the current anticoagulant therapy regimen. Clin Appl Thromb Hemost 2013;19(3):249–55.
26. Goldstein DJ, John R, Salerno C, et al. Algorithm for the diagnosis and management of suspected pump thrombus. J Heart Lung Transplant 2013;32:667–70.
27. Aaronson KD, Slaughter MS, Miller LW, et al. Use of an intrapericardial, continuous-flow, centrifugal pump in patients awaiting heart transplantation. Circulation 2012;125:3191–200.
28. Pagani FD, Miller LW, Russell SD, et al. Extended mechanical circulatory support with a continuous-flow rotary left ventricular assist device. J Am Coll Cardiol 2009;54:312–21.
29. Piccione W. Left ventricular assist device implantation: short and long-term surgical complications. J Heart Lung Transplant 2000;19(Suppl 8):S89–94.
30. Rose EA, Levin HR, Oz MC, et al. Artificial circulatory support with textured interior surfaces. A counterintuitive approach to minimizing thromboembolism. Circulation 1994;90(5 Pt 2):II87–91.
31. Frazier OH, Rose EA, Macmanus Q, et al. Multicenter clinical evaluation of the HeartMate 1000 IP left ventricular assist device. Ann Thorac Surg 1992;53:1080–90.
32. Starling RC, Moazami N, Silvestry SC, et al. Unexpected abrupt increase in left ventricular assist device thrombosis. N Engl J Med 2014;370:33–40.
33. Shah P, Mehta VM, Cowger JA, et al. Diagnosis of hemolysis and device thrombosis with lactate dehydrogenase during left ventricular assist device support. J Heart Lung Transplant 2014;33:102–4.
34. Topilsky Y, Pereira NL, Shah DK, et al. Left ventricular assist device therapy in patients with restrictive and hypertrophic cardiomyopathy. Circ Heart Fail 2011;4:266–75.
35. Holman WL, Park SJ, Long JW, et al. Infection in permanent circulatory support: experience from the REMATCH trial. J Heart Lung Transplant 2004;23:1359–65.
36. Holman WL, Kirklin JK, Naftel DC, et al. Infection after implantation of pulsatile mechanical circulatory support devices. J Thorac Cardiovasc Surg 2010;139:1632–6.e2.
37. Gordon RJ, Weinberg AD, Pagani FD, et al. Prospective, multicenter study of ventricular assist device infections. Circulation 2013;127:691–702.
38. Kalya AV, Tector AJ, Crouch JD, et al. Comparison of Novacor and HeartMate vented electric left ventricular assist devices in a single institution. J Heart Lung Transplant 2005;24:1973–5.

39. Sivaratnam K, Duggan JM. Left ventricular assist device infections: three case reports and a review of the literature. ASAIO J 2002;48:2–7.
40. Sinha P, Chen JM, Flannery M, et al. Infections during left ventricular assist device support do not affect posttransplant outcomes. Circulation 2000;102: III194–9.
41. Aslam S, Hernandez M, Thornby J, et al. Risk factors and outcomes of fungal ventricular-assist device infections. Clin Infect Dis 2010;50:664–71.
42. Shoham S, Shaffer R, Sweet L, et al. Candidemia in patients with ventricular assist devices. Clin Infect Dis 2007;44:e9–12.
43. Bagdasarian NG, Malani AN, Pagani FD, et al. Fungemia associated with left ventricular assist device support. J Card Surg 2009;24:763–5.
44. Chinn R, Dembitsky W, Eaton L, et al. Multicenter experience: prevention and management of left ventricular assist device infections. ASAIO J 2005;51:461–70.
45. Holman WL, Skinner JL, Waites KB, et al. Infection during circulatory support with ventricular assist devices. Ann Thorac Surg 1999;68:711–6.
46. Argenziano M, Catanese KA, Moazami N, et al. The influence of infection on survival and successful transplantation in patients with left ventricular assist devices. J Heart Lung Transplant 1997;16:822–31.
47. Monkowski DH, Axelrod P, Fekete T, et al. Infections associated with ventricular assist devices: epidemiology and effect on prognosis after transplantation. Transpl Infect Dis 2007;9:114–20.
48. Boyle A. Arrhythmias in patients with ventricular assist devices. Curr Opin Cardiol 2012;27:13–8.
49. Pedrotty DM, Rame JE, Margulies KB. Management of ventricular arrhythmias in patients with ventricular assist devices. Curr Opin Cardiol 2013;28:360–8.
50. Oz MC, Rose EA, Slater J, et al. Malignant ventricular arrhythmias are well tolerated in patients receiving long-term left ventricular assist devices. J Am Coll Cardiol 1994;24:1688–91.
51. Vollkron M, Voitl P, Ta J, et al. Suction events during left ventricular support and ventricular arrhythmias. J Heart Lung Transplant 2007;26:819–25.
52. Hoerr HR, Kraemer MF, Williams LJ, et al. In vitro comparison of the blood handling by the constrained vortex and twin roller blood pumps. JECT 1987; 19:316–21.
53. Bennett M, Horton S, Thuys C, et al. Pump-induced haemolysis: a comparison of short-term ventricular assist devices. Perfusion 2004;19:107–11.
54. Iwahashi H, Yuri K, Nosé Y. Development of the oxygenator: past, present, and future. J Artif Organs 2004;7:111–20.
55. Brodie D, Bacchetta M. Extracorporeal membrane oxygenation for ARDS in adults. N Engl J Med 2011;365:1905–14.
56. Peek GJ, Mugford M, Tiruvoipati R, et al. Efficacy and economic assessment of conventional ventilatory support versus extracorporeal membrane oxygenation for severe adult respiratory failure (CESAR): a multicentre randomised controlled trial. Lancet 2009;374(9698):1351–63.
57. Reynolds HR, Hochman JS. Cardiogenic shock: current concepts and improving outcomes. Circulation 2008;117:686–97.
58. Javidfar J, Brodie D, Wang D, et al. Use of bicaval dual-lumen catheter for adult venovenous extracorporeal membrane oxygenation. Ann Thorac Surg 2011;91: 1763–8.
59. Bisdas T, Beutel G, Warnecke G, et al. Vascular complications in patients undergoing femoral cannulation for extracorporeal membrane oxygenation support. Ann Thorac Surg 2011;92:626–31.

60. Gander JW, Fisher JC, Reichstein AR, et al. Limb ischemia after common femoral artery cannulation for venoarterial extracorporeal membrane oxygenation: an unresolved problem. J Pediatr Surg 2010;45:2136–40.
61. Foley PJ, Morris RJ, Woo EY, et al. Limb ischemia during femoral cannulation for cardiopulmonary support. J Vasc Surg 2010;52:850–3.
62. Chauhan S, Subin S. Extracorporeal membrane oxygenation, an anesthesiologist's perspective: physiology and principles. Part 1. Ann Card Anaesth 2011; 14:218–29.
63. Catena E, Tasca G. Role of echocardiography in the perioperative management of mechanical circulatory assistance. Best Pract Res Clin Anaesthesiol 2012;26: 199–216.
64. Bronstein AC, Spyker DA, Cantilena LR Jr, et al. 2010 Annual report of the American Association of Poison Control Centers' National Poison Data System (NPDS): 28th annual report. Clin Toxicol 2011;49:910–41.
65. DeWitt CR, Waksman JC. Pharmacology, pathophysiology and management of calcium channel blocker and beta-blocker toxicity. Toxicol Rev 2004;23: 223–38.
66. Lai MW, Klein-Schwartz W, Rodgers GC, et al. 2005 Annual Report of the American Association of Poison Control Centers' national poisoning and exposure database. Clin Toxicol 2006;44:803–932.
67. Durward A, Guerguerian AM, Lefebvre M, et al. Massive diltiazem overdose treated with extracorporeal membrane oxygenation. Pediatr Crit Care Med 2003;4:372–6.
68. Holzer M, Sterz F, Schoerkhuber W, et al. Successful resuscitation of a verapamil-intoxicated patient with percutaneous cardiopulmonary bypass. Crit Care Med 1999;27:2818–23.
69. Rooney M, Massey KL, Jamali F, et al. Acebutolol overdose treated with hemodialysis and extracorporeal membrane oxygenation. J Clin Pharmacol 1996;36:760–3.
70. Shenoi AN, Gertz SJ, Mikkilineni S, et al. Refractory hypotension from massive bupropion overdose successfully treated with extracorporeal membrane oxygenation. Pediatr Emerg Care 2011;27:43–5.
71. Vivien B, Deye N, Megarbane B, et al. Extracorporeal life support in a case of fatal flecainide and betaxolol poisoning allowing successful cardiac allograft. Ann Emerg Med 2010;56:409–12.
72. Goodwin DA, Lally KP, Null DM Jr. Extracorporeal membrane oxygenation support for cardiac dysfunction from tricyclic antidepressant overdose. Crit Care Med 1993;21:625–7.
73. Ghelani SJ, Spaeder MC, Pastor W, et al. Demographics, trends, and outcomes in pediatric acute myocarditis in the United States, 2006 to 2011. Circ Cardiovasc Qual Outcomes 2012;5:622–7.
74. Sagar S, Liu PP, Cooper LT Jr. Myocarditis. Lancet 2012;379:738–47.
75. Feldman AM, McNamara D. Myocarditis. N Engl J Med 2000;343:1388–98.
76. Saji T, Matsuura H, Hasegawa K, et al. Comparison of the clinical presentation, treatment, and outcome of fulminant and acute myocarditis in children. Circ J 2012;76:1222–8.
77. Teele SA, Allan CK, Laussen PC, et al. Management and outcomes in pediatric patients presenting with acute fulminant myocarditis. J Pediatr 2011;158: 638–43.e1.
78. McNally B, Robb R, Mehta M, et al. Out-of-hospital cardiac arrest surveillance–Cardiac Arrest Registry to Enhance Survival (CARES), United States, October 1, 2005–December 31, 2010. MMWR Surveill Summ 2011;60:1–19.

79. Kudenchuk PJ, Redshaw JD, Stubbs BA, et al. Impact of changes in resuscitation practice on survival and neurological outcome after out-of-hospital cardiac arrest resulting from nonshockable arrhythmias. Circulation 2012;125:1787–94.
80. Belliard G, Catez E, Charron C, et al. Efficacy of therapeutic hypothermia after out-of-hospital cardiac arrest due to ventricular fibrillation. Resuscitation 2007; 75:252–9.
81. Testori C, Sterz F, Holzer M, et al. The beneficial effect of mild therapeutic hypothermia depends on the time of complete circulatory standstill in patients with cardiac arrest. Resuscitation 2012;83:596–601.
82. Sasson C, Rogers MA, Dahl J, et al. Predictors of survival from out-of-hospital cardiac arrest: a systematic review and meta-analysis. Circ Cardiovasc Qual Outcomes 2010;3:63–81.
83. Ewy GA. Cardiocerebral resuscitation: the new cardiopulmonary resuscitation. Circulation 2005;111:2134–42.
84. Kellum MJ, Kennedy KW, Barney R, et al. Cardiocerebral resuscitation improves neurologically intact survival of patients with out-of-hospital cardiac arrest. Ann Emerg Med 2008;52:244–52.
85. Yang CL, Wen J, Li YP, et al. Cardiocerebral resuscitation vs cardiopulmonary resuscitation for cardiac arrest: a systematic review. Am J Emerg Med 2012;30:784–93.
86. Hochman JS, Sleeper LA, Webb JG, et al. Early revascularization and long-term survival in cardiogenic shock complicating acute myocardial infarction. JAMA 2006;295:2511–5.
87. Dumas F, Cariou A, Manzo-Silberman S, et al. Immediate percutaneous coronary intervention is associated with better survival after out-of-hospital cardiac arrest: insights from the PROCAT (Parisian Region Out of hospital Cardiac ArresT) registry. Circ Cardiovasc Interv 2010;3:200–7.
88. Le Guen M, Nicolas-Robin A, Carreira S, et al. Extracorporeal life support following out-of-hospital refractory cardiac arrest. Crit Care 2011;15:R29.
89. Avalli L, Maggioni E, Formica F, et al. Favourable survival of in-hospital compared to out-of-hospital refractory cardiac arrest patients treated with extracorporeal membrane oxygenation: an Italian tertiary care centre experience. Resuscitation 2012;83:579–83.
90. Chen JS, Ko WJ, Yu HY, et al. Analysis of the outcome for patients experiencing myocardial infarction and cardiopulmonary resuscitation refractory to conventional therapies necessitating extracorporeal life support rescue. Crit Care Med 2006;34:950–7.
91. Kagawa E, Inoue I, Kawagoe T, et al. Assessment of outcomes and differences between in- and out-of-hospital cardiac arrest patients treated with cardiopulmonary resuscitation using extracorporeal life support. Resuscitation 2010;81:968–73.
92. Chung SY, Sheu JJ, Lin YJ, et al. Outcome of patients with profound cardiogenic shock after cardiopulmonary resuscitation and prompt extracorporeal membrane oxygenation support: a single-center observational study. Circ J 2012;76:1385–92.
93. Shin TG, Choi JH, Jo IJ, et al. Extracorporeal cardiopulmonary resuscitation in patients with inhospital cardiac arrest: a comparison with conventional cardiopulmonary resuscitation. Crit Care Med 2011;39:17.
94. Bellezzo JM, Shinar Z, Davis DP, et al. Emergency physician-initiated extracorporeal cardiopulmonary resuscitation. Resuscitation 2012;83:966–70.
95. Nagao K, Kikushima K, Watanabe K, et al. Early induction of hypothermia during cardiac arrest improves neurological outcomes in patients with out-of-hospital cardiac arrest who undergo emergency cardiopulmonary bypass and percutaneous coronary intervention. Circ J 2010;74:77–85.

96. Kagawa E, Dote K, Kato M, et al. Should we emergently revascularize occluded coronaries for cardiac arrest? Rapid-response extracorporeal membrane oxygenation and intra-arrest percutaneous coronary intervention. Circulation 2012;126:1605–13.
97. Fagnoul D, Taccone FS, Belhaj A, et al. Extracorporeal life support associated with hypothermia and normoxemia in refractory cardiac arrest. Resuscitation 2013;84:1519–24.

Lung-protective Ventilation Strategies and Adjunctive Treatments for the Emergency Medicine Patient with Acute Respiratory Failure

Brian J. Wright, MD, MPH[a,b,*]

KEYWORDS

- Acute respiratory failure • Acute respiratory distress syndrome
- Mechanical ventilation

KEY POINTS

- Respiratory failure is a frequent disease process encountered in the emergency department.
- There is significant need for improvement in the care of patients on mechanical ventilation. If not contraindicated, lung-protective ventilation strategies should be used.
- Patient specific disease pathophysiology is important to consider when treating patients that are difficult to oxygenate, ventilate or when Pa_{O_2}, Pa_{CO_2}, and/or pH can only be maintained at unsafe ventilator settings.

INTRODUCTION

Invasive mechanical ventilation (MV) is an essential component of critical care and emergency medicine (EM). Successful resuscitation requires an expedient and parallel assessment of airway maintenance, efficiency and effectiveness of breathing mechanics, and adequacy of circulation and perfusion. Management should be directed at ensuring sufficient oxygenation, ventilation, and prompt reversal of the inciting disease process if possible. This article reviews the evidence for safe MV strategies in the critically ill patient in the emergency department (ED) and provides treatment options for patients who are difficult to oxygenate and ventilate or cannot safely be managed with standard MV strategies.

Disclosure: None.

[a] Department of Emergency Medicine, Stony Brook University School of Medicine, 101 Nicolls Road, Stony Brook, NY 11794, USA; [b] Department of Surgery, Stony Brook University School of Medicine, 101 Nicolls Road, Stony Brook, NY 11794, USA

* Corresponding author.

E-mail address: brianjwright1@gmail.com

Emerg Med Clin N Am 32 (2014) 871–887

http://dx.doi.org/10.1016/j.emc.2014.07.012 emed.theclinics.com

EPIDEMIOLOGY/STATEMENT OF THE PROBLEM

Acute respiratory failure (ARF) requiring MV is a common clinical scenario. Wunsch and colleagues[1] suggested that approximately 3% of all hospital admissions in the United States require invasive MV. MV costs approximately $27 billion dollars nationally.[1] Nearly one-third of patients who are placed on MV die in the hospital and among survivors only 30% are discharged home after their admission.[1] Recent data suggest opportunities for improvement because many patients in the ED and intensive care unit (ICU) do not get optimal MV therapy for ARF.[2,3]

PATHOPHYSIOLOGY

Breathing is essential for homeostasis. In critically ill patients the demands for oxygen supply and carbon dioxide removal are often increased. This increased demand can be superimposed on prior impaired cardiopulmonary reserve. In ARF the cardiopulmonary system fails to oxygenate or ventilate adequately or inefficient breathing mechanics put excessive loads on the cardiopulmonary system. MV is used to offload respiratory muscle work and assist in oxygen delivery and ventilation.

OXYGENATION AND HYPEROXIA

Most oxygen is carried by hemoglobin molecules in red blood cells. MV is often used to correct hypoxemia (low oxygen saturation) to improve total blood oxygen content. In emergent situations it is beneficial to increase the fraction of inspired oxygen (Fio_2) to increase blood oxygen content. Increased Fio_2 should only be considered as a temporary fix because there are downsides to high concentrations of Fio_2.

First, in patients with normal lungs, supernormal Fio_2 concentrations lead to hyperoxia or a Pao_2 greater than or equal to 200.[4] Multiple studies suggest that hyperoxia leads to the formation of reactive oxygen species that can cause tissue damage.[4–8] More recent data in brain-injured patients[4,8] and patients after cardiac arrest[9] suggest worse outcomes with hyperoxia versus normal oxygen concentrations. Hyperoxia is an iatrogenic entity that can be avoided by turning the Fio_2 down.

Second, in patients with abnormal lungs, an Fio_2 of 1.0 (100%) can mask the degree of pulmonary dysfunction.[3] A normal oxygen saturation on pulse oximetry can be falsely reassuring.[3] On a Fio_2 of 1.0, a saturation of 100% may correspond with a Pao_2 of between 100 and 500, the latter being normal and the former evidence of significant respiratory dysfunction. Having a through understanding of the magnitude of pulmonary dysfunction may allow better patient care[3] because these patients may be candidates for other adjunctive therapies and lung-protective ventilation strategies (LPVS). Once stabilized and resuscitated through the peri-intubation period, dial down the Fio_2 using pulse oximetry. An oxygen saturation around 95% is sufficient and in certain conditions (chronic obstructive pulmonary disease [COPD], obesity hypoventilation syndrome, and obstructive sleep apnea) a saturation of between 88% and 92% may be more appropriate.[10] Titrating the Fio_2 helps to determine the degree of respiratory dysfunction and helps limit oxygen toxicity.

OXYGEN DELIVERY AND HEART-LUNG INTERACTIONS

Placing a critically ill patient on MV can have serious untoward effects on cardiac output (CO) and oxygen delivery and can lead to adverse events if not appropriately anticipated and managed proactively.[11] In conditions associated with high afterload, MV can be beneficial by decreasing the force opposing left ventricular contraction and left ventricular transmural wall pressure.[11] In preload-dependent states (hypovolemic and distributive shock) and diseases with right ventricular (RV) dysfunction (pulmonary embolism, pericardial tamponade, tension pneumothorax) the increase in intrathoracic pressure and RV afterload during MV can impede venous return to the right side of the heart and CO.[11] This decrease in venous return can manifest as a precipitous decrease in blood pressure and even cardiac arrest after initiation of MV. The reader is referred to recent work by Funk and colleagues[12,13] for a more detailed description of RV function and venous return. Focused bedside echocardiography assessing inferior vena cava collapsibility and RV size and function before intubation (if feasible) may clue the clinician into potential postintubation complications and direct the need for aggressive fluid resuscitation and early vasopressor support during the induction and early MV period.

HYPOXEMIA

Hypoxemia is low arterial oxygen saturation. There are multiple physiologic mechanisms for hypoxemia: hypoventilation (airway obstruction or sedative overdose), low Fio_2 or low partial pressure of O_2 (high altitude), diffusion-limited processes (interstitial lung disease), ventilation/blood flow (V/Q) mismatch (COPD), shunt (pulmonary edema), and low venous oxygen content (shock).[14] During MV, persistent hypoxemia can usually be attributed to a combination of shunt physiology and low venous admixture of blood.[15]

The cardiac and pulmonary systems match ventilation and blood flow. Shunt physiology is a V/Q mismatch in which blood passes from the right to the left side of the heart without participating in gas exchange. Desaturated venous blood mixes with oxygenated arterial blood, decreasing the overall arterial oxygen saturation. Supplemental oxygen only partially corrects hypoxemia or has no effect on systemic oxygen saturation because the shunted blood bypasses the delivered supplemental oxygen.[16]

VENTILATION AND HYPERCAPNEA

Effective MV must provide for adequate CO_2 excretion and O_2 saturation while not exposing the patient to excessive airway pressures (barotrauma) or tidal volumes (T_v) (volutrauma). The clearance of CO_2 depends on the relationship between CO_2 production and alveolar ventilation (V_a)[17]:

$$Paco_2 \approx (CO_2\ \text{production})/(V_a).$$

$$V_a = \text{minute ventilation}\ (V_m) - \text{Dead space ventilation}\ (V_{ds}).$$

The typical MV adjustment to hypercarbia is to increase the V_m by increasing the respiratory rate (RR) or T_v. In most patients this increase in V_m leads to an increase in V_a and lowering of the $Paco_2$. However, in low cardiac output states, acute respiratory distress syndrome (ARDS), advanced COPD, massive pulmonary embolism, and abdominal compartment syndromes,[17] V_{ds} can increase. In these instances, merely adjusting the set V_m may not improve CO_2 clearance if V_a does not improve. Instead, the clinician should attempt to reverse the underlying process if possible and/or attempt to decrease CO_2 production. Rechecking arterial blood gases (ABGs) after MV adjustments is important. Continuous end-tidal CO_2 monitoring ($ETco_2$) is another helpful tool for the patient needing MV but does not obviate ABGs. $ETco_2$ approximates the $Paco_2$. The difference between the $Paco_2$ and $ETco_2$ depend on V_{ds}. Therefore, it is important to obtain an ABG to correct for patient-specific relationships between the $ETco_2$ and $Paco_2$ and not rely solely on the $ETco_2$. The clinician should be cognizant of the value of the $ETco_2$ and actual V_m (not merely the set or prescribed V_m if the patient is breathing spontaneously at more than the set ventilator rate) when the ABG is drawn. A high $ETco_2$ is an assurance of a high $Paco_2$ but a low or normal $ETco_2$ can be seen with a normal $Paco_2$ or an increased $Paco_2$ in the setting of high V_{ds}. Large differences between $Paco_2$ and $ETco_2$ can be seen with excessive V_{ds} or low CO.[18] Changes in clinical condition, severity of illness, or lung mechanics should prompt the clinician to consider whether a repeat ABG is necessary to recalibrate the $ETco_2$ with the $Paco_2$.

ARDS AND LUNG-PROTECTIVE VENTILATION

ARDS was first described by Ashbaugh and colleagues[19] in 1967. They described 12 patients with a diffuse alveolar infiltrative chest radiograph pattern that manifested acute onset of tachypnea, hypoxemia, and cyanosis that was refractory to oxygen therapy. ARDS was defined in 1994,[20] and this definition was revised in 2012 (the Berlin definition[21]) to address some limitations of the earlier definition. The major changes and new ARDS criteria are as follows:

1. The term acute lung injury was eliminated and the 2-tiered model was replaced by a 3-tiered scale based on the degree of hypoxemia as measured by the Pao_2/Fio_2 (P/F) ratio: mild ($\leq$300–200 mm Hg), moderate ($\leq$200–100 mm Hg), and severe ($\leq$100 mm Hg). A minimum continuous positive airway pressure (CPAP) or positive end-expiratory pressure (PEEP) must be present.
2. Onset within 1 week of inciting event.
3. Bilateral opacities consistent with pulmonary edema that are nonhydrostatic or noncardiogenic in origin. A wedge pressure is no longer required, but the respiratory failure must not be fully explained by cardiac failure or fluid overload.[21]

The new severity scale that uses the degree of hypoxemia is the most important change to the new definition. Worsening P/F ratio predicts mortality and duration of MV in survivors and can help triage patients who may benefit from more aggressive therapies.[21]

With a few exceptions, MV is usually required in ARDS. Over the last 5 decades, it has been recognized that MV can be injurious. In the 1970s, ventilator settings were titrated to normalize blood gas values. Clinicians used T_v of 12 to 15 mL/kg of body weight.[22] Gross barotrauma in the form of pneumothorax, pneumomediastinum, and pneumoperitoneum was common, and mortality in severe ARDS was as high as 90%.[23] Work by Amato and colleagues[24] and then the landmark ARDSNet (Acute Respiratory Distress Syndrome Network)[25] trial in 2000 showed improved outcomes with low T_v ventilation strategies (4–6 mL/kg of ideal body weight [IBW]) versus higher traditional T_v (10–12 mL/kg IBW). IBW is determined by the patient's height and sex and predicts lung volume better than actual weight.

A better understanding of ventilator induced lung injury (VILI) in recent years has created a renewed impetus on providing LPVS.[26] LPVS was first shown to be beneficial in patients with ARDS but more recent data suggest that lowering the tidal volume in patients without ARDS may be beneficial.[27–30] There are 4 major theories for ventilator-induced lung injury: barotrauma, volutrauma, atelectrauma, and biotrauma.[27] Barotrauma is lung damage secondary to high airway pressure (ie, pneumothorax or pneumomediastinum). Volutrauma is injury induced by high T_v causing overdistention of alveoli. Atelectrauma is damage from the shear and strain of collapsible lung units opening and closing, and biotrauma is damage from the release of proinflammatory cytokines and immune-mediated injury that occurs when lung tissue is exposed to unphysiologic stress or strain.[26]

SELECTION OF OPTIMAL TIDAL VOLUME

The mainstays of LPVS are to (1) limit tidal volume; (2) limit end-inspiratory plateau pressure (P_{plat}); (3) provide adequate PEEP to keep the lung open and prevent alveolar collapse, and (4) limit Fio_2.[30]

The optimal T_v for patients without ARDS who require MV is not known.[30–32] Animal data suggest that normal T_v for mammals is 6.3 mL/kg.[33] Data from ARDSNet[25] as well as multiple additional trials[27–29] suggest that T_v greater than 10 mL/kg IBW is harmful. Lellouche and colleagues[27] showed a lower incidence of organ failure and shorter ICU length of stay (LOS) when using T_v less than 10 mL/kg IBW in patients having cardiac surgery. The IMPROVE[28] study group similarly showed less postoperative respiratory support, less pneumonia, and shorter hospital LOS among patients receiving low intraoperative T_v (6–8 mL/kg IBW) after abdominal surgery. In addition, Serpa Neto and colleagues[29] performed a meta-analysis of the use of LPVS with low T_v and clinical outcomes among patients without ARDS and showed less subsequent lung injury (RR, 0.33; [0.23–0.47], number needed to treat [NNT], 11), less mortality (RR, 0.64; [0.46–0.89]; NNT, 23), and shorter hospital LOS.

If using LPVS and low T_v, it is imperative that the RR is turned up to maintain an adequate V_m. Adequate V_m is especially important in the ED environment when paralytics like succinylcholine and longer acting agents like rocuronium are used for rapid sequence induction and patients are heavily sedated to facilitate management. In these instances respiratory drive is blunted and patients cannot increase their RR to compensate for low T_v. This can lead to alveolar hypoventilation, hypercarbia, and worsening acidosis. Normal V_m is approximately 100 mL/kg. This requirement is greater in critically ill patients. It is helpful to use the patients pre-intubation respiratory rate and depth of ventilation to gauge the post-intubation V_m requirements. A patient with Kussmaul breathing will need a high RR and appropriate T_v to maintain respiratory compensation for their metabolic acidosis post-intubation. Alternatively, if a patient is on Non-Invasive Ventilation (NIV) prior to intubation, post-intubation V_m can be estimated by using the V_m from the NIV respirator.

Maintaining adequate pH should be weighed against the need to provide safe MV settings and safe airway pressures. In many clinical scenarios the goal should not be to normalize blood gas values but to provide LPVS while accepting permissive hypercapnia and a mild acidosis. Some data even suggest that mild hypercapnea is protective against lung injury[30] and improves red blood cell oxygen delivery.[14] ARDSnet[25] tolerated pH levels down to 7.15. However, in certain clinical scenarios (eg, brain injury with increased intracranial pressure, toxicologic emergencies, refractory shock) an increased $Paco_2$ may not be safe. In addition, in ARDSNet, some patients required bicarbonate drips to maintain pH and the low T_v group had a mean respiratory rate of approximately 30 breaths per minute.[25] Higher respiratory rates shorten the expiratory time. In certain patient populations with increased airway resistance and obstructive lung disease this can potentially lead to air-trapping and auto-PEEP. Auto-PEEP in preload-dependent states can decrease venous return and lead to hemodynamic instability, increased vasopressor and fluid needs, and even cardiovascular collapse in severe cases.

In summary, with regard to T_v selection, in patients who meet criteria for ARDS, a low-T_v strategy that replicates the original ARDSNet trial (4–6 mL/kg IBW) should be used (Appendix 1).[3,25] In patients without ARDS, expert opinion and clinical data suggest that LPVS with a T_v of 6 to 8 mL/kg of IBW is prudent.[31] Using T_v greater than 10 mL/kg of IBW is associated with worse clinical outcomes. Whether the optimal tidal volume is 6 or 8 mL/kg is still open to debate.[32,33] When using LPVS, it is important to ensure an adequate V_m by providing an appropriate RR. ABG, in addition to pulse oximetry and $ETco_2$, should be used to ensure adequate oxygenation and ventilation.

LIMITING INSPIRATORY P_{plat}

An additional goal of LPVS is to limit airway pressure to avoid barotrauma. The inspiratory hold or P_{plat} estimates the pressure distending the alveolus. This maneuver is done by pausing the flow of air at the end of inspiration. There is no definitive safe P_{plat}.[34] In ARDS, the goal should be a P_{plat} less than 30 cm H_2O.[25] Hager and colleagues,[34] in their analysis of the ARDSNet data, saw improved outcomes with lower P_{plat} values. Whether this was causal or coincidental and whether a lower P_{plat} should be actively sought by lowering T_v is currently unclear. In obese patients or patients with stiff chest walls, P_{plat} may not accurately reflect transpulmonary pressure or the pressure distending the alveoli. In these instances it may be acceptable to tolerate higher P_{plat}.[31] In patients without ARDS, targeting a P_{plat} less than 20 cm H_2O is suggested by some experts.[31] Lowering P_{plat} is accomplished primarily by decreasing T_v but, again, acceptable (albeit not necessarily normal) $Paco_2$ and pH should be ensured. In addition to lowering T_v, providing adequate sedation to facilitate patient synchrony, adjusting PEEP to optimal levels, ensuring that auto-PEEP is not present, and ruling out pneumothorax or mucous plugging are other measures that can help lower P_{plat}.

SELECTION OF OPTIMAL PEEP AND OPEN LUNG RECRUITMENT

As stated earlier, most oxygenation problems that occur on MV are secondary to shunt physiology. Shunts are caused by pulmonary (pneumonia, pulmonary contusion, pulmonary edema, and so forth) or cardiac (patent foramen oval, atrial or ventricular septal defects) causes.

The typical treatment of hypoxemia from pulmonary shunts is to attempt to recruit collapsed lung units by increasing PEEP. The optimal PEEP settings, or even the best method to go about choosing PEEP, are controversial.[35,36] To simplify management in the ED, I recommend using the PEEP table provided by ARDSNet[37] because it has been validated and is easy to use[35] (see Appendix 1). There is no evidence favoring a high-PEEP versus a low-PEEP strategy in terms of survival, but a high-PEEP strategy has been associated with improved oxygenation.[38] PEEP goals should be reassessed if vasopressor or fluid requirements increase after increasing PEEP, P_{plat} is greater than 30 to 35 cm H_2O (depending on body habitus and clinical condition), or there is evidence of worsening tissue oxygen delivery or worsening oxygen saturation.

If increasing PEEP fails to correct oxygenation, or oxygenation worsens, it is important for the clinician to troubleshoot and not continue with treatment strategies that do not help and potentially complicate the clinical scenario. Cardiac shunts can worsen with increased PEEP because the increase in RV afterload increases right-to-left shunt.[39] Dessap and colleagues[40] in their cohort of 203 patients with ARDS found a prevalence of a moderate to large patent foramen ovale (PFO) shunt in 19.2% of their patients. These patients had a poorer P/F ratio response to PEEP and had longer ICU and ventilator days compared with their counterparts without PFO shunting. Inhaled pulmonary vasodilators and prone positioning (discussed later) may be a more appropriate treatment option in patients with PFO shunts. A transthoracic echocardiogram (or ideally transesophageal echocardiography) bubble study can help to detect cardiac shunts.

In addition, unilateral lung diseases (pneumonia, mucous plugging, pulmonary contusions, and so forth) may have a paradoxic response to increasing levels of PEEP.[41] In these situations the increased airway pressure from applied PEEP may overdistend healthy lung tissue. This will divert perfusion away from aerated lung and through the shunt worsening oxygenation. These conditions can be difficult to predict, but when a patient has worsening hypoxemia with initiation of MV (ie, after intubation) or with increasing levels of positive airway pressure, it is important for the clinician to consider these disease processes. The treatment of patients with unilateral lung shunts and cardiac shunts is different than the standard open lung recruitment strategies used in most patients with hypoxemic respiratory failure. In these infrequent instances, blindly following a PEEP/Fio_2 table is likely to worsen the clinical scenario. In these patients, limiting PEEP, prone positioning, and pulmonary vasodilators might be more effective techniques.

Fig. 1 summarizes a stepwise strategy for selection of appropriate T_V, RR, Fio_2 and PEEP. In addition to ensuring adequate Pao_2, $Paco_2$, and/or pH, every effort should be made to provide safe LPVS. **Fig. 2** summarizes a stepwise strategy for a patient with a ventilator crisis or with a failure to oxygenate or ventilate.

ADJUNCTIVE MANEUVERS

Multiple new and promising developments that focus on non-MV adjunctive treatment measures for patients with refractory ARDS and respiratory failure have recently been

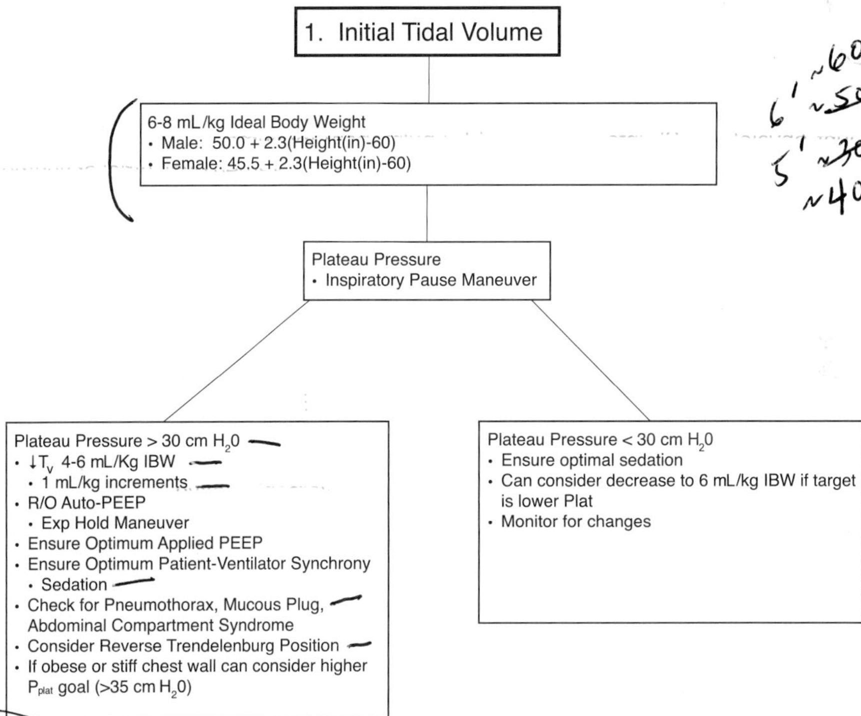

Fig. 1. Algorithm for initiating initial MV settings in the ED. (*Ventilator Waveform from* Santanilla JI, Daniel B, Yeow ME. Mechanical ventilation. Emerg Med Clin N Am 2008;26:849–62. *PEEP table modified from* Haas CF. Lung protective mechanical ventilation in acute respiratory distress syndrome. Respir Care Clin N Am 2003;9(3):363–96. *Adapted from* The Acute Respiratory Distress Syndrome Network. Ventilation with lower tidal volumes compared with traditional tidal volumes for acute lung injury and the acute respiratory distress syndrome. N Engl J Med 2000;342:1301–8 and Slutsky AS, Ranieri VM. Ventilator-induced lung injury. N Engl J Med 2013;369:2126–36.)

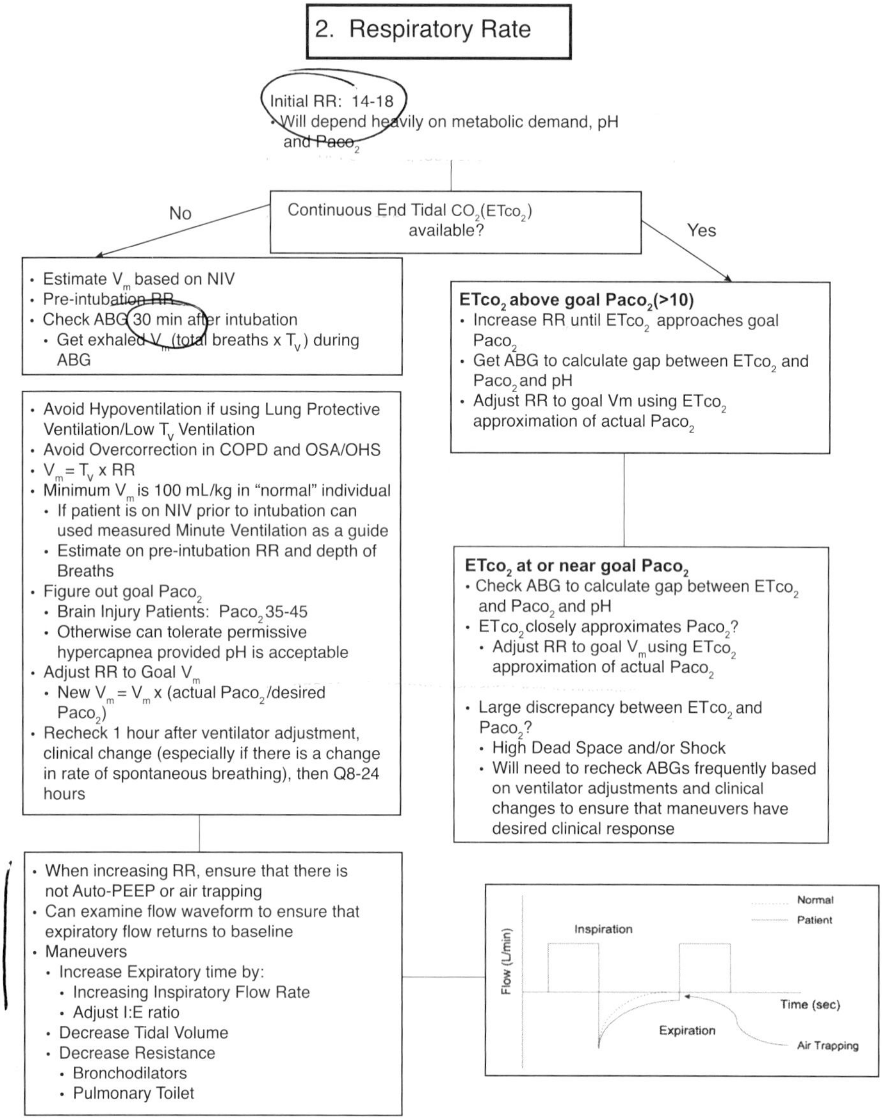

Fig. 1. (*continued*)

developed. These treatments may find a role in the EM management of ARDS and severe respiratory failure. Further information on each can be found in references.[38,42,43]

NEUROMUSCULAR BLOCKING AGENTS

Neuromuscular blocking agents (NMBAs) are used in patients with severe respiratory failure to facilitate ventilator synchrony.[44] A patient who is bucking the ventilator can be exposed to barotrauma, volutrauma from breath stacking, and other serious complications (eg, tube dislodgment). NMBAs have been used to facilitate ventilator synchrony and are associated with improvements in P/F ratio.[31] The rational for this benefit is not fully clear because NMBAs seem to help even in patients who do not

3. Fraction of Inspired Oxygen (Fio_2)

- If acceptable pulse oximetry waveform is present titrate down to lowest possible Fio_2 required for goal Oxygen Saturation (> 95%)
  - COPD, OSA/OHS: 88-92%
- If no lung pathology (ie intubated for airway protection) can do rapidly
- Otherwise ≈ ↓10% Q 10 minutes
- Get ABG to confirm once at goal
- If you can't get Fio_2 less than 50%, see PEEP table below
  - Consider ARDS and other causes of Shunt Physiology and Severe Respiratory Failure

4. Positive End Expiratory Pressure

- Ensure patient is volume resuscitated and monitored
- Adjust PEEP per table to lowest Fio_2 and PEEP value to maintain adequate Spo_2
- Monitor for appropriate response
  - If paradoxical response, ie Oxygen Saturation drops with higher PEEP or initiation of MV consider cardiac shunts and unilateral lung disease and shunt
    - Chest xray and/or Lung US
    - ECHO bubble study
    - Decrease PEEP and consider other treatments for hypoxemia
- If PEEP > 8 is needed consider ARDS and other causes of Shunt Physiology and Severe Respiratory Failure

Fio_2	0.3	0.4	0.4	0.5	0.5	0.6	0.7	0.7	0.7	0.8	0.9	0.9	0.9	1.0
PEEP	5	5	8	8	10	10	10	12	14	14	14	16	18	18-24

Fig. 1. (*continued*)

have ventilator dysynchrony.[31] However, concern for ICU-acquired weakness has limited the use of NMBAs, especially in patients receiving steroids.[44] The ACURASYS study,[45] a multicenter trial, recently assessed the use of cisatracurium in the early management (6–29 hours from diagnosis) of patients with severe ARDS (P/F ratio <150) and showed an improvement in 90-day mortality (hazard ratio, 0.68; confidence interval, 0.48–0.98). The incidence of ICU-acquired weakness did not differ between the two groups.[45] EM physician familiarity with NMBA and the early timing of intervention make this a promising study for the ED; however, it is important to ensure that the patient is adequately sedated before initiating NMBA because it is challenging to assess the level of sedation in a paralyzed patient.

INHALED PULMONARY VASODILATORS

Inhaled nitric oxide (INO) and inhaled prostacyclin (IP) are the inhaled pulmonary vasodilators (IPVs) currently used for salvage therapy in refractory hypoxemia. The

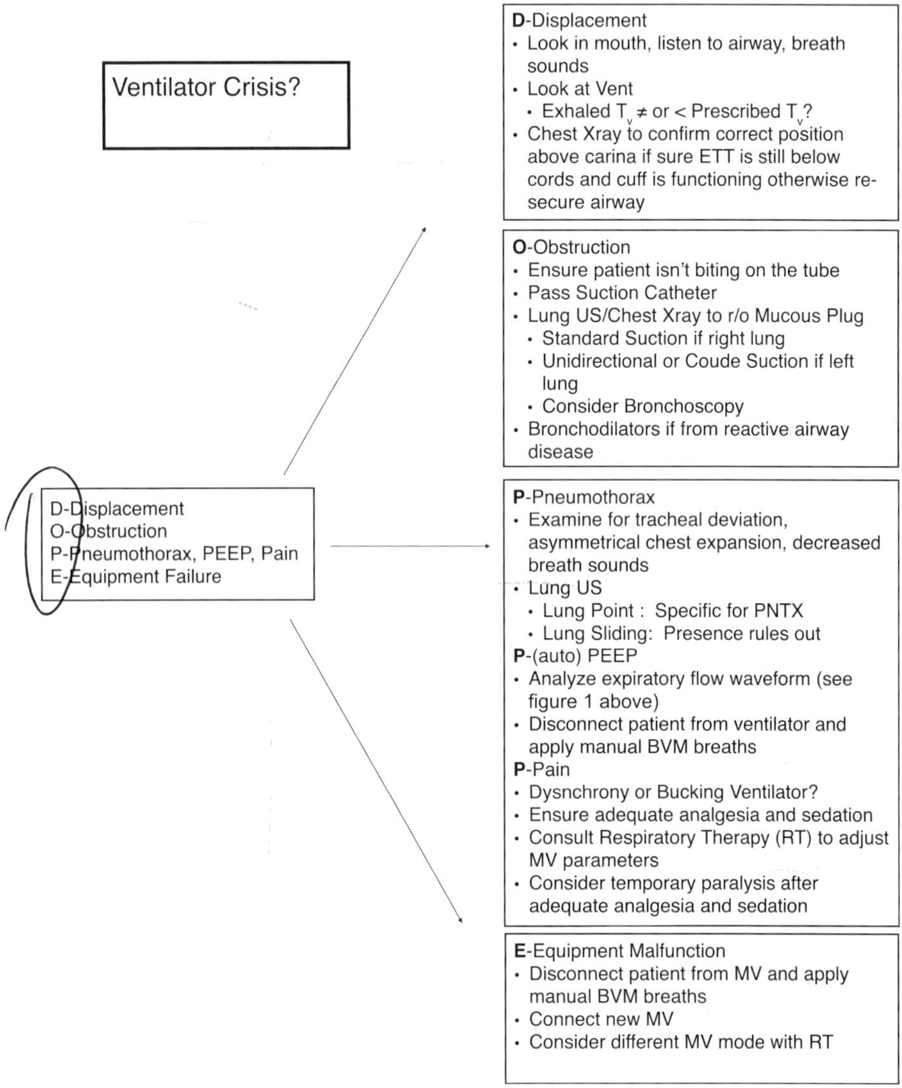

Fig. 2. An algorithm for an approach to the crashing patient on MV. (*Adapted from* Diaz JV, Brower R, Calfee CS, et al. Therapeutic strategies for severe acute lung injury. Crit Care Med 2010;38(8):1646–48.)

reader is encouraged to read a more in-depth review from the clinics series.[46] IPVs work by improving blood flow to ventilated lung units and decreasing shunt magnitude. In many cases this leads to an improvement, albeit transient (24–96 hours), in oxygenation.[42,43,46]

In addition to better V/Q matching, IPV may be beneficial in patients with acute right heart failure (ie, pulmonary embolism) and right-to-left cardiac shunts. **Fig. 2** shows how to titrate INO and IP. The major benefit of IP compared with INO is cost: $275/d versus $3000/d.[46] Tachyphylaxis can occur with both so the lowest effective dose should be used. The beneficial effects should be seen immediately. INO has been

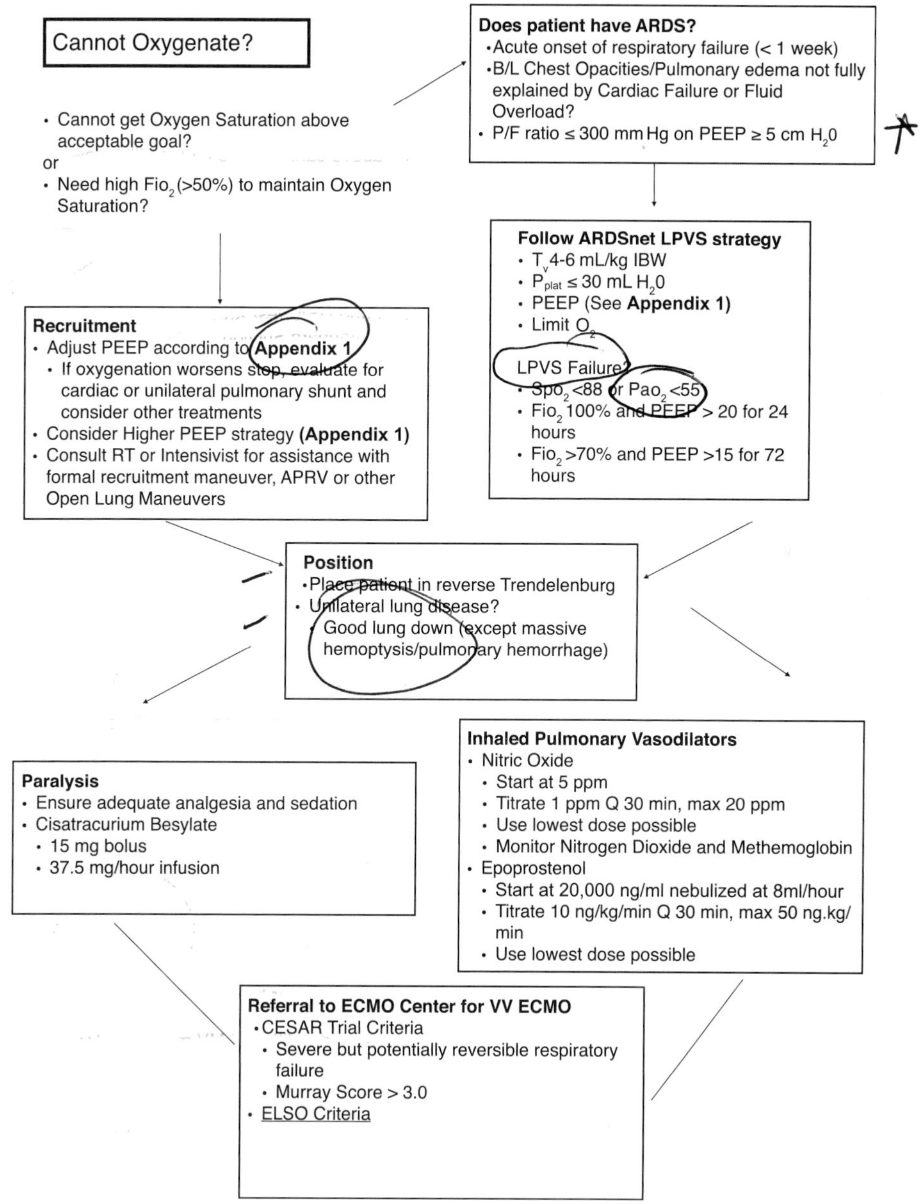

Fig. 2. (*continued*)

more extensively studied for refractory hypoxemia than IP.[42,46] Daily blood methemoglobin and inhaled nitrogen dioxide levels should be checked with INO because these byproducts are toxic.[42,43] IP has a longer half-life than INO so there is a theoretic risk of systemic hypotension from nonselective vasodilation, although this has not been shown in small studies of patients with ARDS.[47,48] Neither medication is US Food and Drug Administration approved for treatment of hypoxemia,[46] and neither medication is associated with improved mortality. However, if faced with refractory

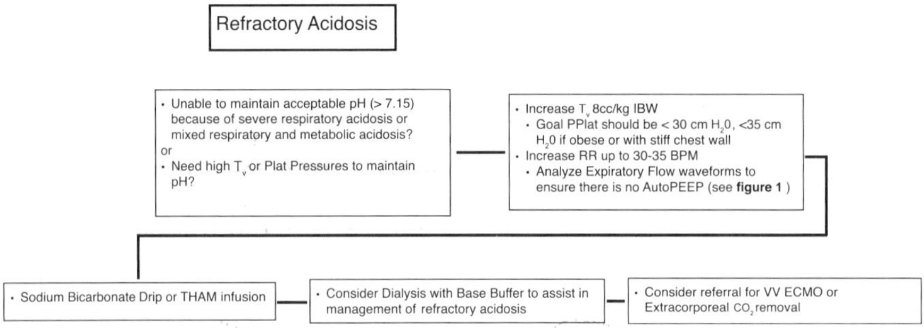

Fig. 2. (*continued*)

hypoxemia, INO and IP can be considered as salvage therapy while planning other interventions (see **Fig. 2**).

PRONE POSITIONING

Prone positioning (PP) involves rotating the patient from the standard supine position to a face-down or prone position. When supine, the inferior and posterior portions of the lung can become atelectatic from compression by the heart, thorax, and diaphragm. Atelectasis can worsen gas exchange, decrease compliance, and increase the risk for volutrauma because the T_V prescribed is now directed to a smaller lung volume. PP in some individuals allows reexpansion of these posterior lung units. Previous data have suggested that PP improved oxygenation and P/F ratio, but did not necessarily improve outcomes across all patients with ARDS.[49–51] However, a trend toward improved survival was seen in the sickest patient with ARDS.[52]

Recent data by the PROSEVA group[53] examined PP in severe ARDS (P/F ratio <150 mm Hg) and found a reduction in 28-day mortality (16.0% vs 32.8%) and no increase in complications in the prone group. The investigators who participated in this trial had significant experience with PP that potentially minimized complications (airway and central line dislodgment, pressure ulcers). They also required a stabilization period of 12 to 24 hours before PP was attempted.

If considering PP, appropriate staff (especially nursing) should be available. If the ICU has experience with this technique they should be consulted for assistance. The reader is encouraged to refer to these practical resources on the logistics of PP and for additional information on indications and contraindications.[53–55] In ED patients with difficult oxygenation, a trial of reverse Trendelenburg or placing the good lung down (provided there is not massive pulmonary hemorrhage) can be attempted.

EXTRACORPOREAL MEMBRANE OXYGENATION

The use of venovenous extracorporeal membrane oxygenation (ECMO) in severe ARDS and refractory hypercarbic respiratory failure has gained renewed interest after recent encouraging data from the United Kingdom[56] and from experience with ARDS during the 2009 H1N1 pandemic.[57] Work from the late twentieth century showed dismal survival[23] and no benefit in patients with ARDS treated with ECMO[58] but improvements in technology have made this a potential modality for severe ARDS.

ECMO has risks and costs so only the sickest patients with potentially reversible lung injury should be considered for this treatment. The Extracorporeal Life Support Organization (ELSO) has guidelines for consideration of ECMO in respiratory failure that can be viewed online (http://elso.org/resources/guidelines).[59] ECMO has risks and costs so only the sickest patients with potentially reversible lung injury should be considered for this treatment. Indications for VV ECMO include: failure to oxygenate, severe CO_2 retention or the ability maintain acceptable CO_2 levels at unsafe airway pressures (PPlat <30 cm H_2O) or severe air leak syndromes.[59]

The CESAR trial[56] is the major trial to date showing the potential benefit of ECMO in ARDS. A controversy surrounding the study is that some of the benefits found in the CESAR trial might be secondary to treatment of ARDS in a high-volume center with experience in providing best-evidence medicine (ie LPVS) to patients with ARDS and not necessarily related solely to treatment with ECMO.[60]

Current expert opinion suggests that clinicians consider referral of adult patients with severe ARDS or severe respiratory failure with high risk of mortality, as defined by CESAR[56] entry criteria or ELSO guidelines,[59] to an ARDS center with ECMO capabilities if available. Prolonged treatment with unacceptable MV strategies (high Fio_2 or P_{plat}) is a contraindication so these patients should be referred early in the disease process.

The main adverse events associated with ECMO are bleeding, hemolysis, disseminated intravascular coagulation, and infection. In addition, there is significant financial cost associated with ECMO.[56,60]

SUMMARY

Respiratory failure is a frequent disease process encountered in the ED. Better care can lead to better outcomes for patients on MV.[61] If not contraindicated, LPVS should be used. It is important to consider disease pathophysiology when formulating treatment strategies in patients that are difficult to oxygenate or ventilate, or when Pao_2, $PaCo_2$, and pH can only be maintained with unsafe ventilator settings. If MV adjustments do not produce the expected clinical outcome then different treatment strategies should be considered. There are multiple adjunctive therapies for ARDS and severe respiratory failure. Some strategies are straightforward and can potentially be applied in the ED (IPV for refractory hypoxemia or NMBA for severe ARDS), whereas other treatments require a collaborative multidisciplinary approach and the assistance of other health care providers (PP and referral to ECMO-capable ARDS centers). Preemptively developing multidisciplinary treatment protocols assists in treating this complicated patient population.

REFERENCES

1. Wunsch H, Linde-Zwirble WT, Angus DC, et al. The epidemiology of mechanical ventilation use in the United States. Crit Care Med 2010;38:1947–53.
2. Fuller BM, Mohr NM, Dettmer M, et al. Mechanical ventilation and acute lung injury in emergency department patients with severe sepsis and septic shock: an observational study. Acad Emerg Med 2013;20(7):659–69.
3. Manoach S. Mechanical ventilation in the emergency department: a call to action in a resource-constrained era. Acad Emerg Med 2013;20(7):746–8.
4. Brenner M, Stein D, Hu P, et al. Association between early hyperoxia and worse outcomes after traumatic brain injury. Arch Surg 2012;147(11):1042–6.
5. Davis WB, Rennard SI, Bitterman PB, et al. Pulmonary oxygen toxicity: early reversible changes in human alveolar structures induced by hyperoxia. N Engl J Med 1983;309(15):878–83.
6. Kistler GS, Caldwell PR, Weibel ER. Development of fine structural damage to alveolar and capillary lining cells in oxygen-poisoned rat lungs. J Cell Biol 1967;32(3):605–28.

7. Yusa T, Beckman JS, Crapo JD, et al. Hyperoxia increases H_2O_2 production by brain in vivo. J Appl Physiol (1985) 1987;63:353–8.
8. Rincon F, Kang J, Maltenfort M, et al. Association between hyperoxia and mortality after stroke: a multicenter cohort study. Crit Care Med 2014;42(2):387–96.
9. Kilgannon JH, Jones AE, Shapiro NI, et al, Emergency Medicine Shock Research Network (EMShockNet) Investigators. Association between arterial hyperoxia following resuscitation from cardiac arrest and in-hospital mortality. JAMA 2010;303:2165–71.
10. O'Driscoll R. Emergency oxygen use. BMJ 2012;345:e6856.
11. Feihl F, Broccard AF. Interactions between respiration and systemic hemodynamics. Part II: practical implications in critical care. Intensive Care Med 2009;35(2):198.
12. Funk DJ, Jacobsohn E, Kumar A. The role of venous return in critical illness and shock—part I: physiology. Crit Care Med 2013;41(1):255–62.
13. Funk DJ, Jacobsohn E, Kumar A. Role of the venous return in critical illness and shock: part II—shock and mechanical ventilation. Crit Care Med 2013;41(2): 573–9.
14. West JB. Pulmonary pathophysiology, the essentials. 7th edition. Philadelphia: Lippincott Williams & Wilkins; 2005.
15. Takala J. Hypoxemia due to increased venous admixture: influence of cardiac output on oxygenation. In: Pinsky MR, Brochard L, Mancebo J, et al, editors. Applied physiology in intensive care medicine 1. Berlin Heidelberg (Germany): Springer; 2012. p. 67–70.
16. Budinger GS, Mutlu GM. Balancing the risks and benefits of oxygen therapy in critically Ill adults. Chest 2013;143(4):1151–62.
17. Schwartzstein RM, Parker MJ. Rising Pa_{CO_2} in the ICU: using a physiologic approach to avoid cognitive biases. Chest 2011;140(6):1638–42.
18. Frankenfield DC, Alam S, Bekteshi E, et al. Predicting dead space ventilation in critically ill patients using clinically available data. Crit Care Med 2010;38(1): 288–91.
19. Ashbaugh DG, Bigelow DB, Petty TL, et al. Acute respiratory distress in adults. Lancet 1967;2(7511):319–23.
20. Bernard GR, Artigas A, Brigham KL, et al. The American-European Consensus Conference on ARDS: definitions, mechanisms, relevant outcomes, and clinical trial coordination. Am J Respir Crit Care Med 1994;149(3 pt 1):818–24.
21. The ARDS Definition Task Force. Acute respiratory distress syndrome. JAMA 2012;307(23):2526–33.
22. Gattinoni L, Vagginelli F, Chiumello D, et al. Physiologic rationale for ventilator setting in acute lung injury/acute respiratory distress syndrome patients. Crit Care Med 2003;31(4 Suppl):S300–4.
23. Zapol WM, Snider MT, Hill JD, et al. Extracorporeal membrane oxygenation in severe acute respiratory failure. A randomized prospective study. JAMA 1979; 242(20):2193–6.
24. Amato MB, Barbas CS, Medeiros DM, et al. Effect of a protective-ventilation strategy on mortality in the acute respiratory distress syndrome. N Engl J Med 1998;338:347–54.
25. The Acute Respiratory Distress Syndrome Network. Ventilation with lower tidal volumes as compared with traditional tidal volumes for acute lung injury and the acute respiratory distress syndrome. N Engl J Med 2000;342:1301–8.
26. Gattinoni L, Protti A, Caironi P, et al. Ventilator-induced lung injury: the anatomical and physiological framework. Crit Care Med 2010;38(10 Suppl):S539–48.

27. Lellouche F, Dionne S, Simard S, et al. High tidal volumes in mechanically ventilated patients increase organ dysfunction after cardiac surgery. Anesthesiology 2012;116(5):1072–82.
28. Futier E, Constantin J-M, Paugam-Burtz C, et al. A trial of intraoperative low-tidal-volume ventilation in abdominal surgery. N Engl J Med 2013;369:428–37.
29. Serpa Neto A, Cardoso SO, Manetta JA, et al. Association between use of lung-protective ventilation with lower tidal volumes and clinical outcomes among patients without acute respiratory distress syndrome: a meta-analysis. JAMA 2012; 308:1651–9.
30. Sinclair SE, Kregenow DA, Lamm WJ, et al. Hypercapnic acidosis is protective in an in vivo model of ventilator-induced lung injury. Am J Respir Crit Care Med 2002;166(3):403–8.
31. Slutsky AS, Ranieri VM. Ventilator-induced lung injury. N Engl J Med 2013;369: 2126–36.
32. Mohr NM, Fuller BM. Low tidal volume ventilation should be the routine ventilation strategy of choice for all emergency department patients. Ann Emerg Med 2012;60(2):215–6.
33. Wright B, Slesinger TL. Low tidal volume should not routinely by used for emergency department patients requiring mechanical ventilation. Ann Emerg Med 2012;60(2):216–7.
34. Hager DN, Krishnan JA, Hayden DL, et al, ARDS Clinical Trials Network. Tidal volume reduction in patients with acute lung injury when plateau pressures are not high. Am J Respir Crit Care Med 2005;172(10):1241.
35. Miller RR, MacIntyre NR, Hite RD, et al. Chest 2012;141(6):1379–82.
36. Schmidt GA. Counterpoint: should positive end-expiratory pressure in patients with ARDS be set based on oxygenation? No. Chest 2012;141(6):1382–4.
37. Available at: http://www.ardsnet.org/system/files/Ventilator Protocol Card.pdf. Accessed on August 22, 2014.
38. Esan A, Hess DR, Raoof S, et al. Severe hypoxemic respiratory failure part 1–ventilatory strategies. Chest 2010;137(5):1203–16.
39. Michard F, Alaya S, Medkour F. Monitoring right-to-left intracardiac shunt in acute respiratory distress syndrome. Crit Care Med 2004;32(1):308–9.
40. Dessap AM, Boissier F, Leon R, et al. Prevalence and prognosis of shunting across patent foramen ovale during acute respiratory distress syndrome. Crit Care Med 2010;38(9):1786–92.
41. Broccard A. Challenges of mechanical ventilation in unilateral pneumonia: is PEEP the answer? Intensive Care Med 2004;30(4):530–2.
42. Raoof S, Goulet K, Esan A, et al. Severe hypoxemic respiratory failure part 2—nonventilatory strategies. Chest 2010;137(6):1437–48.
43. Diaz JV, Brower R, Calfee CS, et al. Therapeutic strategies for severe acute lung injury. Crit Care Med 2010;38(8):1644–50.
44. Puthucheary Z, Rawal J, Ratnayake G, et al. Neuromuscular blockade and skeletal muscle weakness in critically ill patients: time to rethink the evidence? Am J Respir Crit Care Med 2012;185(9):911–7.
45. Papazian L, Forel JM, Gacouin A, et al. Neuromuscular blockers in early acute respiratory distress syndrome. N Engl J Med 2010;363:1107–16.
46. Puri N, Dellinger RP. Inhaled nitric oxide and inhaled prostacyclin in acute respiratory distress syndrome: what is the evidence? Crit Care Clin 2011;27(3): 561–87.
47. van Heerden PV, Barden A, Michalopoulos N, et al. Dose-response to inhaled aerosolized prostacyclin for hypoxemia due to ARDS. Chest 2000;117(3):819–27.

48. Zwissler B, Kemming G, Habler O, et al. Inhaled prostacyclin (PGI2) versus inhaled nitric oxide in adult respiratory distress syndrome. Am J Respir Crit Care Med 1996;154(6):1671–7.
49. Gattinoni L, Tognoni G, Pesenti A, et al. Effect of prone positioning on the survival of patients with acute respiratory failure. N Engl J Med 2001;345:568–73.
50. Sud S, Sud M, Friedrich JO, et al. Effect of mechanical ventilation in the prone position on clinical outcomes in patients with acute hypoxemic respiratory failure: a systematic review and meta-analysis. CMAJ 2008;178(8):1153–61.
51. Taccone P, Pesenti A, Latini R, et al. Prone positioning in patients with moderate and severe acute respiratory distress syndrome: a randomized controlled trial. JAMA 2009;302:1977–84.
52. Gattinoni L, Carlesso E, Taccone P, et al. Prone positioning improves survival in severe ARDS: a pathophysiologic review and individual patient meta-analysis. Minerva Anestesiol 2010;76(6):448–54.
53. Guérin C, Reignier J, Richard JC, et al. Prone positioning in severe acute respiratory distress syndrome. N Engl J Med 2013;368(23):2159–68.
54. Messerole E, Peine P, Wittkopp S, et al. The pragmatics of prone positioning. Am J Respir Crit Care Med 2002;165(10):1359–63.
55. Gattinoni L, Taccone P, Carlesso E, et al. Prone position in acute respiratory distress syndrome: rationale, indications and limits. Am J Respir Crit Care Med 2013;188(11):1286–93.
56. Peek GJ, Mugford M, Tiruvoipati R, et al. Efficacy and economic assessment of conventional ventilatory support versus extracorporeal membrane oxygenation for severe adult respiratory failure (CESAR): a multicentre randomised controlled trial. Lancet 2009;374(9698):1351–63.
57. Davies A, Jones D, Bailey M, et al. Extracorporeal membrane oxygenation for 2009 influenza A (H1N1) acute respiratory distress syndrome. JAMA 2009; 302(17):1888–95.
58. Morris AH, Wallace CJ, Menlove RL, et al. Randomized clinical trial of pressure-controlled inverse ratio ventilation and extracorporeal CO_2 removal for adult respiratory distress syndrome. Am J Respir Crit Care Med 1994;149(2 Pt 1): 295–305.
59. Available at: http://elso.org/resources/guidelines. Accessed on August 22, 2014.
60. Wallace DJ, Milbrandt EB, Boujoukos A. Ave, CESAR, morituri te salutant! (Hail, CESAR, those who are about to die salute you!). Crit Care 2010;14(2):308.
61. Fuller BM, Mohr NM, Hotchkiss RS, et al. Reducing the burden of acute respiratory distress syndrome: the case for early intervention and the potential role of the emergency department. Shock 2014;41(5):378–87.

APPENDIX 1

ARDSnet

NIH NHLBI ARDS Clinical Network
Mechanical Ventilation Protocol Summary

INCLUSION CRITERIA: Acute onset of

1. $Pao_2/Fio_2 \leq 300$ (corrected for altitude)
2. Bilateral (patchy, diffuse, or homogeneous) infiltrates consistent with pulmonary edema
3. No clinical evidence of left atrial hypertension

PART I: VENTILATOR SETUP AND ADJUSTMENT

1. Calculate predicted body weight (PBW)
   Males = 50 + 2.3 [height (inches) - 60]
   Females = 45.5 + 2.3 [height (inches) -60]
2. Select any ventilator mode
3. Set ventilator settings to achieve initial V_T = 8 mL/kg PBW
4. Reduce V_T by 1 mL/kg at intervals ≤ 2 hours until V_T = 6mL/kg PBW.
5. Set initial rate to approximate baseline minute ventilation (not > 35 bpm).
6. Adjust V_T and RR to achieve pH and plateau pressure goals below.

pH GOAL: 7.30-7.45

Acidosis Management: (pH < 7.30)

If pH 7.15-7.30: Increase RR until pH > 7.30 or $PaCo_2$ < 25 (Maximum set RR = 35).

If pH < 7.15: Increase RR to 35.
If pH remains < 7.15, V_T may be increased in 1 mL/kg steps until pH > 7.15 (Pplat target of 30 may be exceeded).
May give $NaHCO_3$

Alkalosis Management: (pH > 7.45) Decrease vent rate if possible.

I: E RATIO GOAL: Recommend that duration of inspiration be ≤ duration of expiration.

PART II: WEANING

A. Conduct a SPONTANEOUS BREATHING TRIAL daily when:

1. $Fio_2 \leq 0.40$ and PEEP ≤ 8.
2. PEEP and Fio_2 ≤ values of previous day.
3. Patient has acceptable spontaneous breathing efforts. (May decrease vent rate by 50% for 5 minutes to detect effort.)
4. Systolic BP ≥ 90 mm Hg without vasopressor support.
5. No neuromuscular blocking agents or blockade.

OXYGENATION GOAL: Pao_2 55-80 mmHg or SpO_2 88-95%
Use a minimum PEEP of 5 cm H_2O. Consider use of incremental Fio_2/PEEP combinations such as shown below (not required) to achieve goal.

Lower PEEP/higher Fio_2

Fio_2	0.3	0.4	0.4	0.5	0.5	0.6	0.7	0.7
PEEP	5	5	8	8	10	10	10	12

Fio_2	0.7	0.8	0.9	0.9	0.9	1.0
PEEP	14	14	14	16	18	18-24

Higher PEEP/lower Fio_2

Fio_2	0.3	0.3	0.3	0.3	0.3	0.4	0.4	0.5
PEEP	5	8	10	12	14	14	16	16

Fio_2	0.5	0.5-0.8	0.8	0.9	1.0	1.0
PEEP	18	20	22	22	22	24

PLATEAU PRESSURE GOAL: ≤ 30 cm H_2O
Check Pplat (0.5 second inspiratory pause), at least q 4h and after each change in PEEP or V_T.
If Pplat > 30 cm H_2O: decrease V_T by 1mL/kg steps (minimum = 4 mL/kg).
If Pplat < 25 cm H_2O and V_T< 6 mL/kg, increase V_T by 1 mL/kg until Pplat > 25 cm H_2O or V_T = 6 mL/kg.
If Pplat < 30 and breath stacking or dys-synchrony occurs: may increase V_T in 1mL/kg increments to 7 or 8 mL/kg if Pplat remains ≤ 30 cm H_2O.

B. SPONTANEOUS BREATHING TRIAL (SBT):
If all above criteria are met and subject has been in the study for at least 12 hours, initiate a trial of UP TO 120 minutes of spontaneous breathing with Fio_2 ≤ 0.5 and PEEP ≤ 5:

1. Place on T-piece, trach collar, or CPAP ≤ 5 cm H_2O with PS ≤ 5
2. Assess for tolerance as below for up to two hours.
   a. SpO_2 ≥ 90: and/or Pao_2 ≥ 60 mm Hg
   b. Spontaneous V_T ≥ 4 mL/kg PBW
   c. RR ≤ 35/min
   d. pH ≥ 7.3
   e. No respiratory distress (distress= 2 or more)
      - HR > 120% of baseline
      - Marked accessory muscle use
      - Abdominal paradox
      - Diaphoresis
      - Marked dyspnea
3. If tolerated for at least 30 minutes, consider extubation.
4. If not tolerated resume pre-weaning settings.

Definition of UNASSISTED BREATHING
(Different from the spontaneous breathing criteria as PS is not allowed)

1. Extubated with face mask, nasal prong oxygen, or room air, OR
2. T-tube breathing, OR
3. Tracheostomy mask breathing, OR
4. CPAP less than or equal to 5 cm H_2O **without pressure support or IMV assistance.**

Neurotrauma

Wan-Tsu W. Chang, MD[a], Neeraj Badjatia, MD, MSc[b,c,d,*]

KEYWORDS

• Neurotrauma • Traumatic brain injury • Traumatic spinal cord injury
• Neuroprotection • Neurocritical care

KEY POINTS

- Resuscitation of the patient with neurotrauma is focused on prevention of secondary injuries. Hypoxia and hypotension are associated with increased morbidity and mortality.
- Management of suspected intracranial hypertension follows a tiered approach. Hyperventilation should only be used transiently in an acute herniation syndrome as a bridge to more definitive therapy.
- The use of steroids for traumatic brain injury and traumatic spinal cord injury is not recommended.
- Care of the critically ill patient with neurologic injury by specialized neurocritical care teams has been shown to reduce hospital length of stay and in-hospital mortality.

INTRODUCTION

Injuries to the central nervous system (the brain and spinal cord) are a heterogeneous group of pathologic disorders. They can be categorized by mechanisms of injury, clinical severity, radiological appearance, or anatomic distribution. Neurologic injury from trauma not only results from the initial physical insult but also continues to occur in the ensuing hours or days. Prevention of primary neurologic injury from trauma is the focus of public health efforts such as the use of helmets and seatbelts. A major component in the management of patients with neurotrauma is the prevention of secondary injury such as ischemia and hypoxia. This article reviews common neurologic injuries associated with trauma, considerations in the critical care management of these patients, and the evidence behind current treatment therapies.

The authors have nothing to disclose.

[a] Department of Emergency Medicine, University of Maryland School of Medicine, 110 South Paca Street, 6th Floor, Suite 200, Baltimore, MD 21201, USA; [b] Department of Neurology, University of Maryland School of Medicine, 110 South Paca Street, 3rd Floor, 072, Baltimore, MD 21201, USA; [c] Department of Anesthesiology, University of Maryland School of Medicine, Baltimore, MD, USA; [d] Department of Neurosurgery, University of Maryland School of Medicine, Baltimore, MD, USA

* Corresponding author. Department of Neurology, University of Maryland School of Medicine, 22 South Greene Street G718, Baltimore, MD 21201.

E-mail address: nbadjatia@som.umaryland.edu

Emerg Med Clin N Am 32 (2014) 889–905
http://dx.doi.org/10.1016/j.emc.2014.07.008 emed.theclinics.com
0733-8627/14/$ – see front matter

EPIDEMIOLOGY

Neurotrauma is a critical public health problem. Injuries remain a leading cause of death worldwide. In the United States, traumatic brain injury (TBI) contributes to nearly one-third of all injury-related deaths.[1] More than 1.3 million US emergency department visits annually are related to TBI, accounting for 4.8% of injury-related visits and 1.4% of all visits. Leading causes of TBI are falls (35.2%), motor vehicle–related injuries (17.3%), blunt impact (16.5%), and assaults (10%).[1] The incidence of blast injury in the US civilian population is low, with a report of 0.2% in a major urban trauma center. However, TBI has been associated in up to one-third of blast injuries.[2] Young children (aged <5 years), adolescents (aged 15–19 years), and the elderly (aged ≥75 years) have higher rates of TBI.[1] Although there has been a decrease in TBI-related deaths, likely reflecting preventive measures such as seat belt and helmet use, at least 3.2 million Americans live with long-term disabilities as a result of TBI.[3] The annual cost of TBI in the United States is estimated at $76.5 billion, including direct medical and rehabilitation costs and indirect societal economic costs.[4]

Traumatic spinal cord injury (SCI) is a rare but potentially severe injury that primarily affects young adults and male patients. Nearly half of all injuries occur between the ages of 16 and 30 years and 80.7% of injuries reported to the national database were in male patients. Leading causes of traumatic SCI are motor vehicle–related injuries (36.5%), falls (28.5%), and acts of violence (14.3%). Despite advances made in early recognition and treatment, less than 1% of patients experience complete neurologic recovery by hospital discharge.[5,6]

COMMON NEUROLOGIC INJURIES ASSOCIATED WITH TRAUMA

Head Injury

Blunt injury

Direct blunt impact of the head results in acceleration and deceleration of the brain within the cranial vault. These mechanical forces cause tissue compression, distortion, and shearing, resulting in parenchymal contusions, extra-axial hematomas, and diffuse axonal injury. Common patterns of brain injury seen with blunt trauma are described in **Table 1**.

Table 1
Common brain injury patterns with blunt trauma

	Pathophysiology	Typical Locations	Characteristics
Parenchymal contusions	Coup/contrecoup injury	Orbitofrontal Anterior temporal	One-third expand within 24 h after injury
Epidural hematoma	Injury to middle meningeal artery, middle meningeal vein, diploic veins, or venous sinuses	Adjacent to skull fracture	Convex (lens shaped) Does not cross skull suture lines
Subdural hematoma	Injury of bridging veins	Cerebral convexities Along tentorium or falx	Concave (crescent shaped) Crosses skull suture lines
Subarachnoid hemorrhage	Injury of pial vessels	Cerebral convexities Basal cistern Ventricles	Can be confined to few sulci and fissures or diffuse
Diffuse axonal injury	Shear injury of axons	Junction between cortex and white matter Midline white matter structures	Axonal swelling with ultimate axotomy

Penetrating injury

Penetrating TBI is less common than blunt TBI but is associated with worse prognosis, with only 9% survival reported in a statewide registry.[7] Most civilian penetrating head injury is caused by firearm injuries. As a projectile penetrates the brain, it lacerates the parenchyma. In the wake of the projectile, tissue compression and expansion in a wavelike pattern cause further tissue injury. The degree of injury depends on the kinetic energy transferred from the projectile to the surrounding tissue; therefore, higher velocity projectiles cause more injury than lower velocity projectiles.

Blast injury

Blast TBI is observed primarily in soldiers exposed to improvised explosive devices. However, any explosion can be associated with transmission of energy through the cranium and blood vessels to the brain. Malignant cerebral edema may occur rapidly (within an hour), as opposed to the more slowly developing edema seen in blunt TBI (hours to days). Cerebral vasospasm may occur in up to 50% of blast TBI. Concomitant blast injuries to the eyes and to the auditory and vestibular systems are often seen.[8]

SCI

Blunt injury

Blunt SCI occurs as a result of cord compression, distraction, or shearing by disc herniation, vertebral fracture, or subluxation. Compromise of the spinal canal also contributes to impedance of blood flow through the spinal arteries, leading to further oligemia and ischemia. Because of the mechanisms of injury, concomitant injuries to the head, chest, and abdomen are common.

Penetrating injury

Penetrating trauma can cause laceration and transection of the spinal cord. Although rare, cervical and thoracic spine is more commonly affected.

Vascular Injury

The incidence of vascular injuries associated with neurotrauma is likely underreported because vascular imaging is usually performed only when injury is suspected. When a liberal screening protocol was implemented at a level I trauma center, an incidence of 1.2% was found.[9] Blunt injuries to the extracranial carotid and vertebral arteries may present with late-onset ischemic strokes. Vertebral artery injury may be common in patients with concomitant cervical spine trauma, although no specific cervical vertebral fracture pattern has a higher association with blunt vertebral artery injury.

Secondary Injuries

Neurotrauma initiates cellular and molecular cascades that exacerbate edema and ischemia, as well as promoting cell death. Many mechanisms underlying these pathways have been studied but no neuroprotection panacea has been found. Cerebral ischemia, intracranial hypertension, systemic hypotension, hypoxia, fever, hypocapnia, and hypoglycemia have all been shown to independently worsen survival after blunt TBI.[10] Coagulopathy associated with TBI may exacerbate ischemic brain injury through microvascular thrombosis and embolism.[11] In traumatic spinal cord injuries, ischemia, inflammation, free radicals, and excitotoxicity similarly contribute to necrotic and apoptotic neuronal death.[12] A large component in the management of patients with neurotrauma is the prevention and reduction of secondary injuries.

GENERAL APPROACH AND RESUSCITATION STRATEGIES FOR THE PATIENT WITH NEUROTRAUMA

Airway, Breathing, and Circulation

Initial management of a patient with neurotrauma should be focused on the assessment and stabilization of the airway, breathing, and circulation, as with any other critically ill patient. For patients with a Glasgow Coma Scale (GCS) less than 8, endotracheal intubation should be considered for airway protection. Rapid sequence intubation with in-line stabilization of the cervical spine is the preferred method of securing the airway in patients with neurologic trauma. Pretreatment with fentanyl (3 μg/kg) may be considered for its attenuating effect on the reflex sympathetic response and associated increase of intracranial pressure (ICP) that can be seen with laryngoscopy.[13] However, evidence for pretreatment with lidocaine is mixed and limited.[14] Awake, fiberoptic intubation may be considered in patients with cervical spine injury to reduce cervical spine motion.

In patients with TBI, hypoxia, defined as Pa_{O_2} less than 60 mm Hg or O_2 saturation less than 90%, is significantly associated with increased morbidity and mortality.[15] Hyperoxygenation with Pa_{O_2} greater than 470 mm Hg is also discouraged.[16] Target Pa_{CO_2} is 35 to 45 mm Hg with target end-tidal CO_2 of 30 to 40 mm Hg.[17] Hyperventilation should be avoided except in the acutely herniating patient as a bridge to more definitive therapies.

Hypotension is similarly associated with a 2-fold increase in mortality compared with matched controls in TBI.[15] In studies of the Traumatic Coma Data Bank (TCDB), a single observation of systolic blood pressure less than 90 mm Hg was one of 5 most powerful predictors of outcome, along with age, admission GCS motor score, pupillary function, and intracranial hypertension.[18] However, systolic pressure greater than 90 mm Hg may be desirable during resuscitation of patients with neurotrauma, but no studies have been performed thus far to determine a resuscitation target. Instead, 90 mm Hg should be considered a threshold to avoid.

Fluid Resuscitation

Fluid resuscitation in a patient with TBI needs special emphasis on the osmolality of the choice of fluid. Hypo-osmotic fluids can increase cerebral edema and ICP in the context of an injured blood-brain barrier. In 2004, 2 large randomized multicenter trials examined the use of albumin and hypertonic saline (HTS) in the resuscitation of patients with TBI. From the Saline versus Albumin Fluid Evaluation (SAFE) study, a post hoc study of 460 patients with TBI revealed that resuscitation with albumin was associated with higher mortality but similar functional outcome in survivors compared with saline.[19] Cooper and colleagues[20] examined the use of HTS in prehospital resuscitation of 229 hypotensive patients with TBI and found no significant difference in survival or neurologic outcome. A similar study by Bulger and colleagues[21] comparing HTS, HTS with dextran, and normal saline in out-of-hospital resuscitation of patients with TBI without hypovolemic shock was terminated for futility.

Resuscitation of the patient with neurogenic shock from SCI may require the use of vasopressors after achieving euvolemia to counteract the loss of sympathetically mediated vascular tone.

ICP

ICP is a function of the volume and compliance of each component of the intracranial compartment: brain tissue, blood, and cerebrospinal fluid (CSF). This concept was described by Alexander Monro and George Kellie, stating that to maintain a state of volume equilibrium in a fixed compartment, any increase in volume of one component must be compensated by a decrease in volume of another. Normal compensation to an increase in intracranial volume (eg, mass, hemorrhage, cerebral edema) is a decrease in cerebral blood volume and egress of CSF into the spinal space. Once these compensatory mechanisms are maximized, the addition of further volume leads to a sharp increase in ICP. Cerebral ischemia can be caused by increased ICP from reduction of cerebral perfusion pressure (CPP), or direct mass effect on cerebral arteries. Intractable intracranial hypertension can lead to compression of the brainstem and herniation syndrome, most classically described by the Cushing triad of widening pulse pressure, irregular respirations, and bradycardia. Inability to attenuate or reverse this process ultimately leads to cardiopulmonary arrest or brain death.

Initial management of suspected intracranial hypertension includes elevating the head of bed, maintaining the neck in neutral position, and avoiding neck constriction such as with poorly fitted cervical collars or circumferential tape or ties used to secure the endotracheal tube. Adequate treatment of pain, agitation, fever, and seizures can also reduce increases of ICP.

Comatose patients with GCS less than or equal to 8 are at highest risk for intracranial hypertension, thus ICP monitoring is recommended by the Brain Trauma Foundation (BTF) for patients with severe TBI. The preferred method for ICP monitoring is an external ventricular drain, because of its ability to provide a more reliable measure of global ICP and immediate effect on increased ICP from CSF drainage. ICP increase greater than 20 mm Hg is treated by the algorithm shown in **Table 2**, using a tiered approach of therapies. When using osmotic agents such as mannitol, clinicians should avoid intravascular volume depletion and hypotension with concurrent replacement of urinary losses with isotonic fluids. Hyperventilation is an effective emergent treatment of intracranial hypertension because CSF alkalosis is a potent vasoconstrictor of cerebral blood flow (CBF). However, it should be used transiently in an acute herniation syndrome as a bridge to more definitive therapy. Sustained and vigorous hyperventilation may result in cerebral ischemia and worse outcome.[22]

Clinical herniation can occur at ICP less than 20 mm Hg, depending on the location of an intracranial mass lesion. Pupillary abnormalities occurring with ICP values as low

Table 2
ICP management by a tiered approach

Tier 0	Head of bed >30° Optimize physiologic parameters Normothermia goal Adequate sedation and analgesia
Tier 1	CSF drainage via ventriculostomy Mannitol 0.5–1 g/kg bolus
Tier 2	Hypertonic saline bolus Propofol bolus and infusion
Tier 3	Decompressive craniectomy Pharmacologic coma Hypothermia Decompressive laparotomy or thoracotomy

Data from Brain Trauma Foundation, American Association of Neurological Surgeons, Congress of Neurological Surgeons, et al. Guidelines for the management of severe traumatic brain injury. Methods. J Neurotrauma 2007;24(Suppl 1):S3–6; and Stevens RD, Huff JS, Duckworth J, et al. Emergency neurological life support: intracranial hypertension and herniation. Neurocrit Care 2012;17(Suppl 1):S60–5.

as 18 mm Hg have been reported.[23] Therefore, management of intracranial hypertension should be correlated with the clinical examination and neuroimaging for each patient.

Cerebral Perfusion

Resuscitation of the injured brain is directed at restoring and maintaining adequate cerebral metabolism by ensuring sufficient delivery of oxygen and glucose to the brain tissue. In the uninjured brain, an autoregulatory mechanism maintains constant CBF across a wide range of CPP through modulation of cerebral vascular diameters (**Fig. 1**). However, autoregulation can be disrupted in brain injury, thus changes in CPP can significantly affect CBF. The use of CPP as a surrogate parameter for CBF therefore assumes that autoregulation is impaired.

Systemic hypotension is highly associated with increased morbidity and mortality in TBI.[24,25] Low CPP is also associated with poor physiologic indices as well as poor clinical outcome.[26] Studies suggest that there is a critical threshold for CPP between 50 and 60 mm Hg. Robertson and colleagues[27] conducted a randomized controlled trial of therapy targeting CPP greater than 70 mm Hg compared with therapy targeting ICP less than or equal to 20 mm Hg while maintaining CPP greater than 50 mm Hg. They found no difference in outcome, but the aggressive CPP target group had a 5-fold incidence of acute respiratory distress syndrome and more frequent use of vasopressor agents. BTF guidelines recommend maintaining CPP between 50 and 70 mm Hg with the goal of avoiding cerebral hypotension rather than aggressive increase of CPP. Optimization of CPP in the normotensive patient with neurotrauma should begin with attempts to lower ICP, because the ICP response to CPP increase is not predictable when autoregulation is compromised.[28]

EVIDENCE FOR CURRENT THERAPIES WITH NEUROTRAUMA

ICP Monitoring

Intracranial hypertension has been correlated with poor outcome in patients with severe TBI. Comatose patients with GCS less than or equal to 8 are at highest risk.[18,29] In

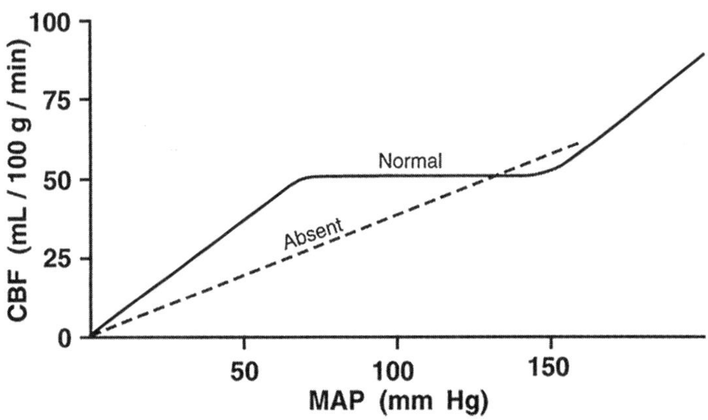

Fig. 1. Cerebral autoregulation. In the normal brain with intact cerebral autoregulation, compensatory mechanisms maintain constant CBF over a range of mean arterial pressures (MAP). In the injured brain with impaired or absent cerebral autoregulation, CBF depends directly on MAP, thus optimization of MAP and associated CPP is critically important. (*Adapted from* Drummond JC, Patel PM. Neurosurgical anesthesia. In: Miller RD, editor. Anesthesia. 5th edition. Philadelphia: Churchill Livingstone; 2000. p. 1901.)

a prospective series of patients with severe TBI, Narayan and colleagues[29] found that comatose patients with abnormal computed tomography (CT) scans have an incidence of intracranial hypertension of 55% to 63% compared with those with normal CT scan at admission (13%). However, the risk of intracranial hypertension was similar for patients with normal CT scans if they had 2 of 3 risk factors: age greater than 40 years, unilateral or bilateral motor posturing, or systolic blood pressure less than 90 mm Hg. In the largest prospective observational study that analyzed ICP in increments of 5 mm Hg, ICP greater than 20 mm Hg had the most predictive value.[18]

ICP monitoring can be the first indicator of worsening intracranial disorder.[30] Without ICP monitoring, CPP cannot be used as a therapeutic target for resuscitation and intervention. A pressure transduction device for ICP monitoring can be placed in the epidural, subdural, subarachnoid, parenchymal, or ventricular location. The ventricular fluid–coupled ICP monitor is the established reference standard for measuring ICP. Parenchymal transducer devices have similar accuracy to ventricular ICP devices but have the potential for drift because of the inability to recalibrate.[31] The 2 most common complications associated with invasive ICP monitoring are infection and intracranial hemorrhage. Although it has been standard of care per recommendations by the BTF guidelines, ICP monitoring has not been shown to improve outcome. In 2012, a multicenter randomized trial of 324 patients with severe TBI found that therapy targeted to maintain ICP less than 20 mm Hg was not superior to therapy based on clinical examination.[32] It would be incorrect to extrapolate results from this study to indicate that ICP monitoring is optional; the results from this randomized controlled trial indicate that more research is needed to better understand the complexities of cerebral hemodynamics. ICP remains a robust predictor of outcome but management of intracranial hypertension should be a clinical decision.

Surgical Decompression

Surgical management of TBI includes evacuation of intracranial mass lesions, repair of depressed skull fractures, as well as decompressive craniectomy for refractory intracranial hypertension. **Table 3** summarizes recommendations for surgical intervention.

The use of decompressive craniectomy for treatment of refractory intracranial hypertension was studied in the multicenter DECRA (Decompressive Craniectomy in Diffuse Traumatic Brain Injury) trial.[33] Bifrontotemporoparietal decompression was performed in randomized patients with severe TBI who failed ICP management with first-tier interventions. Although decompressive craniectomy decreased ICP compared with standard care, the craniectomy group had worse functional outcomes. There have been many discussions and criticisms regarding the DECRA trial.[34–36] However, decompressive craniectomy is an area of ongoing study with the current multicenter RESCUEicp (Randomised Evaluation of Surgery with Craniectomy for Uncontrollable Elevation of Intra-Cranial Pressure) trial.[37]

The timing of surgical management of unstable spinal fractures/subluxations was studied in the Surgical Timing in Acute Spinal Cord Injury Study (STASCIS).[38] Early decompression performed within 24 hours of injury had higher odds of improving neurologic outcome by a 2-grade improvement on the American Spinal Injury Association (ASIA) impairment scale (**Table 4**).

Hyperosmolar Therapies

Hyperosmolar therapy is a key component in the medical management of intracranial hypertension. Both mannitol and HTS are effective in decreasing ICP and improving CPP by their capacity to decrease brain water.[39–41] They also seem to increase CBF in regions of hypoperfusion.[42]

Table 3
Recommendations for surgical management of TBI

	Indications for Surgery
Epidural hematoma	EDH >30 cm^3 GCS <9 with anisocoria
Subdural hematoma	SDH clot thickness >10 mm or midline shift >5 mm, regardless of GCS GCS decline by ≥2 Asymmetric or fixed and dilated pupils ICP >20 mm Hg
Parenchymal lesions	Progressive neurologic deterioration, refractory intracranial hypertension, or signs of mass effect on CT referable to the lesion GCS 6–8 with frontal or temporal contusions >20 cm^3, midline shift ≥5 mm, or cisternal compression on CT Any lesion >50 cm^3
Posterior fossa lesions	Mass effect on CT, neurologic dysfunction or deterioration referable to the lesion
Depressed skull fractures	Open (compound) fractures greater than thickness of cranium Open (compound) fractures with dural penetration, significant intracranial hematoma, depression >1 cm, frontal sinus involvement, gross cosmetic deformity, wound infection, pneumocephalus, or gross wound contamination

Abbreviations: EDH, epidural hematoma; SDH, subdural hematoma.

Data from Bullock MR, Chesnut R, Ghajar J, et al. Guidelines for the surgical management of traumatic brain injury. Neurosurgery 2006;58(Suppl):S2-1–3.

Mannitol has been an osmotic agent in clinical practice for 5 decades, replacing the use of urea and glycerol. Administered as a 20% solution, immediate rheological effects include increased deformability of erythrocytes and decreased blood viscosity, thereby increasing CBF in hypoperfused regions.[43–45] In brain regions with intact autoregulation, compensatory vasoconstriction decreases cerebral blood volume with associated decrease in ICP.[44,46,47] The osmotic effect is delayed while a gradient is established between plasma and cells. Rebound increase in ICP is possible because mannitol is not impermeable to the blood-brain barrier.[48,49] The associated osmotic diuretic effect of mannitol may compromise intravascular volume. There is also a risk of renal failure with cumulative doses of mannitol.[50]

Table 4
ASIA impairment scale

ASIA A	Complete injury	No sensory or motor function preserved in sacral segments S4–S5
ASIA B	Incomplete sensory injury	Sensory but not motor function preserved below neurologic level and includes sacral segments (motor complete)
ASIA C	Incomplete motor injury	Motor function preserved below neurologic level and more than half of key muscles below neurologic level have muscle grade <3 (motor useless)
ASIA D	Incomplete motor injury	Motor function preserved below neurologic level and more than half of key muscles below neurologic level have muscle grade ≥3 (motor useful)
ASIA E	Normal function	—

Worksheet for dermatomes and grading of muscle function and ASIA scale is available at www.asia-spinalinjury.org.

The use of HTS for intracranial hypertension was discovered from studies on small-volume resuscitation in patients with polytrauma with hemorrhagic shock in which the TBI subgroup had the greatest benefit in survival.[51] HTS can be given in concentrations ranging from 2% to 23.4% solutions. It has similar rheological effects that improve CBF[52–54] and osmotic effects that decrease brain water content.[41,55] Because sodium chloride is impermeable to the intact blood-brain barrier, the theoretic risk of rebound increase in ICP is less than that of mannitol. Although HTS also has a diuretic effect through stimulation of atrial natriuretic peptide release, the risk of hypovolemia is less. The most common adverse effect with the use of HTS containing chloride is hyperchloremic metabolic acidemia.

There are few clinical studies that directly compare hyperosmolar therapies in brain injury in a randomized fashion. A retrospective review of patients with TBI treated with mannitol and 23.4% HTS showed a longer duration of ICP reduction with 23.4% HTS despite a smaller osmotic load administered.[56] HTS effectively lowered ICP in those who that were refractory to mannitol.[57,58] Compared as isovolume interventions, 7% HTS was superior to mannitol in ICP reduction.[59] However, compared as equimolar interventions, both mannitol and 7.45% HTS were effective in decreasing ICP, although mannitol was also observed to improve CPP.[60]

Steroids

Steroids were introduced in the early 1960s as treatment of brain edema from experimental evidence that showed restoration of altered vascular permeability, reduction of CSF production, and attenuation of free radical production.[61,62] For many years, steroids became common in the treatment of head injury. However, several studies have called into question the benefit of glucocorticoid therapy in TBI. In 2004, the multicenter international CRASH (Corticosteroid Randomization After Significant Head Injury) trial changed the landscape of steroid therapy in TBI. This study of 10,008 patients from 239 hospitals in 49 countries was stopped early because interim analysis showed an increased risk of death in the steroid group, even when patients were adjusted for extracranial injuries.[63] When the CRASH trial results are included in a meta-analysis, the absolute risk of death with corticosteroids in TBI is 2%.

The use of steroids in SCI is controversial. The National Acute Spinal Cord Injury Studies (NASCIS)[64,65] suggested that high-dose methylprednisolone given within 8 hours of injury for a duration of 24 hours improved neurologic recovery. Criticisms of these studies included that these conclusions were reached by post hoc analyses. A multicenter study by Otani and colleagues was also flawed by the lack of blinding.[66] Current guidelines by the American Association of Neurologic Surgeons (AANS) and the Congress of Neurologic Surgeons (CNS) do not recommend the use of steroids in SCI.[67]

Induced Hypertension

Cardiovascular instability can be seen in patients with acute SCI above the level of T4 caused by the loss of sympathetic tone. This autonomic instability is most common during the first week after injury.[68] Hemodynamic augmentation with volume resuscitation and vasopressors to maintain a mean arterial pressure goal greater than or equal to 85 mm Hg is commonly used in practice per recommendations by the AANS/CNS guidelines.[67] However, complications including arrhythmias, electrocardiogram/troponin changes, and acidosis have been reported with vasopressor use in SCI.[69] Further studies are necessary to determine whether blood pressure augmentation has an impact on outcomes following SCI and the most appropriate threshold and duration of therapy.

Pharmacologic Coma

Barbiturates have been shown to reduce ICP in patients with refractory intracranial hypertension.[70] Their ICP reducing and cerebral protective effects have been attributed to alterations in vascular resistance, suppression of cerebral metabolism, and inhibition of neuronal excitotoxicity.[71,72] High-dose barbiturates have risks and can cause numerous complications including hypotension, gastroparesis, and immunosuppression.[73,74] A Cochrane Review in 2012 did not find any evidence that barbiturates improved outcome in patients with severe TBI. Instead, barbiturate therapy resulted in a decrease in blood pressure in 1 in 4 treated patients.[75]

Hypothermia

Prophylactic hypothermia, used irrespective of ICP, has been studied as a potential neuroprotectant. Despite promising data from small single-center studies, a Cochrane Review in 2009 found no benefit in mortality or outcome.[76] A follow-up multicenter study was terminated for futility in adults with severe TBI.[77] A meta-analysis of 13 trials with a total of 1339 randomized patients found nonsignificant improvements in mortality and neurologic outcome, but the benefits were greatest when cooling was maintained for more than 48 hours and in patients who were not receiving barbiturates for ICP management.[78]

In contrast, therapeutic hypothermia has been shown to be effective in reducing intracranial hypertension. The beneficial effect on ICP is seen in patients with severe TBI,[79] malignant stroke,[80] and even acute hepatic failure.[81] Fever is a strong independent predictor of worse clinical outcome across a variety of brain injuries.[82–84] Targeted temperature management reduces cerebral metabolic rate[85] and posttraumatic release of excitatory neurotransmitters,[86] and attenuates the opening of the blood-brain barrier.[87] Failure of this beneficial effect to translate to improved neurologic outcomes may be caused by rebound ICP increases associated with rewarming.[80]

Hypothermia has also been promising in SCI in preclinical studies.[88] It is currently an experimental clinical therapy. A multicenter trial is being planned to evaluate its effects.

Seizure Prophylaxis

Seizures occur in 10% to 30% of patients with TBI, with the incidence close to 50% in penetrating brain injury. Posttraumatic seizures (PTS) are classified as early, occurring within 7 days of injury, or late, occurring after 7 days following injury. In the acute post-injury period, seizures may worsen outcome by increasing cerebral metabolism and ICP, resulting in excess neurotransmitter release and potential cerebral ischemia. **Table 5** presents risk factors for development of PTS.

Temkin and colleagues[89] conducted a large randomized controlled trial of 404 patients with TBI evaluating the effect of phenytoin on early and late PTS. Treatment with phenytoin had a significant reduction in the incidence of early but not late PTS. Other antiepileptic drugs have also been studied in the prophylaxis of PTS. Compared with phenytoin, valproate is as effective for prophylaxis of PTS, but there was a trend toward higher mortality in patients treated with valproate.[90] An equal rate of early PTS was found when levetiracetam was compared with phenytoin.[91]

From these studies, BTF recommends the use of antiepileptic medications for 1 week following injury to decrease the incidence of early PTS. However, the available evidence does not show that prevention of PTS improves outcome.

Table 5
Risk factors for PTS

Risk Factors for Early PTS	Risk Factors for Late PTS
GCS $\leq$10	Early PTS
Immediate seizures	Cortical contusion
Cortical contusion	Loss of consciousness
Depressed skull fracture	Posttraumatic amnesia lasting >24 h
Penetrating head injury	Acute intracerebral hematoma
No or brief loss of consciousness	Age >65 y
Posttraumatic amnesia lasting >30 min	
Subdural, epidural, or intracerebral hematoma	
Age $\leq$65 y	

Data from Torbic H, Forni A, Anger KE, et al. Use of antiepileptics for seizure prophylaxis after traumatic brain injury. Am J Heal Pharm 2013;70(9):759–66.

Infection Prophylaxis

Infections contribute to morbidity, mortality, and increased hospital length of stay of any critically ill patient, including patients with neurotrauma. Patients with severe TBI are at risk for infections associated with ICP monitoring as with any other invasive monitoring. The incidence of infection with ICP monitors is reported to be as high as 22%, but this depends on the method of detection.[92] In a cohort of 584 patients with severe TBI, Holloway and colleagues[93] found the risk of external ventricular drain (EVD) infection increased over the first 10 days but there was no difference in the infection rate with routine catheter exchange. There is limited and conflicting evidence for prophylactic antibiotics throughout the duration of use of an EVD.[94] In a multicenter trial, Zabramski and colleagues[95] found that catheters impregnated with minocycline and rifampin reduced CSF infection rates and catheter colonization. There is no consensus on the use of prophylactic antibiotics with ICP monitoring, but periprocedural antibiotics are commonly used.[96]

Because basilar skull fractures and CSF leakage have been associated with the risk of meningitis, antibiotics are often given prophylactically. However, a Cochrane Review in 2011 did not support this practice.[97] The common use of prophylactic antibiotics for compound skull fractures has also been based on limited evidence.[98]

FUTURE OF NEUROCRITICAL CARE

Care of the critically ill patient with neurologic injury has grown into a specialty of neurocritical care. Practitioners have multidisciplinary backgrounds and are content experts in both critical care and neurologic disorders. Implementation of a specialized neurocritical care team has been shown to reduce hospital length of stay and in-hospital mortality of neurocritically ill patients.[99] Research in neurocritical care includes neuroprotection; however, to date, no single medication has proved beneficial in the outcome of the patient with neurologic injury. Research in advanced magnetic resonance imaging may improve prognostic accuracy. Real-time bedside monitoring of cerebral physiology may provide more relevant physiologic end points for resuscitation of the critically ill patient with neurologic injury.

SUMMARY

Neurotrauma continues to be a significant cause of morbidity and mortality. Prevention of primary neurologic injury is a critical public health concern. Early and thorough assessment of the patient with neurotrauma with high index of suspicion of traumatic spinal cord injuries and traumatic vascular injuries requires a multidisciplinary approach involving prehospital providers, emergency physicians, neurosurgeons, and neurointensivists. Critical care management of the patient with neurotrauma is focused on the prevention of secondary injuries. Much research is still needed for potential neuroprotection therapies.

REFERENCES

1. Faul M, Xu L, Wald MM, et al. Traumatic brain injury in the United States: emergency department visits, hospitalizations and deaths 2002–2006. Atlanta (GA): Centers for Disease Control and Prevention, National Center for Injury Prevention and Control; 2010.
2. Bochicchio GV, Lumpkins K, O'Connor J, et al. Blast injury in a civilian trauma setting is associated with a delay in diagnosis of traumatic brain injury. Am Surg 2008;74(3):267–70.
3. Coronado VG, Xu L, Basavaraju SV, et al. Surveillance for traumatic brain injury-related deaths – United States, 1997-2007. MMWR Surveill Summ 2011;60(5):1–32.
4. Centers for Disease Control and Prevention NC for IP and C. Traumatic brain injury: statistics. 2013. Available at: http://www.cdc.gov/traumaticbraininjury/statistics.html. Accessed on November 25, 2013.
5. Center NSCIS. Spinal cord injury facts and figures at a glance. Birmingham (AL); 2013. Available at: https://www.nscisc.uab.edu/PublicDocuments/fact_figures_docs/Facts 2013.pdf. Accessed on November 25, 2013.
6. Devivo MJ. Epidemiology of traumatic spinal cord injury: trends and future implications. Spinal Cord 2012;50(5):365–72.
7. Aarabi B, Tofighi B, Kufera JA, et al. Predictors of outcome in civilian gunshot wounds to the head. J Neurosurg 2014;120(5):1138–46.
8. Magnuson J, Leonessa F, Ling GS. Neuropathology of explosive blast traumatic brain injury. Curr Neurol Neurosci Rep 2012;12(5):570–9.
9. Stein DM, Boswell S, Sliker CW, et al. Blunt cerebrovascular injuries: does treatment always matter? J Trauma 2009;66(1):132–43 [discussion: 143–4].
10. McHugh GS, Engel DC, Butcher I, et al. Prognostic value of secondary insults in traumatic brain injury: results from the IMPACT study. J Neurotrauma 2007;24(2):287–93.
11. Stein SC, Smith DH. Coagulopathy in traumatic brain injury. Neurocrit Care 2004;1(4):479–88.
12. Faden A, Simon R. A potential role for excitotoxins in the pathophysiology of spinal cord injury. Ann Neurol 1988;23(6):623–6.
13. Kim JT, Shim JK, Kim SH, et al. Remifentanil vs. lignocaine for attenuating the haemodynamic response during rapid sequence induction using propofol: double-blind randomised clinical trial. Anaesth Intensive Care 2007;35(1):20–3.
14. Robinson N, Clancy M. In patients with head injury undergoing rapid sequence intubation, does pretreatment with intravenous lignocaine/lidocaine lead to an improved neurological outcome? A review of the literature. Emerg Med J 2001;18(6):453–7.
15. Chesnut RM, Marshall LF, Klauber MR, et al. The role of secondary brain injury in determining outcome from severe head injury. J Trauma 1993;34(2):216–22.
16. Davis DP, Meade W, Sise MJ, et al. Both hypoxemia and extreme hyperoxemia may be detrimental in patients with severe traumatic brain injury. J Neurotrauma 2009;26(12):2217–23.

17. Seder DB, Riker RR, Jagoda A, et al. Emergency neurological life support: airway, ventilation, and sedation. Neurocrit Care 2012;17(Suppl 1):S4–20.
18. Marmarou A, Anderson RL, Ward JD, et al. Impact of ICP instability and hypotension on outcome in patients with severe head trauma. J Neurosurg 1991; 75(Suppl):S59–66.
19. Myburgh J, Cooper DJ, Finfer S, et al. Saline or albumin for fluid resuscitation in patients with traumatic brain injury. N Engl J Med 2007;357(9):874–84.
20. Cooper DJ, Myles PS, McDermott FT, et al. Prehospital hypertonic saline resuscitation of patients with hypotension and severe traumatic brain injury. JAMA 2004;291(11):1350–7.
21. Bulger EM, May S, Brasel KJ, et al. Out-of-hospital hypertonic resuscitation following severe traumatic brain injury. JAMA 2010;304(13):1455–64.
22. Muizelaar JP, Marmarou A, Ward JD, et al. Adverse effects of prolonged hyperventilation in patients with severe head injury: a randomized clinical trial. J Neurosurg 1991;75(5):731–9.
23. Marshall LF, Barba D, Toole BM, et al. The oval pupil: clinical significance and relationship to intracranial hypertension. J Neurosurg 1983;58(4):566–8.
24. Pietropaoli J, Rogers F, Shackford S, et al. The deleterious effects of intraoperative hypotension on outcome in patients with severe head injuries. J Trauma 1992;33(3):403–7.
25. Chesnut RM. Avoidance of hypotension: conditio sine qua non of successful severe head-injury management. J Trauma 1997;42(5S):4S–9S.
26. Nordström C, Reinstrup P, Xu W, et al. Assessment of the lower limit for cerebral perfusion pressure in severe head injuries by bedside monitoring of regional energy metabolism. Anesthesiology 2003;98(4):809–14.
27. Robertson C, Valadka A, Hannay H, et al. Prevention of secondary ischemic insults after severe head injury. Crit Care Med 1999;27(10):2086–95.
28. Bouma GJ, Muizelaar JP. Relationship between cardiac output and cerebral blood flow in patients with intact and with impaired autoregulation. J Neurosurg 1990; 73(3):368–74.
29. Narayan RK, Kishore PR, Becker DP, et al. Intracranial pressure: to monitor or not to monitor? J Neurosurg 1982;56(56):650–9.
30. Servadei F, Antonelli V, Giuliani G, et al. Evolving lesions in traumatic subarachnoid hemorrhage: prospective study of 110 patients with emphasis on the role of ICP monitoring. Acta Neurochir Suppl 2002;81:81–4.
31. Al-Tamimi YZ, Helmy A, Bavetta S, et al. Assessment of zero drift in the Codman intracranial pressure monitor: a study from 2 neurointensive care units. Neurosurgery 2009;64(1):94–8 [discussion: 98–9].
32. Chesnut RM, Temkin N, Carney N, et al. A trial of intracranial-pressure monitoring in traumatic brain injury. N Engl J Med 2012;367(26):2471–81.
33. Cooper DJ, Rosenfeld JV, Murray L, et al. Decompressive craniectomy in diffuse traumatic brain injury. N Engl J Med 2011;364(16):1493–502.
34. Honeybul S, Ho KM, Lind CR. What can be learned from the DECRA study. World Neurosurg 2013;79(1):159–61.
35. Sahuquillo J, Martínez-Ricarte F, Poca MA. Decompressive craniectomy in traumatic brain injury after the DECRA trial. Where do we stand? Curr Opin Crit Care 2013;19(2):101–6.
36. Bohman LE, Schuster JM. Decompressive craniectomy for management of traumatic brain injury: an update. Curr Neurol Neurosci Rep 2013;13(11):392.
37. Hutchinson P, Kolias A, Timofeev I, et al. Update on the RESCUEicp decompressive craniectomy trial. Crit Care 2011;15(Suppl 1):P312.

38. Fehlings MG, Vaccaro A, Wilson JR, et al. Early versus delayed decompression for traumatic cervical spinal cord injury: results of the surgical timing in acute spinal cord injury study (STASCIS). PLoS One 2012;7(2):e32037.
39. Freshman S, Battistella F, Matteucci M, et al. Hypertonic saline (7.5%) versus mannitol: a comparison for treatment of acute head injuries. J Trauma 1993; 35(3):344–8.
40. Thenuwara K, Todd MM, Brian JE. Effect of mannitol and furosemide on plasma osmolality and brain water. Anesthesiology 2002;96(2):416–21.
41. Wang LC, Papangelou A, Lin C, et al. Comparison of equivolume, equiosmolar solutions of mannitol and hypertonic saline with or without furosemide on brain water content in normal rats. Anesthesiology 2013;118(4):903–13.
42. Scalfani M, Dhar R, Zazulia A, et al. Effect of osmotic agents on regional blood flow in traumatic brain injury. J Crit Care 2012;27(5):526.e7–12.
43. Kassell N, Baumann K, Hitchon P, et al. The effects of high dose mannitol on cerebral blood flow in dogs with normal intracranial pressure. Stroke 1982;13(1): 59–61.
44. Muizelaar JP, Wei EP, Kontos HA, et al. Mannitol causes compensatory cerebral vasoconstriction and vasodilation in response to blood viscosity changes. J Neurosurg 1983;59(5):822–8.
45. Mendelow AD, Teasdale GM, Russell T, et al. Effect of mannitol on cerebral blood flow and cerebral perfusion pressure in human head injury. J Neurosurg 1985; 63(1):43–8.
46. Muizelaar JP, Lutz HA, Becker DP. Effect of mannitol on ICP and CBF and correlation with pressure autoregulation in severely head-injured patients. J Neurosurg 1984;61(4):700–6.
47. Rosner M, Coley I. Cerebral perfusion pressure: a hemodynamic mechanism of mannitol and the postmannitol hemogram. Neurosurgery 1987;21(2):147–56.
48. McManus M, Soriano S. Rebound swelling of astroglial cells exposed to hypertonic mannitol. Anesthesiology 1998;88(6):1586–91.
49. Palma L, Bruni G, Fiaschi A, et al. Passage of mannitol into the brain around gliomas: a potential cause of rebound phenomenon. A study on 21 patients. J Neurosurg Sci 2006;50(3):63–6.
50. Fang L, You H, Chen B, et al. Mannitol is an independent risk factor of acute kidney injury after cerebral trauma: a case-control study. Ren Fail 2010;32(6):673–9.
51. Wade C, Grady J, Kramer G, et al. Individual patient cohort analysis of the efficacy of hypertonic saline/dextran in patients with traumatic brain injury and hypotension. J Trauma 1998;42(Suppl 5):S61–5.
52. Prough DS, Whiteley JM, Taylor CL, et al. Regional CBF following resuscitation from hemorrhagic shock with HTS influence of a subdural mass. Anesthesiology 1991;75(2):319–27.
53. Shackford SR, Zhuang J, Schmoker J. Intravenous fluid tonicity: effect on intracranial pressure, cerebral blood flow, and cerebral oxygen delivery in focal brain injury. J Neurosurg 1992;76(1):91–8.
54. Shackford S, Schmoker J, Zhuang J. The effect of hypertonic resuscitation on pial arteriolar tone after brain injury and shock. J Trauma 1994;37(6):899–908.
55. Hartl R, Schurer L, Goetz C, et al. The effect of hypertonic fluid resuscitation on brain edema in rabbits subjected to brain injury and hemorrhagic shock. Shock 1995;3(4):274–9.
56. Ware ML, Nemani VM, Meeker M, et al. Effects of 23.4% sodium chloride solution in reducing intracranial pressure in patients with traumatic brain injury: a preliminary study. Neurosurgery 2005;57(4):727–36.

57. Schatzmann C, Heissler H, Konig K, et al. Treatment of elevated intracranial pressure by infusions of 10% saline in severely head injured patients. Acta Neurochir Suppl 1998;71:31–3.
58. Horn P, Munch E, Vajkoczy P, et al. Hypertonic saline solution for control of elevated intracranial pressure in patients with exhausted response to mannitol and barbiturates. Neurol Res 1999;21(8):758–64.
59. Vialet R, Albanèse J, Thomachot L, et al. Isovolume hypertonic solutes (sodium chloride or mannitol) in the treatment of refractory posttraumatic intracranial hypertension: 2 mL/kg 7.5% saline is more effective than 2 mL/kg 20% mannitol. Crit Care Med 2003;31(6):1683–7.
60. Francony G, Fauvage B, Falcon D, et al. Equimolar doses of mannitol and hypertonic saline in the treatment of increased intracranial pressure. Crit Care Med 2008;36(3):795–800.
61. Maxwell RE, Long DM, French LA. The effects of glucosteroids on experimental cold-induced brain edema. Gross morphological alterations and vascular permeability changes. J Neurosurg 1971;34(4):477–87.
62. Hall ED. The neuroprotective pharmacology of methylprednisolone. J Neurosurg 1992;76(1):13–22.
63. Roberts I, Yates D, Sandercock P, et al. Effect of intravenous corticosteroids on death within 14 days in 10008 adults with clinically significant head injury (MRC CRASH trial): randomised placebo-controlled trial. Lancet 2004;364(9442): 1321–8.
64. Bracken M, Shepard M, Collins W, et al. A randomized, controlled trial of methylprednisolone or naloxone in the treatment of acute spinal-cord injury. Results of the Second National Acute Spinal Cord Injury Study. N Engl J Med 1990; 322(20):1405–11.
65. Bracken MB, Shepard MJ, Holford TR, et al. Administration of methylprednisolone for 24 or 48 hours or tirilazad mesylate for 48 hours in the treatment of acute spinal cord injury. JAMA 1997;277(20):1597–604.
66. Bracken M. Steroids for acute spinal cord injury. Cochrane Database Syst Rev 2012;(1):CD001046.
67. Hadley MN, Walters BC, Aarabi B, et al. Guidelines for the management of acute cervical spine and spinal cord injuries. Neurosurgery 2013;72(Suppl 2): 1–259.
68. Piepmeier JM, Lehmann KB, Lane JG. Cardiovascular instability following acute cervical spinal cord trauma. Cent Nerv Syst Trauma 1985;2(3):153–61.
69. Inoue T, Manley GT, Patel N, et al. Medical and surgical management after spinal cord injury: vasopressor usage, early surgerys, and complications. J Neurotrauma 2014;31(3):284–91.
70. Eisenberg HM, Frankowski RF, Contant CF, et al. High-dose barbiturate control of elevated intracranial pressure in patients with severe head injury. J Neurosurg 1988;69(1):15–23.
71. Kassell N, Hitchon P, Gerk M, et al. Alterations in cerebral blood flow, oxygen metabolism, and electrical activity produced by high dose sodium thiopental. Neurosurgery 1980;7(6):598–603.
72. Goodman JC, Valadka AB, Gopinath SP, et al. Lactate and excitatory amino acids measured by microdialysis are decreased by pentobarbital coma in head-injured patients. J Neurotrauma 1996;13(10):549–56.
73. Stover JF, Stocker R. Barbiturate coma may promote reversible bone marrow suppression in patients with severe isolated traumatic brain injury. Eur J Clin Pharmacol 1998;54(7):529–34.

74. Bochicchio GV, Bochicchio K, Nehman S, et al. Tolerance and efficacy of enteral nutrition in traumatic brain-injured patients induced into barbiturate coma. JPEN J Parenter Enteral Nutr 2006;30(6):503–6.
75. Roberts I, Sydenham E. Barbiturates for acute traumatic brain injury. Cochrane Database Syst Rev 2012;(12):CD000033.
76. Sydenham E, Roberts I, Alderson P. Hypothermia for traumatic head injury. Cochrane Database Syst Rev 2009;(2):CD001048.
77. Clifton GL, Valadka A, Zygun D, et al. Very early hypothermia induction in patients with severe brain injury (the National Acute Brain Injury Study: Hypothermia II): a randomised trial. Lancet Neurol 2011;10(2):131–9.
78. Peterson K, Carson S, Carney N. Hypothermia treatment for traumatic brain injury: a systematic review and meta-analysis. J Neurotrauma 2008;25(1):62–71.
79. Sadaka F, Veremakis C. Therapeutic hypothermia for the management of intracranial hypertension in severe traumatic brain injury: a systematic review. Brain Inj 2012;26(7–8):899–908.
80. Schwab S, Georgiadis D, Berrouschot J, et al. Feasibility and safety of moderate hypothermia after massive hemispheric infarction. Stroke 2001;32(9):2033–5.
81. Jalan R, Olde Damink SW, Deutz NE, et al. Moderate hypothermia in patients with acute liver failure and uncontrolled intracranial hypertension. Gastroenterology 2004;127(5):1338–46.
82. Rossi S, Zanier ER, Mauri I, et al. Brain temperature, body core temperature, and intracranial pressure in acute cerebral damage. J Neurol Neurosurg Psychiatr 2001;71(4):448–54.
83. Diringer MN, Reaven NL, Funk SE, et al. Elevated body temperature independently contributes to increased length of stay in neurologic intensive care unit patients. Crit Care Med 2004;32(7):1489–95.
84. Rincon F, Patel U, Schorr C, et al. Brain injury as a risk factor for fever upon admission to the intensive care unit and association with in-hospital case fatality: a matched cohort study. J Intensive Care Med 2013. [Epub ahead of print].
85. Bering E. Effect of body temperature change on cerebral oxygen consumption of the intact monkey. Am J Physiol 1961;200(3):417–9.
86. Busto R, Globus MY, Dietrich WD, et al. Effect of mild hypothermia on ischemia-induced release of neurotransmitters and free fatty acids in rat brain. Stroke 1989;20(7):904–10.
87. Smith SL, Hall ED. Mild pre- and posttraumatic hypothermia attenuates blood-brain barrier damage following controlled cortical impact injury in the rat. J Neurotrauma 1996;13(1):1–9.
88. Dietrich WD, Levi AD, Wang M, et al. Hypothermic treatment for acute spinal cord injury. Neurotherapeutics 2011;8(2):229–39.
89. Temkin NR, Dikmen SS, Wilensky AJ, et al. Randomized, double-blind study of phenytoin for the prevention of post-traumatic seizures. N Engl J Med 1990;323(8):497–502.
90. Temkin NR, Dikmen SS, Anderson GD, et al. Valproate therapy for prevention of posttraumatic seizures: a randomized trial. J Neurosurg 1999;91(4):593–600.
91. Inaba K, Menaker J, Branco BC, et al. A prospective multicenter comparison of levetiracetam versus phenytoin for early posttraumatic seizure prophylaxis. J Trauma Acute Care Surg 2013;74(3):766–71 [discussion: 771–3].
92. Lozier AP, Sciacca RR, Romagnoli MF, et al. Ventriculostomy-related infections: a critical review of the literature. Neurosurgery 2002;51(1):170–82.

93. Holloway KL, Barnes T, Choi S, et al. Ventriculostomy infections: the effect of monitoring duration and catheter exchange in 584 patients. J Neurosurg 1996;85(3):419–24.
94. Sonabend AM, Korenfeld Y, Crisman C, et al. Prevention of ventriculostomy-related infections with prophylactic antibiotics and antibiotic-coated external ventricular drains: a systematic review. Neurosurgery 2011;68(4):996–1005.
95. Zabramski JM, Whiting D, Darouiche RO, et al. Efficacy of antimicrobial-impregnated external ventricular drain catheters: a prospective, randomized, controlled trial. J Neurosurg 2003;98(4):725–30.
96. McCarthy PJ, Patil S, Conrad SA, et al. International and specialty trends in the use of prophylactic antibiotics to prevent infectious complications after insertion of external ventricular drainage devices. Neurocrit Care 2010;12(2):220–4.
97. Ratilal B, Costa J, Sampaio C, et al. Antibiotic prophylaxis for preventing meningitis in patients with basilar skull fractures. Cochrane Database Syst Rev 2011;(8):CD004884.
98. Ali B, Ghosh A, Mackway-Jones K. Antibiotics in compound depressed skull fractures. Emerg Med J 2002;19:552–3.
99. Suarez JI, Zaidat OO, Suri MF, et al. Length of stay and mortality in neurocritically ill patients: impact of a specialized neurocritical care team. Crit Care Med 2004;32(11):2311–7.

Critical Care Ultrasonography

Daniel Peterson, BSc, MD, PhD, FRCPC[a], Robert T. Arntfield, MD, FRCPC[b,c,*]

KEYWORDS

• Critical care • Ultrasonography • Point of care • Resuscitative medicine

KEY POINTS

- The use of point-of-care ultrasonography (POCUS) has become an integral part of critical care and resuscitative medicine in recent years.
- A major accelerant of the POCUS revolution, across all clinical domains, has been the miniaturization of ultrasonography machines, allowing them to be brought to patients easily, rather than requiring patients to be transported away from their clinical environment to be imaged.
- Whether in a prehospital setting, the emergency department, or the intensive care unit, patients at risk of deterioration and/or death benefit most from the timely, multisystem bedside analysis provided by POCUS.

INTRODUCTION

Resuscitation scenarios require rapid diagnostic and therapeutic decisions tailored to a patient's underlying condition and evolving physiology. Diagnostic and monitoring tools that can reliably reveal organ failure or life-threatening conditions at the bedside are of the utmost value in these often overwhelming situations.

The use of point-of-care ultrasonography (POCUS) has become an integral part of critical care and resuscitative medicine in recent years. A major accelerant of the POCUS revolution, across all clinical domains, has been the miniaturization of ultrasonography machines, allowing them to be brought to patients easily, rather than requiring patients to be transported away from their clinical environments to be imaged. Nowhere has this paradigm shift been more beneficial to patients and providers than with the critically ill patient. Whether in a prehospital setting, the emergency department (ED), or the intensive care unit (ICU), patients at risk of deterioration

Disclosure: None.

[a] University of Calgary, 1403 29 St NW Calgary, Alberta T2N 2T9, Canada; [b] Division of Emergency Medicine, London Health Sciences Centre, Western University, 800 Commissioners Road East, London, Ontario N6A 5W9, Canada; [c] Division of Critical Care Medicine, London Health Sciences Centre, Western University, 800 Commissioners Road East, London, Ontario N6A 5W9, Canada

* Corresponding author. Division of Emergency Medicine, London Health Sciences Centre, Western University, 800 Commissioners Road East, London, Ontario N6A 5W9, Canada.

E-mail address: robert.arntfield@gmail.com

Emerg Med Clin N Am 32 (2014) 907–926

http://dx.doi.org/10.1016/j.emc.2014.07.011 emed.theclinics.com

0733-8627/14/$ – see front matter

and/or death benefit most from the timely, multisystem bedside analysis provided by POCUS.

From its origins in the trauma bay in the assessment for hemopericardium[1,2] and hemoperitoneum,[3,4] POCUS for the critically ill patient has a growing list of applications. Some applications are the foundation of resuscitation, such as the cause of shock in the undifferentiated patient, whereas other, newer concepts, like intracranial pressure determination from optic nerve sheath diameter, require more time to determine their clinical value. This article reviews the contemporary applications of POCUS that are most relevant to resuscitation.

Before discussing ultrasonography related to the care of the critically ill, a distinction should be made between what has classically been referred to as critical care ultrasonography as described by the American College of Chest Physicians (ACCP) in 2009 and resuscitative ultrasonography, as discussed here. Critical care ultrasonography has been described as a specific set of skills used in the ICU setting involving thoracic, abdominal, vascular, and cardiac ultrasonography and requiring a minimum standard of competence outlined by the ACCP.[5] Resuscitative ultrasonography encompasses a wide range of practitioners of various skill levels using ultrasonography to assist with resuscitation across a variety of clinical settings. Although resuscitative ultrasonography in the ED is frequently labeled critical care ultrasonography, we therefore favor the more descriptive and nonpartisan term of resuscitative ultrasonography.

APPLICATION 1: DIFFERENTIATING SHOCK STATES

Multisystem Protocols

One of the most powerful applications of POCUS is in the rapid differentiation of shock states, which has been an area of intense clinical and academic interest over the past decade with the advent of several multisystem scanning protocols (**Table 1**) for shock published in the literature.[6–11] The published protocols encourage the routine use of a systematic, multiorgan approach when assessing patients with undifferentiated hypotension. Because no single protocol has proved superior to another, it is the common systematic, multiorgan approach they all endorse, rather than the details of their exact execution that should be emphasized. In general, in the face of undifferentiated shock or hypotension, the following ultrasonography examination elements should be executed: focused point-of-care echocardiography, thoracic (lung and pleural) ultrasonography, inferior vena cava (IVC) assessment, abdominal free fluid, and aortic aneurysm assessments. Shock differentiation is fundamental to resuscitative ultrasonography and worthy of further organ-by-organ discussion.

Assessment for Cardiogenic Causes of Shock

Evaluation of the heart with POCUS during shock can alter a patient's treatment trajectory in a matter of seconds. In typical goal-directed echocardiography, a phased-array transducer is used to generate 4 standard echocardiographic views of the heart: the parasternal long axis (PLAX) and parasternal short axis (PSAX), the apical 4-chamber (A4C), and subxiphoid (SUBX) views. Each view provides new or complementary information about the relevant cardiac chambers' size and function, gross valvular disorders, as well as the state of the pericardium. Imaging findings are rapidly synthesized to fit in to one of several clinical syndromes. A summary of the clinical syndromes and corresponding imaging details that are of interest in resuscitation are summarized in **Table 2**.

Assessment of the patient's left ventricular function begins with obtaining the PLAX and PSAX views of the heart. The PLAX is often referred to as the scout view of the

Table 1
Examples of protocols published for multiorgan ultrasonography assessment for undifferentiated hypotension

Protocol Name	Organs Assessed	Patient Population	Comment/Notes
Undifferentiated hypotensive patient ultrasonography protocol	Abdomen, aorta	ED	The first standardized ultrasonography protocol for ED patients using 3 accepted POCUS applications. No quantitative data provided
Focused echocardiographic evaluation in life support	Cardiac	Prehospital	Limited echocardiography performed by an emergency physician in periresuscitation scenarios alters management in 78% of cases
Focused echocardiographic evaluation in resuscitation	Cardiac	ED, ICU	Proposed protocol for incorporating limited echocardiography assessment into ACLS with the goal of identifying reversible causes of cardiac arrest. Feasibility of limited echocardiography during CPR was shown
Abdominal and cardiac evaluation with sonography	Cardiac, IVC, aorta, abdomen, pleura	ED	Six-view structured approach to assess hypotensive patient with sonography. Examples of how results would change management are given, but no outcome data presented. Protocol remains to be validated
RUSH	Cardiac, IVC, abdomen, pleura, aorta	ED	Three-step bedside physiologic assessment of the pump, tank, and pipes of a hypotensive patient. Components of RUSH protocol studied previously, not the complete RUSH protocol
Echocardiography-guided life support	Cardiac, lung, IVC	ED, ICU	An algorithmic approach to optimizing early management of critically ill patients based on answering several clinical questions with ultrasonography. Incorporates aspects of several previously published protocols

Abbreviations: ACLS, advanced cardiac life support; CPR, cardiopulmonary resuscitation; IVC, inferior vena cava; RUSH, rapid ultrasonography in shock.

Data from Refs.[6–11]

heart, providing a broad overview of most relevant structures of interest. Most of the left ventricle (LV) is seen in this view, along with the right ventricular outflow tract, the left atrium, the aortic root, the pericardium, the descending aorta, and the mitral and aortic valves (**Fig. 1**A).

The PSAX view of the heart is orthogonal to the PLAX and although there are 5 levels of assessment in the short axis the level of the papillary muscles is the most representative of global left ventricular function and therefore is the preferred view when

Table 2
Clinical syndromes and corresponding echo details of interest in resuscitation

Clinical Syndrome	Relevant Cardiac Ultrasonography Views	Findings	Pitfalls and Pearls
Hypovolemic shock	IVC, PSAX	IVC: narrow diameter, respiratory variation. PSAX: hyperdynamic function, kissing papillary muscles	Off-axis imaging falsely portraying narrow IVC or apical PSAX showing falsely hyperdynamic function
LV systolic failure	PLAX, PSAX, IVC	PLAX: hypocontractility, reduced EPSS PSAX: hypocontractility	Off-axis imaging may show falsely normal function
RV failure	PSAX, A4C, IVC	PSAX: D-shaped septum A4C: increased RV size IVC: plethoric	Off-axis imaging may show an elliptical RV and mimic a flattened septum
Catastrophic valvulopathy	PLAX, A4C	PLAX/A4C: vegetation on valves, chordae tendonae rupture, massive regurgitation with color Doppler	Color Doppler assessment best done when flow is toward or away from the transducer (ie, A4C)
Tamponade	PLAX, A4C, IVC	PLAX: large, circumferential effusion A4V: right atrial/ventricular collapse IVC: dilated	Patients in shock with a nontrivial effusion and dilated IVC should be considered to have tamponade until proved otherwise
Circulatory arrest	SUBX	In cardiac standstill: no myocardial thickening. Valve fluttering may be seen	Best position to obtain view is SUBX. Standstill predictive of poor outcome
Vasodilatory (eg, septic) shock	PLAX, PSAX, A4C, IVC	Normal to hyperdynamic LV in all views; IVC of variable size. Otherwise normal examination	Early hyperdynamic state of the LV has been shown to be specific for ultimate diagnosis of sepsis[5]

Abbreviations: EPSS, E point septal separation; LV, left ventricle; RV, right ventricle.

performing POCUS. The LV is seen as a thick circular ring of cardiac muscle with the smaller, thin-walled, and crescent-shaped right ventricle (RV) next to it. Also visible in the short axis is the echogenic pericardium (**Fig. 2**A).

Determining quantitative measures of left ventricular systolic function using POCUS is neither necessary nor practical. Estimating gross left ventricular function visually at the bedside has been studied and endorsed by both intensivists and emergency physicians.[12–15] Although left ventricular function is a continuous variable, it is more clinically relevant to categorize the LV into broader gradations of function: normal, hyperdynamic, depressed, and severely depressed. Although this 4-category approach is arbitrary, many clinicians find that this approach strikes an appropriate balance between too few categories (resulting in overgeneralizations of function) and too many categories (resulting in clinically insignificant distinctions of function).

In the PLAX and PSAX views, a normal heart shows that the cardiac muscle thickens and contracts in unison during systole. The walls of the LV should contract toward the

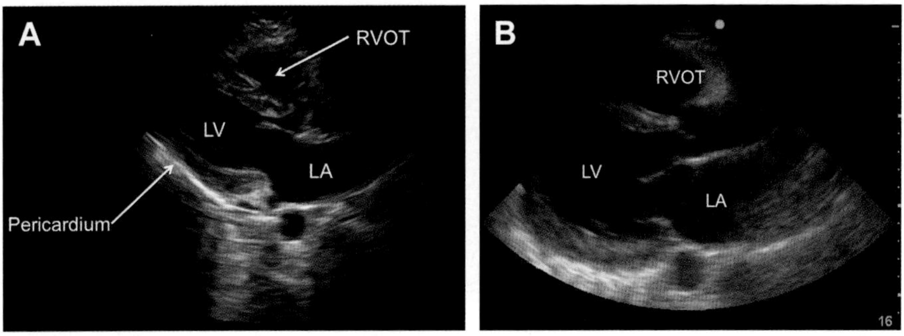

Fig. 1. (*A*) Normal PLAX view. (*B*) Dilated LV in the PLAX with decreased E point septal separation.

center of the LV cavity. In addition, the distance between the anterior leaflet of the mitral valve and the septum can also provide important information in the PLAX view regarding gross left ventricular function (a parameter known as E point septal separation [EPSS]). Under normal conditions, the anterior mitral valve leaflet should open vigorously and nearly meet the septum during diastole. When left ventricular function is reduced, wall thickening and contraction of the ventricular free walls and septum are reduced and the mitral valve does not open with the same vigor as in a normal heart (see **Fig. 1**B). If this EPSS distance is more than 1 cm, it is almost certain that the LV has depressed function.[16] Severely decreased left ventricular function is characterized by an LV that shows further progression of the diminished muscle excursion and thickening seen in the depressed category. In addition, a hyperdynamic LV is one that is seen to be contracting overly vigorously, typically in the context of hypovolemia and/or low afterload conditions like septic shock. The walls of the ventricle are observed to collapse vigorously toward the center of the LV and often touch, or kiss, at the end of systole. Off-axis imaging, either in the PLAX or the PSAX view, can falsely mimic a hyperdynamic state, so attention to imaging through the middle of the LV cavity (PLAX) and avoiding being apically displaced (PSAX) help to avoid overestimating left ventricular function. Overall, grading LV function in a qualitative fashion is straightforward to do after acquiring appropriate experience.

Assessing the pericardium for pericardial effusion can be done in any of the 4 basic echocardiographic views of the heart, although many favor the PLAX view because it offers an ideal view for the posterior pericardium, in which even small pericardial

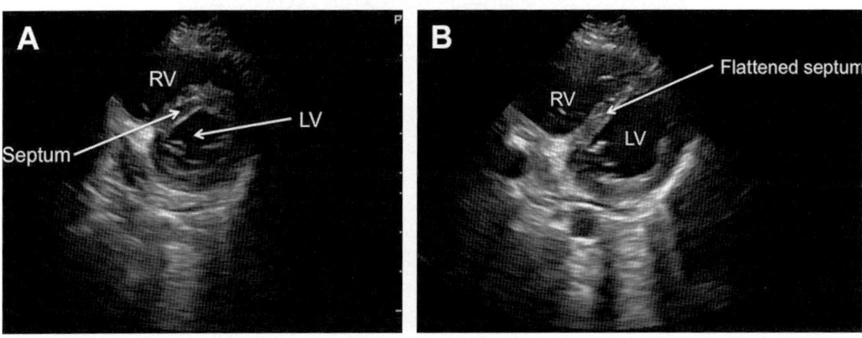

Fig. 2. (*A*) Normal PSAX view. (*B*) D-shaped LV as a result of increased right-sided pressure.

effusions may be observed in supine patients (**Fig. 3**). An effusion is seen as an anechoic collection between the bright echogenic layers of the pericardium. Most are free flowing around the pericardium, although loculated effusions are common after cardiac procedures, increasing the complexity of the assessment in this population. The hemodynamic influence of any given pericardial effusion depends on a variety of factors, including speed of accumulation, size, and the volume status of the patient.

If pericardial pressure exceeds right-sided filling pressures, cardiac tamponade ensues. In a patient with shock in whom a nontrivial pericardial effusion is identified, providers should generally assume that tamponade physiology is present until proved otherwise. For advanced sonographers, appreciation of the echocardiography findings of tamponade physiology, including right atrial or right ventricular collapse (**Fig. 4**) or variation in mitral inflow Doppler patterns, may be possible and further boosts diagnostic confidence and influences management accordingly.[17] Although these features of tamponade physiology are commonly described, the diagnostic performance of these findings outside of controlled echocardiography laboratories is unknown. It is therefore proposed that a more useful adjuvant tool in the context of a pericardial effusion is assessment of IVC size and respiratory variation. When tamponade is present, the IVC must be dilated. Because the IVC is easily imaged by POCUS, a nondilated IVC can be an effective bedside tool for ruling out tamponade physiology with high sensitivity.[18] POCUS also provides the opportunity to guide and visualize pericardiocentesis in real time, aiming for the area of the largest collection of pericardial fluid while avoiding overlying lung.

The presence or absence of right ventricular failure can radically alter the therapeutic decisions and prognosis of critically ill patients.[19–22] Acute cor pulmonale is usually the result of a pulmonary embolism or an exacerbation of a chronic lung condition causing increased right-sided pressures. Assessment for right ventricular failure with POCUS should start with determining the size of the RV compared its larger neighbor, the LV. This determination is best done using the PSAX and A4C views. In the short axis, increased right-sided heart pressure results in an enlargement of the RV and a flattening of the usually rounded interventricular septum, creating a D-shaped LV (see **Fig. 2**B). In the A4C view, the RV should be seen to be no more than two-thirds the size of the LV during diastole. Further, under normal conditions, the LV should dominate the apex (**Fig. 5**A). In acute cor pulmonale, the weaker RV

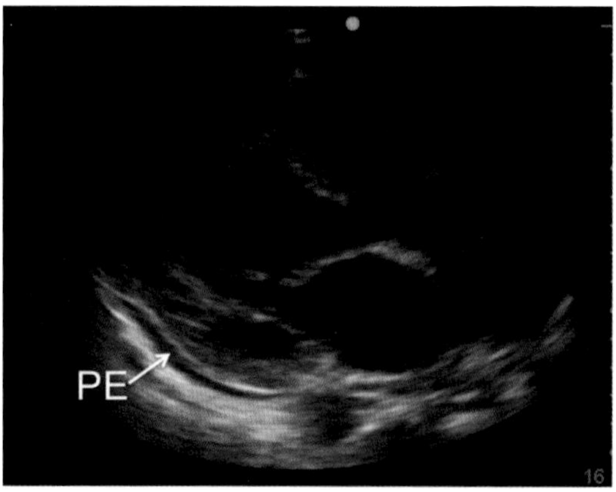

Fig. 3. Small posterior pericardial effusion (PE) in the PLAX.

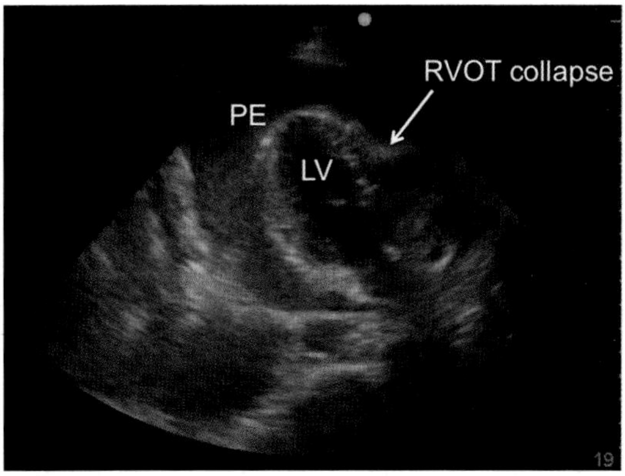

Fig. 4. Cardiac tamponade; right ventricular outflow collapse in the PLAX. RVOT, right ventricular outflow tract.

quickly becomes overwhelmed and increases in size to become moderately dilated (more than two-thirds the size of the LV) or severely dilated (larger than the LV) and may displace the LV and occupy most of the apex (see **Fig. 5**B). Right ventricular dysfunction is an area of intense study in the resuscitation literature. In turn, precise and well-accepted management strategies for a failing or strained RV are not discussed in this article.

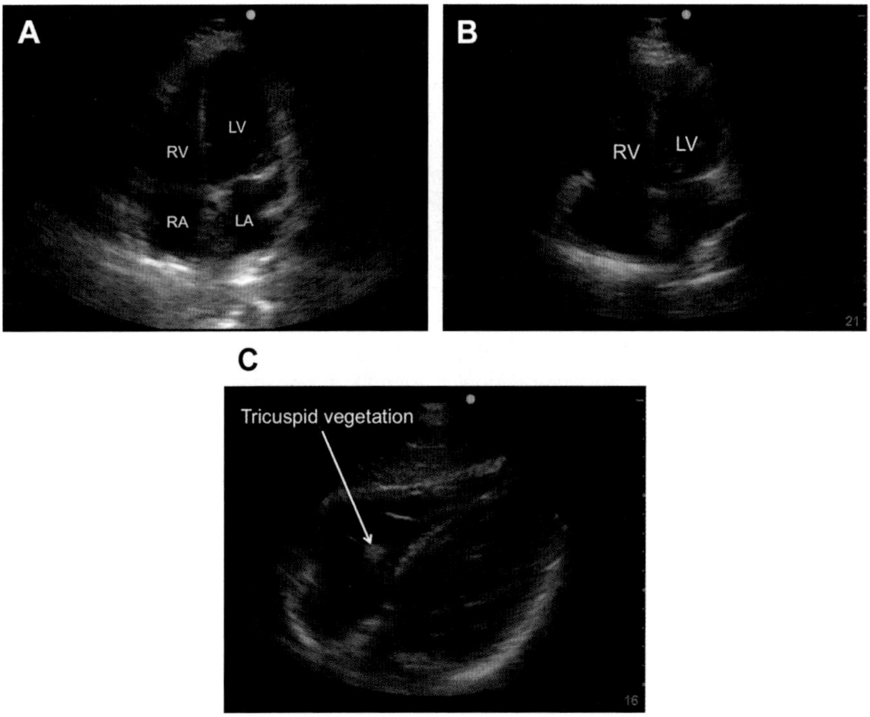

Fig. 5. (*A*) Normal apical 4-chamber view. (*B*) Right ventricular enlargement in the apical 4-chamber view. (*C*) Tricuspid valve vegetation; subxiphoid view.

Acute valvular regurgitation may be the cause of, or may complicate, a patient's shock state and should form part of a thorough point-of-care echocardiogram. Although valvular heart disease and the Doppler applications required for accurate valvular analysis are complex, color Doppler may be used to crudely screen across the tricuspid valve (TV) or mitral valves (MV) in the A4C or the aortic valve (AV) in the neighboring apical 5-chamber view for severe regurgitation. Important causes of severe regurgitation include endocarditis (MV, AV, and TV; see **Fig. 5**C), ischemia (MV), aortic dissection (AV), or acute cor pulmonale (TV).

Identification of any of the constellation of cardiac findings discussed earlier is of little value until they are appropriately clinically integrated. A one-size-fits-all algorithm for incorporation of these findings into clinical care is not realistic; however, there are some important points worth mentioning.

Identifying a hyperdynamic LV has been shown to be associated with early sepsis or hypovolemia, both of which are amenable to rapid fluid administration.[23] Depressed or severely depressed left ventricular function may be associated with late sepsis, toxins, or cardiogenic shock, in which case moving toward administration of inotropic medications earlier may be of benefit as well as transferring the patient for cardiac catheterization if the clinical situation is more likely cardiac in origin. Identification of pericardial effusions and cardiac tamponade at the bedside allows more rapid initiation of a potentially life-saving pericardiocentesis. Recognizing patients with right heart strain or acute cor pulmonale is valuable because it often represents an acute pulmonary embolus that requires anticoagulation, thrombolysis, or potentially surgery. Patients with right heart strain on POCUS should undergo further evaluation with computed tomography (CT) pulmonary angiogram, if stable enough, or transesophageal echocardiography (TEE) or potentially thrombolysis if the patient continues to deteriorate or has cardiac arrest.

POCUS allows for frequent reassessment of a patient's hemodynamic status as their clinical situation progresses. Those septic patients with an initially hyperdynamic LV may progress to an LV with depressed function as their conditions evolve. It is also useful to monitor the effects of interventions, whether these are intravenous fluids, pharmacologic (eg, vasopressors), or a physical intervention such as insertion of an intra-aortic balloon pump. Frequent monitoring with POCUS is advantageous because there is no radiation exposure, it is portable and noninvasive, and it offers real-time evaluation of important physiology in the critically ill patient.

Estimating Fluid Responsiveness Using the IVC

A long-axis view of the IVC, obtained from the subcostal window, can provide information about volume status and, occasionally, volume responsiveness. Through interpretation of its absolute size as well as how it varies with respiratory efforts, approximations of central venous pressure (CVP) can be made (in spontaneously breathing patients) and predictions of volume responsiveness can accurately be made in patients who are passively mechanically ventilated. When assessing the size and variation of the IVC, attention should be directed to the confluence of the vertically oriented hepatic vein and the IVC, or about 2 cm distal to the right atrium–IVC junction (**Fig. 6**).

IVC examination can help corroborate additional cardiac findings. For instance, in the context of a hyperdynamic LV for which the cause could be multifactorial (vasodilatory shock, right ventricular obstruction, hypovolemic shock, or high-output states), a small IVC (<1.0 cm in a spontaneous breathing patient) suggest a hypovolemic state.

Although imaging the IVC is easy, its interpretation requires thoughtful reflection by the provider regarding the respiratory physiology of the patient and the way it

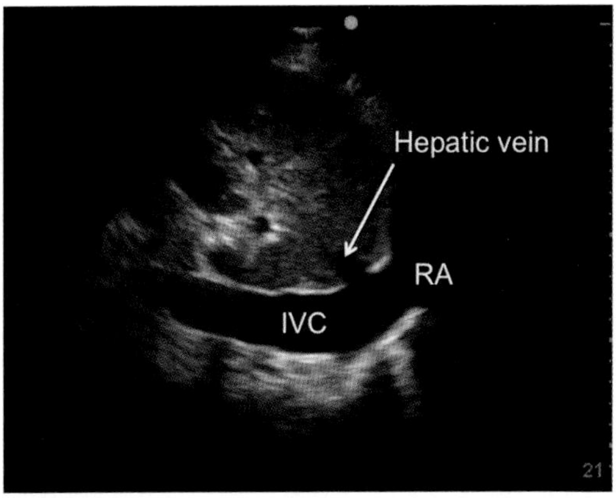

Fig. 6. Dilated IVC in the long axis. RA, right atrium.

influences the IVC. The strongest evidence for use of IVC ultrasonography comes from mechanical ventilated patients who are passively (ie, not triggering) being ventilated.[24,25] In these patients, distention of between 12% and 18% of the IVC during inspiration predicts volume responsiveness.

Because of the variable respiratory effort with all other states of spontaneously breathing physiology, it has not been possible for research to provide a similar level of evidence or a single algorithm to predict volume responsiveness using the IVC. However, the IVC has been shown to predict CVP and, in keeping with this, many clinicians advocate that an IVC showing greater than 50% collapse (corresponding with a CVP of 0–5 mm Hg) under spontaneously breathing physiology can support fluid administration. Despite the reliance on CVP in prominent resuscitative guidelines,[26] it has never been proved to predict volume responsiveness and therefore relying on CVP for fluid management, no matter how it is derived, is coming under increasing scrutiny.[27]

Despite the ease of imaging the IVC, it cannot be applied in the same fashion or with the same value across all critically ill patients. Alternative, more laborious and advanced ultrasonography approaches have been explored. Common to many of these advanced techniques is reliance on spectral Doppler profiles from various sites in the body, including the left ventricular outflow tract and the brachial or carotid arteries.[28,29] The variation of the amplitude of the stroke volume envelope that is displayed (known as the velocity time integral) can be measured, in response to respiratory efforts, volume administration, or passive leg raising (**Fig. 7**). Various thresholds of variation exist to predict volume responsiveness.

The use of a more complex Doppler tissue method of determining increased left atrial pressure by determining the ratio (E/E′) of transmitral pulsed-wave Doppler flow (E) to the relaxation velocity of the LV (E′) has promise but uptake is limited by expertise and time demands.[30,31]

Assessment of the Abdomen and Aorta as Potential Causes of Shock

Assessing the abdominal compartment for free fluid and the aorta for an abdominal aortic aneurysm (AAA) are fundamental POCUS skills for any emergency physician. There is strong evidence supporting the accuracy and speed with which this examination can be performed in the ED in the setting of trauma (focused assessment with sonography for trauma [FAST]) or suspected aneurysm.[32–34]

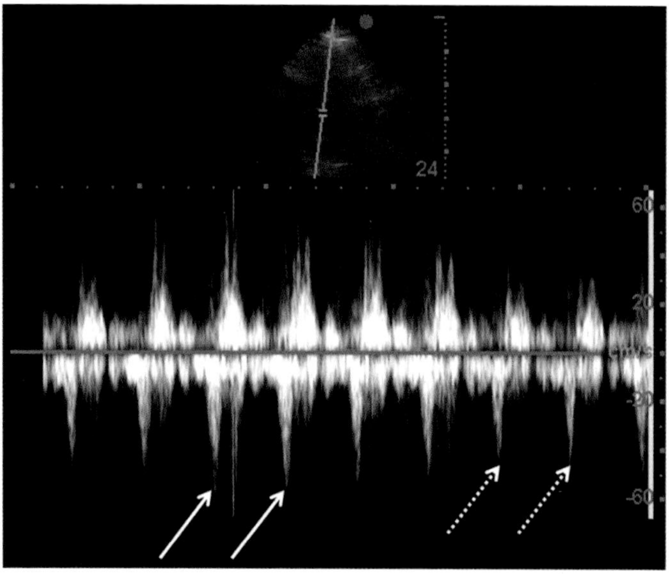

Fig. 7. Pulsed-wave Doppler of the left ventricular outflow tract showing respiratory variation in stroke volume from end expiration (*solid arrows*) and end inspiration (*dashed arrows*) in a spontaneously breathing patient, suggesting volume responsiveness.

Aortic dissection remains a diagnostic challenge for emergency physicians. Diagnosis of a type B or extensive type A dissection is occasionally made through abdominal aorta assessment when an intimal flap is revealed (**Fig. 8**). In an unstable patient, too sick to go to a CT scanner, an examination of the AV, aortic root, and proximal ascending aorta (with the PLAX view) and the pericardium should immediately be undertaken to assess for features supportive of a type A aortic dissection such as severe aortic regurgitation, a dissection flap in the proximal aorta, and hemopericardium.

Examination of the gallbladder in a hypotensive septic patient that is otherwise undifferentiated may occasionally reveal cholangitis as the cause. The sonographic

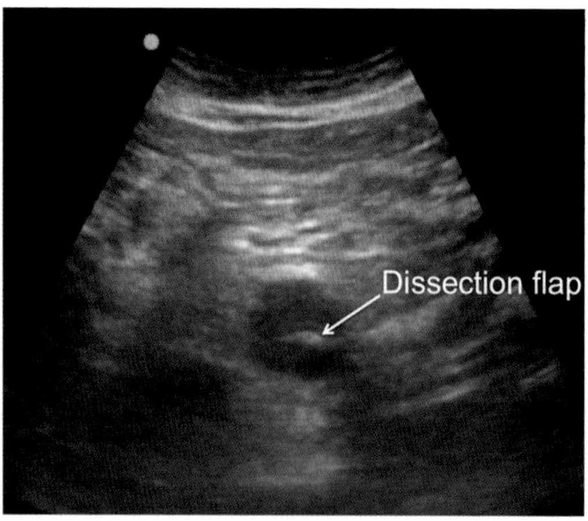

Fig. 8. Aortic dissection flap seen in cross section.

changes associated with an infected gallbladder include any combination of the presence of gallstones, a sonographic Murphy sign, a thick gallbladder wall (>3 mm), pericholecystic fluid, or a dilated common bile duct (**Fig. 9**).[35,36] Given the need for early, invasive source control, the benefits of identifying or excluding an abdominal source of septic shock, such as cholangitis, cannot be overstated.

Hemothorax and Pneumothorax as Causes for Hypotension

Particularly in the setting of trauma, the pleural space may conceal a hemodynamically important amount of blood that can be readily be identified with ultrasonography.[37] Hemothorax typically appears as an anechoic free space cranial to the diaphragm and may look similar to a simple medical effusion. However, a hemothorax may show some distinguishing features such as fibrin or clot formation (**Fig. 10**) or the so-called hematocrit sign as red cells separate from plasma. Nontraumatic causes of hemothorax, such as thoracic aneurysm rupture, are plausible but uncommon to reach hospital.

Pneumothorax, particularly tension pneumothorax, is a commonly implicated cause for shock in the setting of trauma, after a procedure, or during mechanical ventilation. With the diagnostic performance of supine chest radiograph leaving much to be desired (sensitivity of 28%–79%), lung ultrasonography offers a significant diagnostic advantage (sensitivity of 82%–98%) and is much faster to acquire than an urgent portable chest film.[38–40] Assessing for pneumothorax involves identifying reliable artifacts produced by the contact of the visceral and parietal pleural membranes, which are referred to as lung sliding (or shimmering), comet-tails (or B lines), and lung-point (**Fig. 11**).[41–43] In particular, it should be emphasized that the sensitivity of lung ultrasonography makes it an excellent tool to rule out pneumothorax. Tension pneumothorax is rare compared with other causes of hypotension or shock that are commonly lumped with the so-called Hs and Ts of the advanced cardiac life support dogma and the ability of lung ultrasonography to eliminate this distracting diagnosis from a list of more plausible causes makes it an exceptional tool in the rapidly evolving shock or cardiac arrest state.

CAUSES OF RESPIRATORY FAILURE

There is increasing literature advocating the use of lung ultrasonography to assist the clinician in determining a diagnosis at the bedside of an acutely dyspneic patient. The

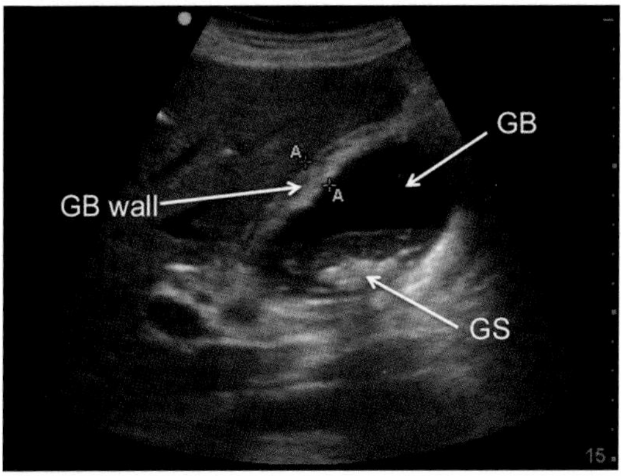

Fig. 9. Gallbladder (GB) with multiple gallstones (GS) and a thick wall (1.16 cm).

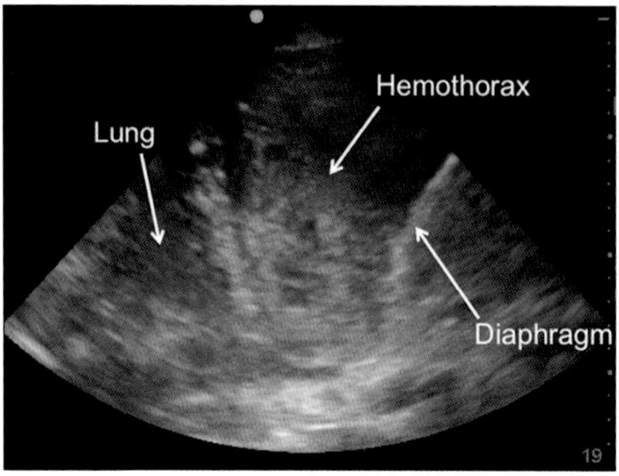

Fig. 10. Large left-sided hemothorax caused by an aortic injury. The effusion is showing a more isoechoic density caused by the early clotting.

air-filled lungs provide reliable artifact patterns in health and in various disease states that allow, with some training and reflective integration, the categorization of most patients in to a lung profile. The study and protocol best showing the feasibility and diagnostic accuracy of this approach was Lichtenstein and Meziere's[44] BLUE protocol study.

The BLUE protocol requires the clinician to perform an ultrasonography scan of the anterior and anterolateral thorax bilaterally, as well as 2 dedicated views of the pleural space, looking for specific lung artifact patterns: sliding lung, A lines (horizontal reverberation artifact) or B lines (vertical, hyperechoic lines that descend from pleural line to bottom of the ultrasonography screen), pleural effusion, or consolidation pattern (hepatized lung, suggesting atelectasis or pneumonia). Three or more B lines in a single rib space (B+ lines) indicates the interstitial syndrome, consistent most commonly in the ED with pulmonary edema but also seen with acute respiratory distress syndrome and lung fibrosis. An A/B pattern of lung artifacts consists of one hemithorax with an A-line pattern and the contralateral hemithorax with a B-line pattern, and indicates pneumonia. The C profile is characterized by anterior consolidation and indicates pneumonia as well. The use of this protocol allowed the investigators to correctly diagnose the cause of a patient's respiratory failure in 90.5% of 260 cases (**Table 3**).[44]

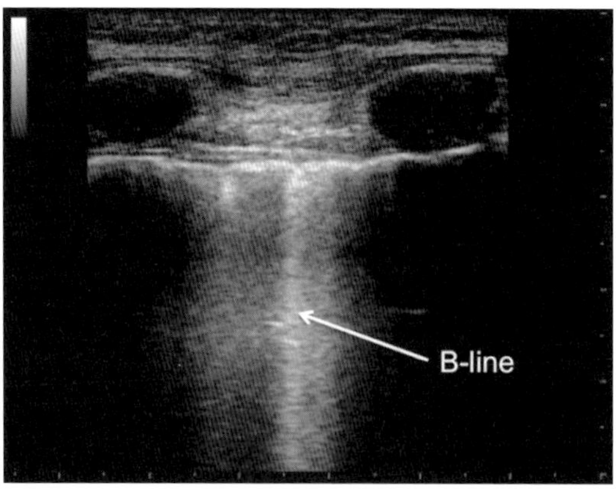

Fig. 11. B-line artifact arising from the pleural line.

Table 3
Causes of respiratory failure

Clinical Syndrome	Lung Ultrasonography Pattern	Additional Sonographic Findings	Image
Pulmonary edema	Diffuse B-line pattern	+ Lung sliding	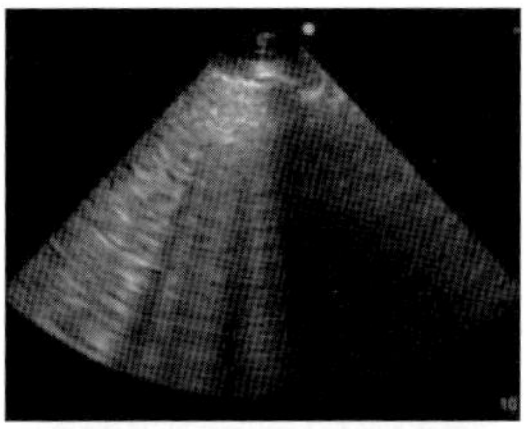
COPD Asthma PE Pneumothorax	A-line pattern A-line pattern A-line pattern A-line pattern	± Lung sliding + Lung sliding + Lung sliding + DVT – Lung sliding	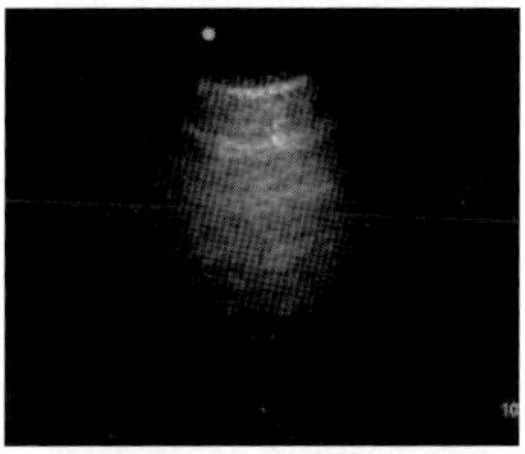
Pneumonia	A/B pattern	+ PLAPS ± Lung sliding	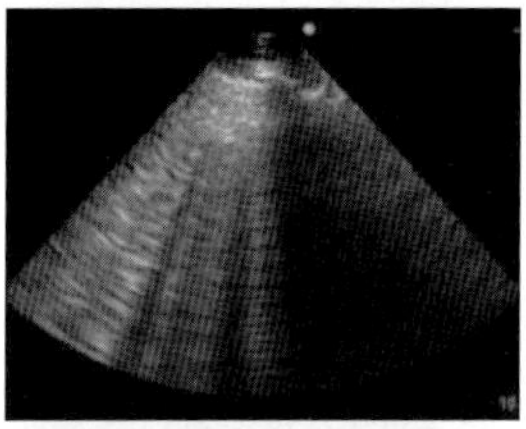 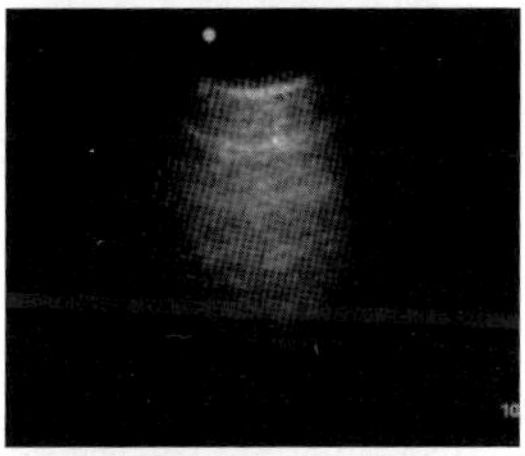
Pneumonia	C pattern	—	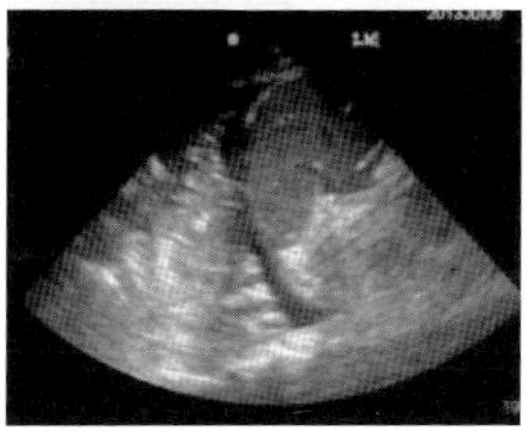

Abbreviations: COPD, chronic obstructive pulmonary disease; DVT, deep vein thrombosis; PE, pericardial effusion; PLAPS, posterolateral alveolar and/or pleural syndrome.

RESUSCITATIVE END POINTS

Under-resuscitation and over-resuscitation for circulatory failure can both contribute to excess mortality.[45,46] Serologic values (such as lactate and central venous oxygen saturation) and invasive measures (CVP) remain endorsed by the Surviving Sepsis Campaign Guidelines[26] and are measures of preload and oxygen delivery that are frequently used in the ED. There has been a natural enthusiasm for the ability of ultrasonography to either complement or replace some of these measures in guiding the intensity of resuscitation. As earlier, relying on the IVC for assessing a patient's fluid status and potential fluid responsiveness has many pitfalls. It is thus important to consider other methods by which clinicians can tailor resuscitation and identify, in particular, when volume resuscitation remains indicated and when further volume may cause harm.

Lichtenstein and Karakitsos[47] advocated looking at the main vital organ (the lung) rather than following indirect parameters such as changes in the LV or IVC size. Lichtenstein and Karakitsos's[47] fluid administration limited by lung sonography (FALLS) protocol can be used to guide fluid administration strategies during resuscitation scenarios using lung ultrasonography. Pulmonary edema is a classic resuscitation end point that is easily assessed for using POCUS. The FALLS protocol advocates for frequent imaging of the thorax throughout a resuscitation, looking for an evolving B-line pattern indicating pulmonary edema. A diffuse B-line pattern, with persistent shock, signals the resuscitationist to alter the management strategy (ie, vasopressors) because continued fluid administration may be harmful. This strategy works best when the initial lung ultrasonography reveals an A-line pattern (**Fig. 12**). If patients present with an initial diffuse B-profile on lung ultrasonography, then alternate strategies must be used to assess potential fluid responsiveness, as discussed earlier.

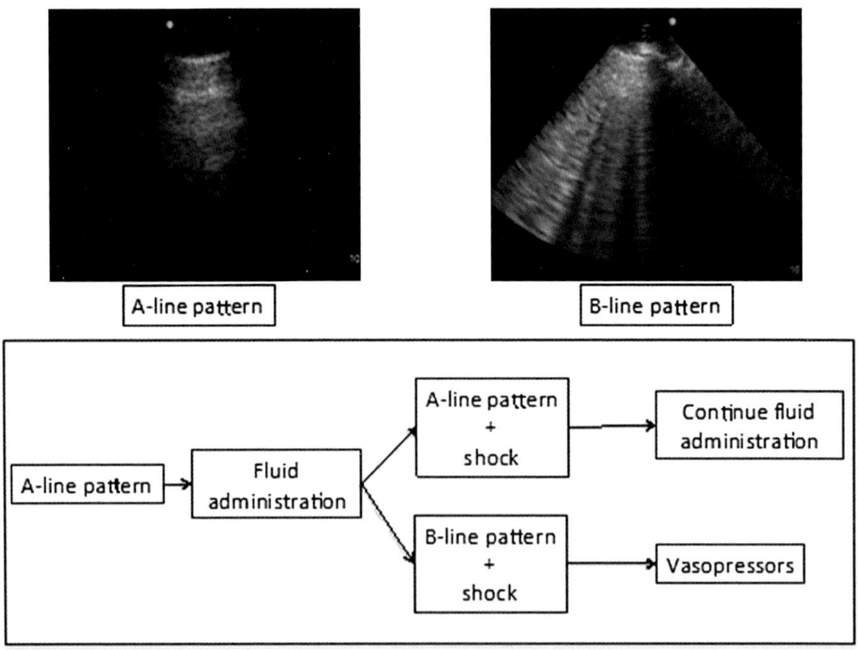

Fig. 12. Simplified FALLS fluid administration protocol.

It is readily apparent that there are several important aspects to assessing a patient in shock with POCUS when evaluating for potential causes, as well as potential therapeutic interventions. Integrating information gleaned from cardiac, lung, and IVC ultrasonography at the patient's bedside aids the astute clinician in managing these complex patients. Again, one of the strongest advantages of POCUS when treating critical patients is the ability to repeat the examination at various stages of treatment in determining not only the potential cause of the shock state but in initiating appropriate and potentially life-saving interventions.

NEUROLOGIC APPLICATIONS

Altered mental status and lateralizing features of brain dysfunction are easily recognized on cursory physical examination in the ED. Unlike other organs, little else can be done in the ED via laboratory or plain radiograph to further characterize or exclude anatomic causes of CNS failure, which frequently results in the need to transport critically ill patients out of the resuscitation room for CT scans of the head. Because of the time and risk of transport, the role of ultrasonography to image the brain at the point of care is attractive. Despite the sonographically impenetrable nature of bone, there are 2 distinct areas of the head (in an adult) where acoustic windows exist and create the opportunity for assessment: (1) the ocular window, imaging through the globe of the eye; and (2) the transcranial windows at the perimeter of the skull.

Identifying increased intracranial pressure (ICP) through imaging the optic nerve sheath diameter (ONSD) has received considerable attention. The optic nerve has a sheath that is fenestrated and, under conditions of increased ICP, the diameter of the nerve increases. Measurements more than 5 mm in width in the ED have been shown to correlate with increased ICP[48] and in a prospective trial showed 100% sensitivity for the identification of increased ICP, with a specificity of 63%.[49] The high-sensitivity 5-mm cut value for ONSD provides a helpful binary tool for the resuscitation physician to assist in ruling out increased ICP as the cause of an altered mental status in a critically ill patient (**Fig. 13**). ONSD is much less useful when increased because there are many false-positives (low specificity) and these patients all require CT scanning. Further, in true-positives with increased ONSD and increased ICP, what is needed is the ICP value to help guide blood pressure and corresponding cerebral perfusion pressure (CPP) titration.

Transcranial Doppler (TCD) ultrasonography makes use of transcranial windows (typically transtemporal) to measure velocity and resistance profiles of blood flow, typically via the middle cerebral artery. This Doppler information may be applied to determine the presence or absence of increased ICP given the reliable effect that increased ICP has on systolic (increased) and diastolic (reduced) velocities (**Fig. 14**). This modality has shown feasibility for use in an ED setting to identify both increased ICP and midline shift successfully.[50] However, TCD outperforms ONSD in its ability to provide real-time feedback in response to therapy for increased ICP. In an ED study on traumatic brain injury, a goal-directed protocol using TCD to guide blood pressure (and thus CPP), TCD was able to show normalization of systolic and diastolic velocities in response to a corrected CPP.[51] Despite the advantages that TCD may offer, TCD requires additional expertise in image acquisition and a good understanding of Doppler and its pitfalls, and is not routinely part of ultrasonography training in North America.

FUTURE DIRECTIONS

TEE for critically ill patients is a powerful tool in answering hemodynamic and anatomic questions regarding circulatory failure.[52] TEE has several advantages compared with

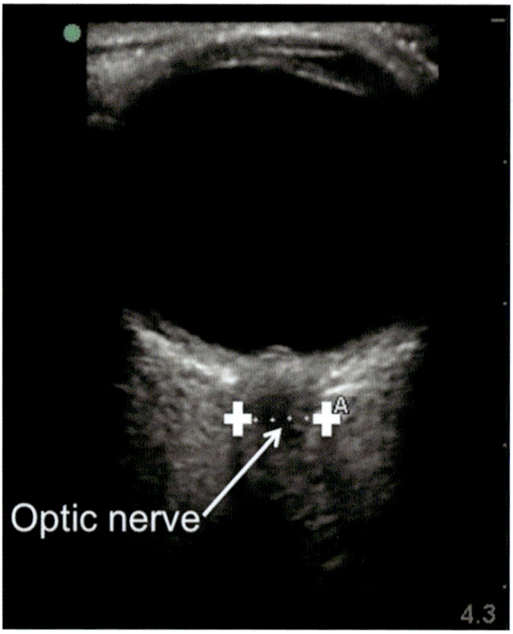

Fig. 13. Ultrasonography of the optic nerve sheath in a patient with traumatic brain injury. Caliper measurements show an optic nerve diameter of 6.5 mm, suggesting increased ICP.

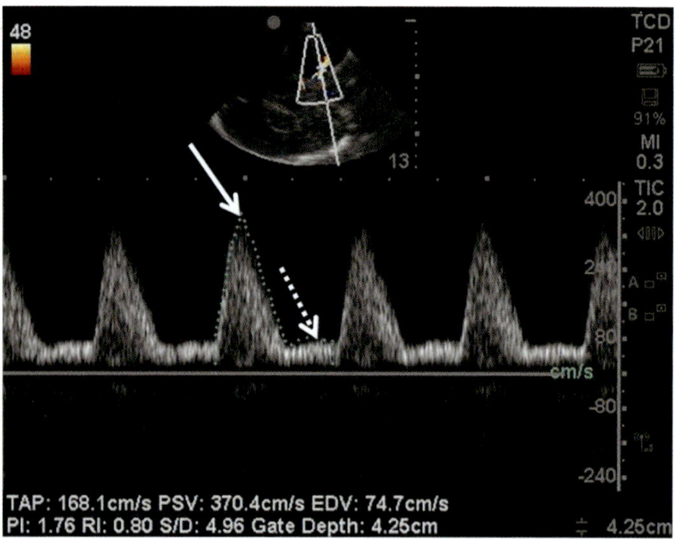

Fig. 14. Transcranial Doppler profile of the left middle cerebral artery as obtained in the ED from a patient with increased ICP that corresponds here subjectively with a heightened difference between the peak systolic velocity (*solid arrow*) and the diastolic velocity (*dashed arrow*) or, more objectively, a resistive index (systolic velocity – diastolic velocity/systolic velocity) of 0.80 (normal: <0.60).

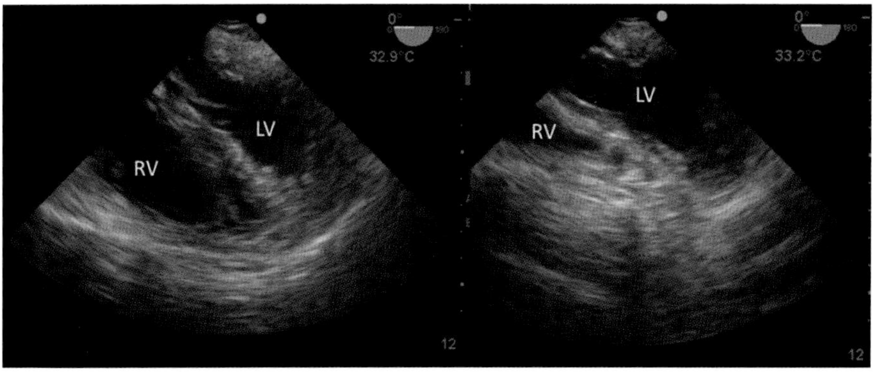

Fig. 15. Transesophageal echocardiography images obtained from a patient undergoing CPR in the ED. The view is from the midesophagus during CPR. On the right image, compression of the heart (RV in particular) is evident during active compressions.

the transthoracic approach, including more reliable, high-quality images and its indwelling location that enables continuous monitoring of the heart during resuscitation, including cardiopulmonary resuscitation (CPR) (**Fig. 15**). Despite these advantages, uptake in the ED has been limited to this point, largely because of the cost and limited training opportunities. It is anticipated that, with the advent of high-fidelity TEE simulators and the increased uptake of emergency physicians with critical care training, TEE use in the ED for critically ill patients will continue to increase.

SUMMARY

Resuscitative ultrasonography provides rapid, repeatable, and multisystem assessment to guide diagnosis and management of critically ill patients in the ED. Cardiac ultrasonography offers new anatomic and hemodynamic information, previously unavailable in an ED setting, whereas other applications match or exceed the speed and utility of existing tests such as chest radiograph (thoracic ultrasonography) or CVP determination (IVC ultrasonography). Evolving areas of resuscitative ultrasonography, including neurologic assessment and TEE, are increasing, further maximizing the ability for ultrasonography to enhance the provision of critical care in the ED.

REFERENCES

1. Plummer D, Brunette D, Asinger R, et al. Emergency department echocardiography improves outcome in penetrating cardiac injury. Ann Emerg Med 1992;21:709–12.
2. Rozycki GS, Feliciano DV, Ochsner MG, et al. The role of ultrasound in patients with possible penetrating cardiac wounds: a prospective multicenter study. J Trauma 1999;46:543–51.
3. Kimura A, Otsuka T. Emergency center ultrasonography in the evaluation of hematoperitoneum: a prospective study. J Trauma 1991;31:20–3.
4. Rozycki GS, Ochsner MG, Jaffin JH, et al. Prospective evaluation of surgeons' use of ultrasound in the evaluation of the trauma patient. J Trauma 1993;34:516–27.
5. Mayo PH, Beaulieu Y, Doelken P, et al. American College Of Chest Physicians/la Société de Reanimation de Langue Française statement on competence in critical care ultrasonography. Chest 2009;135:1050–60.

6. Rose JS, Bair AE, Manavia D, et al. The UHP protocol: a novel ultrasound approach to the empiric evaluation of the undifferentiated hypotensive patient. Am J Emerg Med 2001;19:299–302.
7. Breitkreutz R, Walcher F, Seegar FH. Focused echocardiographic evaluation in resuscitation management: concept of an advanced life support-confirmed algorithm. Crit Care Med 2007;35:S150–61.
8. Atkinson PR, McAuley DJ, Kendall RJ, et al. Abdominal and cardiac evaluation with sonography in shock (ACES): an approach by emergency physicians for the use of ultrasound in patients with undifferentiated hypotension. Emerg Med J 2009;26:87–91.
9. Perera P, Mailhot T, Riley D, et al. The RUSH exam: rapid ultrasound in shock in the evaluation of the critically ill. Emerg Med Clin North Am 2010;28:29–56.
10. Breitkreutz R, Price S, Steiger HV, et al. Focused echocardiographic evaluation in life support and peri-resuscitation of emergency patients: a prospective trial. Resuscitation 2010;81:1527–33.
11. Lanctôt JF, Valois M, Beaulieu Y. EGLS: echo-guided life support. Crit Ultrasound J 2011;3:123–9.
12. Melamed R, Sprenkle MD, Ulstad VK, et al. Assessment of left ventricular function by intensivists using hand-held echocardiography. Chest 2009;135:1416–20.
13. Moore CL, Rose GA, Tayal VS, et al. Determination of left ventricular function by emergency physician echocardiography of hypotensive patients. Acad Emerg Med 2002;9:186–93.
14. Pershad J, Myers S, Plouman C, et al. Bedside limited echocardiography by the emergency physician is accurate during evaluation of the critically ill patient. Pediatrics 2004;114:e667–71.
15. Randazzo MR, Snoey ER, Levitt MA, et al. Accuracy of emergency physician assessment of left ventricular ejection fraction and central venous pressure using echocardiography. Acad Emerg Med 2003;10:973–7.
16. Kimura BJ, Yogo N, O'Connell C, et al. A cardiopulmonary limited ultrasound examination for "quick-look" bedside application. Am J Cardiol 2011;108(4):586–90.
17. Singh S, Wann LS, Schuchard GH, et al. Right ventricular and right atrial collapse in patients with cardiac tamponade—a combined echocardiographic and hemodynamic study. Circulation 1984;70:966–71.
18. Himelman RB, Kircher B, Rockey DC, et al. Inferior vena cava plethora with blunted respiratory response: a sensitive echocardiography sign of cardiac tamponade. J Am Coll Cardiol 1988;12(6):1470–7.
19. Kimchi A, Ellrodt AG, Berman DS, et al. Right ventricular performance in septic shock: a combined radionuclide and hemodynamic study. J Am Coll Cardiol 1984;4(5):945–51.
20. Ghio S, Gavazzi A, Campana C, et al. Independent and additive prognostic value of right ventricular systolic function and pulmonary artery pressure in patients with chronic heart failure. J Am Coll Cardiol 2001;37:183–8.
21. Torbicki A, Perrier A, Konstantinides S, et al. The Task Force for the Diagnosis and Management of Acute Pulmonary Embolism of the European Society of Cardiology. Guidelines on the diagnosis and management of acute pulmonary embolism. Eur Heart J 2008;29:276–315.
22. Osman D, Monnet X, Castelain V, et al. Incidence and prognostic value of right ventricular failure in acute respiratory distress syndrome. Intensive Care Med 2009;35:69–76.

23. Jones AE, Craddock PA, Tayal VS, et al. Diagnostic accuracy of left ventricular function for identifying sepsis among emergency department patients with nontraumatic symptomatic undifferentiated hypotension. Shock 2005;24(6): 513–7.
24. Barbier C, Loubières Y, Schmit C, et al. Respiratory changes in inferior vena cava diameter are helpful in predicting fluid responsiveness in ventilated septic patients. Intensive Care Med 2004;30:1740–6.
25. Feissel M, Michard F, Faller JP, et al. The respiratory variation in inferior vena cava diameter as a guide to fluid therapy. Intensive Care Med 2004;30:1834–7.
26. Dellinger RP, Levy MM, Rhodes A, et al. Surviving sepsis campaign: international guidelines for management of severe sepsis and septic shock, 2012. Intensive Care Med 2013;39(2):165–228.
27. Marik PE, Cavallazzi R. Does the central venous pressure predict fluid responsiveness? An updated meta-analysis and a plea for some common sense. Crit Care Med 2013;41:1774–81.
28. Feissel M, Michard F, Mangin I, et al. Respiratory changes in aortic blood velocity as an indicator of fluid responsiveness in ventilated patients with septic shock. Chest 2001;119:867–73.
29. Brennan JM, Blair JE, Hampole C, et al. Radial artery pulse pressure variation correlates with brachial artery peak velocity variation in ventilated subjects when measured by internal medicine residents using hand-carried ultrasound devices. Chest 2007;131:1301–7.
30. Ommen SR, Nishimura RA, Appleton CP, et al. Clinical utility of Doppler echocardiography and tissue Doppler imaging in the estimation of left ventricular filling pressures a comparative simultaneous Doppler-catheterization study. Circulation 2000;102:1788–94.
31. Moore CL, Tham ET, Samuels KJ, et al. Tissue Doppler of early mitral filling correlates with simulated volume loss in healthy subjects. Acad Emerg Med 2010; 17:1162–8.
32. Stengel D, Bauwens K, Rademacher G, et al. Association between compliance with methodological standards of diagnostic research and reported test accuracy: meta-analysis of focused assessment of US for trauma. Radiology 2005; 236:102–11.
33. Cosantino TG, Bruno EC, Handly N, et al. Accuracy of emergency medicine ultrasound in the evaluation of abdominal aortic aneurysm. J Emerg Med 2005;29: 455–60.
34. Dent B, Kendall RJ, Boyle AA, et al. Emergency ultrasound of the abdominal aorta by UK emergency physicians: a prospective cohort study. Emerg Med J 2007;24:547–9.
35. Ralls PW, Colletti PM, Lapin SA, et al. Real-time sonography in suspected acute cholecystitis: prospective evaluation of primary and secondary signs. Radiology 1985;155:767–71.
36. Handler SJ. Ultrasound of gallbladder wall thickening and its relation to cholecystitis. AJR Am J Roentgenol 1979;132:581–5.
37. Kirkpatrick AW, Sirois M, Laupland KB, et al. Hand-held thoracic sonography for detecting post-traumatic pneumothoraces: the extended focused assessment with sonography for trauma (EFAST). J Trauma 2004;57:288–95.
38. Nandipati KC, Allamaneni S, Kakarla R, et al. Extended focused assessment with sonography for trauma (EFAST) in the diagnosis of pneumothorax: experience at a community based level I trauma center. Injury 2010;42: 511–4.

39. Wilkerson G, Stone MB. Sensitivity of bedside ultrasound and supine anteroposterior chest radiographs for the identification of pneumothorax after blunt trauma. Acad Emerg Med 2010;17:11–7.
40. Nagarsheth K, Kurek S. Ultrasound detection of pneumothorax compared with chest x-ray and computed tomography scan. Am Surg 2011;77:480–4.
41. Lichtenstein DA, Menu Y. A bedside ultrasound sign ruling out pneumothorax in the critically ill: lung sliding. Chest 1995;108:1345–8.
42. Lichtenstein DA, Meziére G, Biderman P, et al. The comet-tail artifact: an ultrasound sign ruling out pneumothorax. Intensive Care Med 1999;25:383–8.
43. Lichtenstein DA, Meziére G, Biderman P, et al. The "lung point": an ultrasound sign specific to pneumothorax. Intensive Care Med 2000;26:1434–40.
44. Lichtenstein DA, Meziere GA. Relevance of lung ultrasound in the diagnosis of acute respiratory failure: the BLUE protocol. Chest 2008;134:117–25.
45. Boyd JH, Forbes J, Nakada T, et al. Fluid resuscitation in septic shock: a positive fluid balance and elevated central venous pressure are associated with increased mortality. Crit Care Med 2011;39:259–65.
46. Rivers E, Nguyen B, Havstad S, et al. Early goal-directed therapy in the treatment of severe sepsis and septic shock. N Engl J Med 2001;345:1368–77.
47. Lichtenstein DA, Karakitsos D. Integrating lung ultrasound in the hemodynamic evaluation of acute circulatory failure (the Fluid Administration Limited by Lung Sonography protocol). J Crit Care 2012;27:533.e11–9.
48. Blaivas M, Theodoro D, Sierzenski PR. Elevated intracranial pressure detected by bedside emergency ultrasonography of the optic nerve sheath. Acad Emerg Med 2003;10:376–81.
49. Tayal VS, Neulander M, Norton HJ, et al. Emergency department sonographic measurement of optic nerve sheath diameter to detect findings of increased intracranial pressure in adult head injury patients. Ann Emerg Med 2007;49:508–14.
50. Shafé M, Blaivas M, Hooker E, et al. Noninvasive intracranial cerebral flow velocity evaluation in the emergency department by emergency physicians. Acad Emerg Med 2004;11:774–7.
51. Ract C, Le Moigno S, Bruder N, et al. Transcranial Doppler ultrasound goal-directed therapy for the early management of severe traumatic brain injury. Intensive Care Med 2007;33:645–51.
52. Vignon P, Mentec H, Terré S, et al. Diagnostic accuracy and therapeutic impact of transthoracic and transesophageal echocardiography in mechanically ventilated patients in the ICU. Chest 1994;106(6):1829–34.

Select Topics in Neurocritical Care

Anthony Noto, MD, Evie Marcolini, MD*

KEYWORDS

- Neurocritical care • Myasthenia gravis • Guillain-Barre syndrome • Meningitis • Encephalitis • Rhombencephalitis

KEY POINTS

- The most important determinant of the need for intensive care in neuromuscular disease is pending respiratory failure.
- Clinical presentation can differentiate meningitis from encephalitis.
- The most common cause of immune-mediated encephalitis in adults is antibody mediated encephalitis.
- Guillian Barre syndrome is a commonly missed diagnosis in the ED which may progress to significant morbidity.

INTRODUCTION

Neurocritical care aims to improve outcomes in patients with life-threatening neurologic illness. The scope of neurocritical care extends beyond the more commonly encountered and important field of cerebrovascular disease, as described previously.[1,2] This article focuses on neuromuscular, neuroinfectious, and neuroimmunologic conditions that are significant causes of morbidity and mortality in the acutely neurologically ill patient. As understanding continues to increase regarding the physiology of these conditions and the best treatment, rapid identification, triage, and treatment of these patients in the emergency department (ED) is paramount.

NEUROMUSCULAR DISEASE

Unlike those in the central nervous system, lesions in the peripheral nervous system can be difficult to localize and may delay diagnosis, with detrimental effects. The 2 main categories of neuromuscular disease that frequently require intensive care are peripheral demyelinating disease (Guillain-Barre syndrome [GBS]) and neuromuscular junction disease (myasthenia gravis). The clinical course can be highly variable, ranging from strictly outpatient treatment to prolonged ventilator dependence in an intensive care unit (ICU) setting, therefore appropriate early triage is important.

Divisions of Neurocritical Care and Emergency Neurology and Surgical Critical Care, Departments of Emergency Medicine and Neurology, Yale University School of Medicine, 464 Congress St. Suite 260, New Haven, CT 06519, USA

* Corresponding author.

E-mail address: emarcolini@gmail.com

Emerg Med Clin N Am 32 (2014) 927–938
http://dx.doi.org/10.1016/j.emc.2014.07.015 emed.theclinics.com
0733-8627/14/$ – see front matter

Peripheral Demyelinating Disease

With an estimated incidence of 1 to 4 per 100,000, GBS and its variants are rare but represent the most common cause of acute paralysis.[3] Guillain-Barre syndrome typically presents with ascending weakness, paresthesias, and areflexia, but at least 4 subtypes have been described with variable presentations. Miller-Fisher syndrome accounts for roughly 5% of GBS cases and presents with ataxia, ophthalmoplegia, and areflexia. Acute motor axonal neuropathy and acute motor sensory axonal neuropathy are differentiated by severe damage to peripheral nerve axons in addition to demyelination, and present as acute paralysis and loss of reflexes with or without sensory loss. Finally, acute panautonomic neuropathy is a rare variant that can be rapidly fatal, and presents with encephalopathy and autonomic instability.[4]

Pathophysiology

Guillain-Barre syndrome is an autoimmune disease with antibodies directed against targets on peripheral nerves. These antibodies usually form 4 to 7 days after an antecedent infection. Most common infections include *Campylobacter jejuni* and cytomegalovirus.[5] Although an association between GBS and influenza has been reported, specifically after the swine flu in the late 1970s, more recent studies have shown no specific correlation.[6] The typical course of GBS progresses through 4 phases: (1) interval between the inciting illness and onset of neuromuscular symptoms, (2) progressive weakness lasting less than a month, (3) plateau, and (4) recovery. Quadriplegia may occur in a rapidly progressive form of GBS, in which onset of respiratory failure can occur within 48 hours.[5]

Clinical presentation and diagnosis

Generalized weakness is a common complaint in the emergency department, and therefore a high index of suspicion is needed to correctly diagnose GBS. A retrospective case series of 20 patients with GBS over 5 years in a large ED found that only 25% were accurately diagnosed during their first visit and on average 2 visits were needed for diagnosis.[4] In patients presenting with ascending weakness or parasthesia after an illness, a neurologic examination is needed to specifically focus on ocular movement abnormalities and absent reflexes. A lumbar puncture should also be performed to assess for albuminocytologic dissociation, in which an elevated protein level is seen (>100 mg/dL) without an elevation in cell count.[3] Electromyography can eventually be helpful to determine the extent and type of damage but it is typically normal in the acute setting and not performed urgently in the ED.

Neuromuscular Junction Disorders

Disorders of the neuromuscular junction refer to interruptions in the transmission of acetylcholine from the nerve terminal to the muscle cell. In developed countries, the most common neuromuscular junction disorder is myasthenia gravis with an incidence of 1 to 3 per 1 million people. As with GBS, the variability of clinical presentation and disease course is significant and a high index of suspicion is needed for diagnosis. A higher incidence of myasthenia gravis is seen in women, with the peak onset occurring in childbearing years. Up to 20% of patients with myasthenia gravis will have a myasthenic crisis, characterized by the need for mechanical ventilation, within 2 years of diagnosis.[7]

Pathophysiology

Myasthenia gravis is an autoimmune disorder with antibodies most commonly directed toward the acetylcholine receptor on the muscle cell membrane. The binding, blocking, and modulating antiacetylcholine receptor antibodies are frequently tested with the binding antibody present in 90% of cases.[7] Medications of many classes that are commonly used in the ED may transform a mild exacerbation into a crisis, and should be avoided (**Table 1**).

Clinical presentation and diagnosis

As in GBS, the chief complaint with myasthenia gravis is often generalized weakness. Muscle fatigability and ocular involvement are the key features of the syndrome. Other symptoms include diplopia, ptosis, dysphagia, dysarthria, proximal weakness, fatigue, and shortness of breath.[7] Conversely, autonomic dysfunction should not be present, because the neuromuscular junction in smooth muscle does not use acetylcholine for signal transmission. Ultimately, electromyography can be helpful to document decreasing muscle response after repetitive nerve stimulation.[7]

Progression to Acute Respiratory Failure in Neuromuscular Disease

Most relevant to neurocritical care is identifying the patients who present with neuromuscular disease that will progress to respiratory failure. Although most patients require hospitalization for treatment of GBS, roughly one-third will require mechanical ventilation at some point during their clinical course.[8] Similarly, in myasthenia gravis, 15% to 27% of patients experience a myasthenic crisis. The general mechanism of acute respiratory failure in neuromuscular disease is a combination of inspiratory and expiratory muscle weakness, resulting in small tidal volumes, atelectasis, hypoxemia, and aspiration.[9] The goal is to identify at-risk patients for admission to the ICU and early, planned intubation rather than emergent after-hours intubation (48% in one study).[10]

A secondary analysis conducted on patients with GBS enrolled in 2 randomized controlled trials found that rapid progression (<7 days from onset to admission), inability to cough, stand, lift elbows or head, and elevated liver enzymes required intubation in greater than 85% of cases with more than 4 predictors.[10] A second retrospective study also identified bulbar dysfunction (impaired gag, dysarthria, dysphagia) and autonomic dysfunction (blood pressure fluctuation and bowel/bladder involvement) as statistically significant predictors of respiratory failure.[10]

Respiratory physiologic measurements can also be helpful to identify early signs of respiratory decline in patients with GBS. Classically, vital capacity (VC) has been the gold standard, with a cutoff of less than 20 mL/kg as an indication for intubation. Serial vital capacity measurements should be performed during the initial assessment, because a greater than 30% reduction is indicative of impending respiratory failure.[11] Maximal inspiratory pressure (PI_{max}) and expiratory pressure (PE_{max}) can supplement decision making, because a PI_{max} of less than −30 cm H_2O or a PE_{max} of less than 40 cm H_2O is indicative of respiratory failure, as applied in the "20/30/40 rule" describing the cutoffs for VC, PI_{max}, and PE_{max}. Maximal inspiratory pressure is the maximum negative pressure that a person can generate during inspiration, and is

Table 1
Medications with risk for exacerbation of myasthenia gravis crisis

Class	
Hormonal	Steroids, thyroid hormone, oral contraceptives
Antibiotics	Aminoglycosides, tetracyclines, ciprofloxacin, clindamycin, erythromycin, bacitracin
Antiarrhythmics	Procainamide, quinidine, lidocaine
Antihypertensives	Beta blockers, calcium channel blockers
Neuromuscular blockers	Magnesium, botulinum toxin
Other	Phenytoin, lithium, carbamazepine, magnesium

an indirect measure of diaphragm strength. Maximal inspiratory pressure is the maximum positive pressure that a person can create after a full inhalation. Both are measured using a mechanical pressure gauge. Vital capacity, measured with a spirometer, is the maximum volume of air that can be expelled after a full inspiration. Although it has been postulated[12] that the decrease in muscle strength (PI_{max}) might be an earlier indicator of respiratory failure than the decrease in lung volume (PE_{max}), Prigent and colleagues[13] found this not to provide any sensitivity benefit.

Overall, multiple clinical and physiologic parameters, taken together with objective respiratory parameters, have been shown to predict acute respiratory decline in neuromuscular disease (**Box 1**).

Treatment of respiratory failure

When impending respiratory failure is recognized, intubation is typically the first-line treatment in neuromuscular conditions rather than noninvasive positive pressure ventilation (NPPV), because concern for aspiration. Only one study examined the outcome of patients with myasthenia gravis treated with NPPV[14]; cases retrospectively reviewed found that intubation was prevented 70% of the time.[15] The cases in which NPPV failed were found to correlate only with initial hypercapnia with a P_{CO_2} greater than 50 mm Hg, and not bulbar weakness as would be expected. Further research is needed to recommend routine use of NPPV. When intubating patients with GBS, extra care should be taken to prevent dysautonomia (cardiac arrhythmia or blood pressure fluctuations) using sedatives, and potentially fatal[16] hyperkalemia using depolarizing paralytics. Nondepolarizing agents, such as rocuronium or vecuronium, may be used in place of succinylcholine in most cases.[17] Initial ventilator settings should focus on lung expansion and counteracting fatigue. Lower tidal volumes and higher respiratory rates have been shown to avoid lung injury, with frequent intermittent recruitment maneuvers (1.5 times tidal volume hold for a brief period) to decrease atelectasis.[7] After intubation, the length of ventilator dependence ranges from median of 18 to 27 days in GBS and 6 to 14 days in myasthenia gravis.[16]

Box 1
Signs and symptoms of pending respiratory failure in neuromuscular disease

Signs

- Generalized weakness
- Oropharyngeal weakness
- Difficulty clearing secretions
- Dysphonia
- Dyspnea on exertion and at rest

Symptoms

- Rapid shallow breathing
- Tachycardia
- Weak cough
- Accessory muscle use
- Shortness of breath when supine
- Neck weakness
- Inability to count to 50 in a single breath

Despite whether the patient with neuromuscular disease requires intubation, they should be admitted to a higher level of nursing care, because the rapidity of progression is not reliably predictable and these patients warrant close monitoring.

Neuroinfectious Disease

One of the most serious and life-threatening conditions that presents to the ED is infection of the central nervous system. Both meningitis (viral and bacterial) and encephalitis have the potential to be rapidly fatal if not triaged and treated urgently. Meningitis is inflammation of the meninges, whereas encephalitis is inflammation of the brain parenchyma itself. Rhombencephalitis, a subset of encephalitis, is an inflammatory and infectious disease involving the brainstem only. Clinical presentation can be used to differentiate meningitis from encephalitis, because patients with meningitis alone will have pain or altered mental status, but should not present with seizure, aphasia, or focal neurologic deficits. The prevalence of meningitis and encephalitis is difficult to estimate because of the wide variation in pathogens and clinical course. The term *meningoencephalitis* refers to a group of systemic infections that cause inflammation affecting both the brain and the meninges. Causative agents include viral, bacterial, tick-borne, and fungal pathogens.

Diagnosis

In the ED, any patient with headache, neck stiffness, fever, and altered mental status should be suspected of having a central nervous system infection, and, as one study validated, at least 95% of patients with infectious meningitis have 2 of these 4 signs.[18] In the past, Kernig and Brudzinski signs have been used to support or refute the diagnosis of bacterial meningitis, but the sensitivity and specificity of these tests were unknown based on a review from 1999 and 2002.[19,20] A recent observational study showed that Kernig and Brudzinski signs, and nuchal rigidity have moderate positive predictive value, whereas jolt accentuation did not.[21] The test for the Kernig is performed by having the patient extend the knee while sitting upright to assess for back pain, whereas the Brudzinski sign is elicited by flexing the patient's neck to assess for reflex flexion at the hips and knees.

To make a definitive diagnosis and determine the cause, a lumbar puncture should be performed urgently. However, nothing should delay empiric treatment. If the neurologic examination is focal or abnormal, or is the patient is immunocompromised, an image of the brain must first be obtained to ensure a lumbar puncture will be safe to perform. With large supratentorial mass lesions such as abscess, a lumbar puncture may precipitate herniation (**Table 2**).

Table 2
Common cerebrospinal fluid results and associated causes in meningitis

	Normal	Bacterial	Viral	Fungal	Tuberculous
Opening pressure (mm H_2O)	<180	200–500	N/A	>250	N/A
WBC (mm^3)	0–5	100–20,000	5–500	20–2000	5–2000
WBC differential	None	>80% PMN	>50% Lymph, <20% PMN	>50% Lymph	>80% Lymph
Protein	15–50	100–500	30–150	40–150	>50
Glucose	45–100 (67% of serum)	<40 (<40% of serum)	30–70	30–70	<40

General Management Strategies

The Neurocritical Care Society Emergency Neurologic Life Support guidelines proposed the flowchart for early triage and management, which is applicable to emergency department providers (**Fig. 1**).[22]

Bacterial meningitis/encephalitis

With a suspected diagnosis of bacterial meningitis, dexamethasone must be initiated urgently, followed by empiric antibiotic therapy. The efficacy of administering dexamethasone (10 mg intravenously) before antibiotic therapy for bacterial meningitis, specifically *Streptococcus pneumonia*, was verified by a 2002 European study.[23] The antibiotics used must have high central nervous system penetration and cover common gram-positive and gram-negative organisms. The most common bacterial causes in adults include *S pneumoniae, Neisseria meningitides*, and *Listeria monocytogenes.* Empiric antibiotics used typically include a third-generation cephalosporin, ampicillin for coverage of *Listeria* in the elderly and immunosuppressed, and vancomycin.

Bacterial meningitis and encephalitis can lead to significant brain edema and increased intracranial pressure, which should be managed aggressively to prevent secondary brain injury. A small cohort study examined the use of lumbar drainage for bacterial meningitis and found reduced mortality in a small subset of patients.[24] Additionally, 5% of adult patients with bacterial meningitis may develop hydrocephalus,

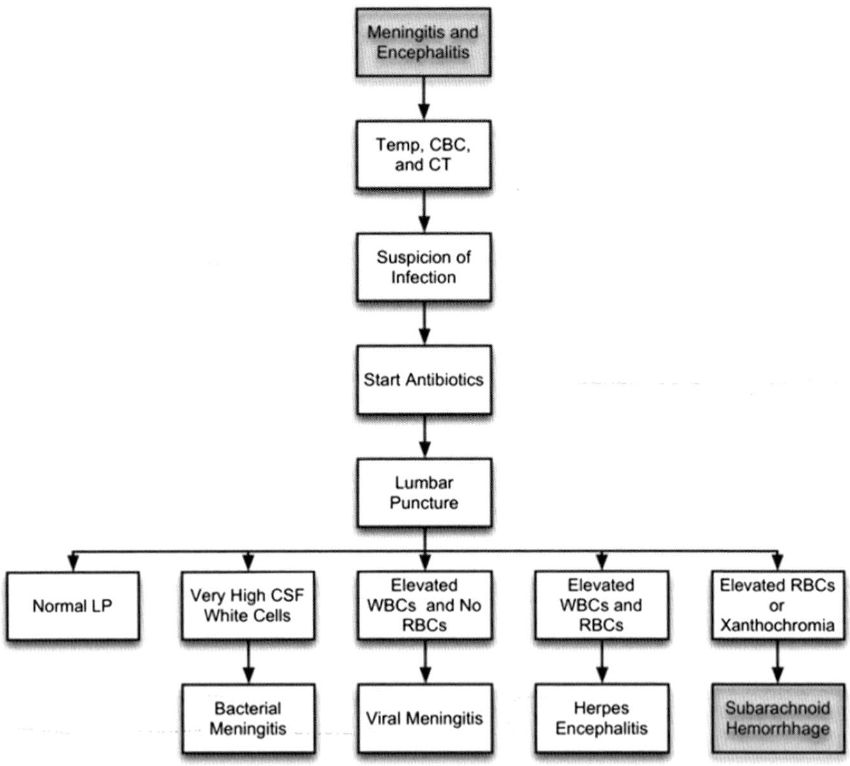

Fig. 1. Management strategies for early triage and management of meningitis and encephalitis. (*From* Gaieski DF, Nathan BR, Weingart SD, et al. Emergency neurologic life support: meningitis and encephalitis. Neurocrit Care 2012;17(Suppl 1):S67; with permission.)

with 69% having hydrocephalus on presentation.[25] The emergency physician should consider ventricular drainage in patients with obstructive hydrocephalus, evolving midline shift, or meningitis and a decline in consciousness.[25] Despite shunting, these patients are at high risk for morbidity and mortality, and in one study hydrocephalus was identified as being a significant independent predictor of death from bacterial meningitis.[25] Septic shock associated with bacterial meningitis is common, and aggressive volume resuscitation is needed per the "Surviving Sepsis Campaign Guidelines for the Management of Severe Sepsis and Septic Shock."[26] Overall, these patients often require ICU care for monitoring and management of increased intracranial pressure and septic shock.

Brain abscesses occur through either seeding from cranial structures, such as ears, paranasal sinuses, osteomyelitic skull lesions, penetrating cranial injuries, or congenital sinus tracts, or through hematogenous spread and septic emboli. The causal pathogen is often *Staphylococcus aureus* or *S pneumoniae*, because these bacteria induce an inflammatory response in glial cells that create a wall around the infected tissue, forming an abscess.[27] Abscesses cause significant edema and mass effect with focal neurologic deficits and can be mistaken for tumor. If multiple abscesses are present, left-sided endocarditis should be suspected. Presentation in the ED is often a first-time seizure or headache, and these patients will usually not appear septic because the infection is contained. In addition to long-term antibiotics, patients require neurosurgical drainage to identify the causative organism and determine definitive treatment.[28] Lumbar puncture is contraindicated because of herniation risk and results are often negative. In one large prospective multicenter observational study (ENDO-REA), 7% of patients with left-sided endocarditis developed abscesses.[29] Although hundreds of types of agents can cause intracranial infection, and the suspected localization of the lesion most effectively guides the protocolling of an imaging study, a few general concepts should be considered. It is prudent to begin with a noncontrast computed tomography (CT) scan to identify large lesions or postinflammatory changes, followed if necessary by contrast-enhanced CT, or magnetic resonance imaging (MRI) with gadolinium if not contraindicated. Abnormal or nonexistent blood-brain barrier causes enhancement of intracranial contrast.[30]

Viral encephalitis

Although viral meningitis is often treated on an outpatient basis with oral antivirals, encephalitis should be managed in an intensive care setting because of significant risk for increased intracranial pressure, status epilepticus, neurogenic shock, and respiratory failure. Currently, the only treatable forms of viral encephalitis are caused by the herpes simplex viruses (HSV) or varicella zoster virus (VZV).[31] Intravenous acyclovir is often started empirically for any concern of encephalitis, and continued until confirmatory testing on cerebrospinal fluid is performed. If HSV is confirmed and there is no response to treatment with acyclovir, especially in immunocompromised hosts, switching to foscarnet is appropriate, because acyclovir-resistant strains of HSV are becoming more common. Specifically for HSV encephalitis, seizures are a major component of presentation, because the temporal lobes are preferentially affected. Initial seizure management begins with the airway, and patients will often need mechanical ventilation and continuous infusion of an antiepileptic, such as propofol or midazolam, or antiepileptic medication.[32] If available, long-term video electroencephalographic monitoring can be useful to determine whether a patient is in refractory nonconvulsive status epilepticus and to gauge efficacy of current treatment. In cases of viral encephalitis not caused by HSV or VZV, management is otherwise focused on supportive care.

Rhombencephalitis

When a patient presents with fever, multiple cranial nerve deficits, ataxia, and altered mental status, suspicion should be raised for infection of the brainstem (rhombencephalon). Several pathogens specifically target the areas of the pons, cerebellum, and medulla. The most common infectious cause is *Listeria monocytogenes*. Other less common infectious origins include enterovirus type 71, Japanese encephalitis, *Mycobacterium tuberculosis*, Epstein-Barr virus, West Nile virus, and *Aspergillus*. Information about rhombencephalitis from these agents is available on an individual case report basis and beyond the scope of this article.

Unlike with central nervous system listeriosis, 80% of patients with listeria rhombencephalitis are healthy immunocompetent adults with a mean age of 48 years, based on one large case series.[32] All cases in this series had unilateral cranial nerve involvement, most often the facial and/or abducens nerve. Lumbar puncture results are often negative and listeria is only present in 33% of cerebrospinal fluid cultures because it is an intracellular organism. With multiple lumbar punctures, the detection rate increases to only 50%. A high index of suspicion is necessary and empiric treatment with ampicillin should begin as soon as possible. In this study, imaging revealed MRI T2 signal abnormalities isolated to the posterior fossa without any supratentorial involvement. Unfortunately, outcomes for listeria rhombencephalitis are poor, with a mortality rate of 20% to 30%, and 55% of patients developing residual neurologic sequelae despite treatment with ampicillin.[33]

NEUROIMMUNOLOGY

When the immune system targets the central nervous system, either through an innate or humoral immune response, the diverse clinical syndrome that results can be difficult to diagnose, especially on first presentation in the ED. Although most neuroimmunologic conditions, including multiple sclerosis, Behçet syndrome, neurosarcoidosis, and paraneoplastic syndrome, can be diagnosed and treated on an outpatient basis or on a general medicine ward, a small subset of these conditions cause rapid neurologic decline and can be fatal if not identified and treated aggressively. As in infectious encephalitis, these emergent cases typically present with acute onset of altered mental status, fever, headache, seizures, and focal neurologic deficits. The standard workup includes advanced brain imaging and lumbar puncture, but often the cause is not readily identified and appropriate management becomes a challenge. The topic of unknown encephalitis was reviewed in one meta-analysis and the proportion of cases of unknown origin was found to be greater than 50% in 26 of 41 studies.[34] These cases are thought to be the result of undiscovered pathogens and antibodies. Within the past decade, new antibody-mediated syndromes targeting voltage-gated potassium channels (VGKC) and *N*-methyl-D-aspartate receptors (NMDAR) have been described and are more frequently recognized as a significant cause of antibody-mediated encephalitis.[35,36] However, the most common cause of immune-mediated encephalitis remains fulminant demyelinating disease, specifically acute disseminated encephalomyelitis (ADEM).[37]

Antibody Mediated Encephalitis

Six commonly described paraneoplastic or antibody-mediated neurologic syndromes exist: pure-sensory neuropathy, cerebellar degeneration, opsoclonus-myoclonus syndrome, Lambert-Eaton myasthenic syndrome, and limbic encephalitis. Of these conditions, limbic encephalitis is the most likely to result in admission to the ICU, because seizures and altered mental status are the predominant clinical features. Of the antibodies known to cause limbic encephalitis, anti-NMDAR encephalitis and anti-VGKC encephalitis are the most common.

Fulminant Demyelinating Disease

Variants of fulminant demyelinating disease requiring aggressive care include ADEM, acute hemorrhagic leukoencephalitis (AHLE), tumefactive multiple sclerosis, and neuromyelitis optica. Treatment strategies for fulminant demyelinating disease include high-dose steroids for 5 days or 7 plasma exchanges for acute illness, and chemotherapy for chronic illness.

Concern for ADEM should be raised in patients with a history of a viral respiratory illness or who received a vaccination 1 to 3 weeks before presentation, because this history is present in up to 70% of cases of ADEM based on one large series.[38] Although ADEM is most typically seen in children and adolescents, it can also affect adults with an incidence of 8 per 1 million people per year.[39] Presentation after vaccination has been discussed extensively in the literature, but only the rabies vaccine has been shown to be clearly associated.[39] Although the clinical presentation can be highly variable, patients may present with significant lethargy to the extent of coma, hemiparesis or paraparesis, seizures, and cranial nerve deficits. Fever is also a presenting component of ADEM, making it difficult to differentiate from infectious origins.[39] Magnetic resonance imaging is particularly helpful for diagnosis and reveals scattered gray and white matter T2/fluid-attenuated inversion recovery hyperintense lesions with poorly defined margins and variable contrast enhancement.

Treatment consists of high-dose corticosteroids and may include either plasma exchange or intravenous immunoglobulin in refractory cases.[39] Unfortunately, no randomized controlled studies of ADEM treatment have been performed. The mortality rate despite treatment is estimated at 5% overall and is typically attributed to respiratory failure or refractory increased intracranial pressure.[38] In one series of 20 adult patients in the ICU with ADEM, 70% required mechanical ventilation and the mortality rate was 25%.[38]

As a severe form of ADEM occurring in up to 2% of patients and therefore rare, AHLE, is characterized by extensive necrosis and hemorrhage through breakdown of the blood-brain barrier.[40] Although AHLE also occurs after viral illness, it has also been reported after gram-negative sepsis and methanol poisoning.[40] It remains rapidly fatal in up to 70% of cases despite aggressive treatment, and survivors often experience significant neurologic sequelae.[40] As with ADEM, early treatment with high-dose corticosteroids and management of secondary seizures and increased intracranial pressure is required. Imaging in AHLE differs in that the T2 hyperintensities are diffusion-weighted imaging–positive and apparent diffusion coefficient–negative, suggesting irreversible neuronal loss.

Tumefactive multiple sclerosis

As a rare variant of multiple sclerosis, tumefactive multiple sclerosis has an estimated incidence of 3 per million per year.[37] The demographics are similar to multiple sclerosis, with women aged 20 to 30 years most often affected. Clinical suspicion for this would be triggered by headache, cognitive abnormalities, confusion, aphasia, apraxia, and seizures. In one case series, 70% of patients with biopsy-proven tumefactive multiple sclerosis had multiple lesions that were typically larger than 2 cm in diameter with significant mass effect.[41] After high-dose corticosteroids and plasma exchange, which may shrink the lesions and reduce mass effect, these multiple sclerosis variants require disease-modifying therapy with interferons, natalizumab, or cyclophosphamide to prevent recurrence.

Neuromyelitis optica

Neuromyelitis optica is a demyelinating variant that preferentially affects the optic nerves and the spinal cord. The typical presentation is unilateral or bilateral blindness followed or preceded by a severe transverse or ascending myelitis. It is an autoantibody-mediated disease against the aquaporin 4 channels on astrocytes.[42] In extreme cases, patients may present with blindness caused by bilateral optic nerve involvement, and quadriparesis caused by longitudinally extensive spinal cord demyelination. Magnetic resonance imaging of the spine and antibody testing of either cerebrospinal fluid or plasma confirm the diagnosis. With all fulminant demyelinating diseases, high-dose corticosteroids, intravenous immunoglobulin, and plasma exchange are the mainstay of treatment along with supportive care, including mechanical ventilation if needed.

Neurologic diseases span a wide variety of presentations and pathologies. In the ED, it is useful to narrow the differential to disorders involving weakness or infectious and/or immunologic origins and to have an organized approach to each category. In this way, the workup can be complete but not superfluous. Patients with neuromuscular disease will benefit from prompt diagnosis and treatment, such as in the case of respiratory failure. Neurologic diseases with neuroinfectious sources require rapid attention for accurate and effective antibiosis; those with neuroimmunologic issues require recognition of signs/symptoms and effective diagnostic testing and imaging.

The astute emergency physician will be able to hone in on the important components of the neurologic examination and combine the clinical information for diagnostic and therapeutic improvement.

REFERENCES

1. Burns JD, Green DM, Metivier K, et al. Intensive care management of acute ischemic stroke. Emerg Med Clin North Am 2012;30(3):713–44.
2. Caceres JA, Goldstein JN. Intracranial hemorrhage. Emerg Med Clin North Am 2012;30(3):771–94.
3. Ropper AH. The Guillain-Barre syndrome. N Engl J Med 1992;326(17):1130–6.
4. Suarez GA, Fealey RD, Camilleri M, et al. Idiopathic autonomic neuropathy: clinical, neurophysiologic, and follow-up studies on 27 patients. Neurology 1994;44(9): 1675–82.
5. McGillicuddy DC, Walker O, Shapiro NI, et al. Guillain-Barre syndrome in the emergency department. Ann Emerg Med 2006;47(4):390–3.
6. Lehmann HC, Hartung HP, Kieseier BC, et al. Guillain-Barre syndrome after exposure to influenza virus. Lancet Infect Dis 2010;10(9):643–51.
7. Bershad EM, Feen ES, Suarez JI. Myasthenia gravis crisis. South Med J 2008; 101(1):63–9.
8. Guptill JT, Sanders DB, Evoli A. Anti-MuSK antibody myasthenia gravis: clinical findings and response to treatment in two large cohorts. Muscle Nerve 2011; 44(1):36–40.
9. Mehta S. Neuromuscular disease causing acute respiratory failure. Respir Care 2006;51(9):1016–21 [discussion: 1021–3].
10. Lawn ND, Fletcher DD, Henderson RD, et al. Anticipating mechanical ventilation in Guillain-Barre syndrome. Arch Neurol 2001;58(6):893–8.
11. Orlikowski D, Prigent H, Sharshar T, et al. Respiratory dysfunction in Guillain-Barre syndrome. Neurocrit Care 2004;1(4):415–22.
12. American Thoracic Society/European Respiratory Society. ATS/ERS statement on respiratory muscle testing. Am J Respir Crit Care 2002;166(4):518–624.

13. Prigent H, Orlikowski D, Letilly N, et al. Vital capacity versus maximal inspiratory pressure in patients with Guillain-Barre syndrome and myasthenia gravis. Neurocrit Care 2012;17(2):236–9.
14. Sharshar T, Chevret S, Bourdain F, et al, French Cooperative Group on Plasma Exchange in Guillain-Barre Syndrome. Early predictors of mechanical ventilation in Guillain-Barre syndrome. Crit Care Med 2003;31(1):278–83.
15. Rabinstein A, Wijdicks EF. BiPAP in acute respiratory failure due to myasthenic crisis may prevent intubation. Neurology 2002;59(10):1647–9.
16. Hor JY. Cardiac arrhythmia after succinylcholine administration in a patient with Guillain-Barre syndrome–a case report. Middle East J Anesthesiol 2010;20(6): 881–3.
17. Roppolo LP, Walters K. Airway management in neurological emergencies. Neurocrit Care 2004;1(4):405–14.
18. van de Beek D, de Gans J, Spanjaard L, et al. Clinical features and prognostic factors in adults with bacterial meningitis. N Engl J Med 2004;351(18):1849–59.
19. Attia J, Hatala R, Cook DJ, et al. The rational clinical examination. Does this adult patient have acute meningitis? JAMA 1999;282(2):175–81.
20. Thomas KE, Hasbun R, Jekel J, et al. The diagnostic accuracy of Kernig's sign, Brudzinski's sign, and nuchal rigidity in adults with suspected meningitis. Clin Infect Dis 2002;35(1):46–52.
21. Nakao JH, Jafri FN, Shah K, et al. Jolt accentuation of headache and other clinical signs: poor predictors of meningitis in adults. Am J Emerg Med 2014;32(1):24–8.
22. Gaieski DF, Nathan BR, Weingart SD, et al. Emergency neurologic life support: meningitis and encephalitis. Neurocrit Care 2012;17(Suppl 1):S66–72.
23. de Gans J, van de Beek D, European Dexamethasone in Adulthood Bacterial Meningitis Study Investigators. Dexamethasone in adults with bacterial meningitis. N Engl J Med 2002;347(20):1549–56.
24. Abulhasan YB, Al-Jehani H, Valiquette MA, et al. Lumbar drainage for the treatment of severe bacterial meningitis. Neurocrit Care 2013;19(2):199–205.
25. Kasanmoentalib ES, Brouwer MC, van der Ende A, et al. Hydrocephalus in adults with community-acquired bacterial meningitis. Neurology 2010;75(10):918–23.
26. Dellinger RP, Levy MM, Carlet JM, et al. Surviving sepsis campaign: international guidelines for management of severe sepsis and septic shock: 2008. Intensive Care Med 2008;34(1):17–60.
27. Kielian T. Immunopathogenesis of brain abscess. J Neuroinflammation 2004;1(1):16.
28. Mathisen GE, Johnson JP. Brain abscess. Clin Infect Dis 1997;25(4):763–79 [quiz: 780–1].
29. Sonneville R, Mirabel M, Hajage D, et al. Neurologic complications and outcomes of infective endocarditis in critically ill patients: the ENDOcardite en REAnimation prospective multicenter study. Crit Care Med 2011;39(6):1474–81.
30. Mullins ME. Emergent neuroimaging of intracranial infection/inflammation. Radiol Clin North Am 2011;49(1):47–62.
31. Solomon T, Michael BD, Smith PE, et al. Management of suspected viral encephalitis in adults—Association of British Neurologists and British Infection Association National Guidelines. J Infect 2012;64(4):347–73.
32. Sabah M, Mulcahy J, Zeman A. Herpes simplex encephalitis. BMJ 2012;344: e3166.
33. Armstrong RW, Fung PC. Brainstem encephalitis (rhombencephalitis) due to Listeria monocytogenes: case report and review. Clin Infect Dis 1993;16(5):689–702.
34. Granerod J, Tam CC, Crowcroft NS, et al. Challenge of the unknown. A systematic review of acute encephalitis in non-outbreak situations. Neurology 2010;75(10):924–32.

35. Vincent A, Buckley C, Schott JM, et al. Potassium channel antibody-associated encephalopathy: a potentially immunotherapy-responsive form of limbic encephalitis. Brain 2004;127(Pt 3):701–12.
36. Dalmau J, Gleichman AJ, Hughes EG, et al. Anti-NMDA-receptor encephalitis: case series and analysis of the effects of antibodies. Lancet Neurol 2008;7(12):1091–8.
37. Johnson RT. The virology of demyelinating diseases. Ann Neurol 1994;36(Suppl): S54–60.
38. Sonneville R, Demeret S, Klein I, et al. Acute disseminated encephalomyelitis in the intensive care unit: clinical features and outcome of 20 adults. Intensive Care Med 2008;34(3):528–32.
39. Menge T, Kieseier BC, Nessler S, et al. Acute disseminated encephalomyelitis: an acute hit against the brain. Curr Opin Neurol 2007;20(3):247–54.
40. Ryan LJ, Bowman R, Zantek ND, et al. Use of therapeutic plasma exchange in the management of acute hemorrhagic leukoencephalitis: a case report and review of the literature. Transfusion 2007;47(6):981–6.
41. Lucchinetti CF, Gavrilova RH, Metz I, et al. Clinical and radiographic spectrum of pathologically confirmed tumefactive multiple sclerosis. Brain 2008;131(Pt 7): 1759–75.
42. Rahmlow MR, Kantarci O. Fulminant demyelinating diseases. Neurohospitalist 2013;3(2):81–91.

Pediatric Critical Care

Emily Rose, MD, Ilene Claudius, MD*

KEYWORDS

- Resuscitation • Sepsis • Status epilepticus • Trauma • Rapid sequence intubation
- Difficult airway • Needle cricothyrotomy • Intraosseous access

KEY POINTS

- The differential diagnosis of the ill neonate includes sepsis, metabolic disease, ductal-dependent cardiac disease, and gastrointestinal disasters.
- Initiate algorithm of status epilepticus in greater than 5 minutes of seizure activity.
- Injury is the most common cause of death in children, and anatomic differences place them at unique risk for injury.
- Respiratory arrest accounts for greater than 95% of pediatric cardiac arrest; rigorous airway support must be maintained in children.
- Intraosseous lines are the fastest and easiest access in the critically ill child.

GENERAL APPROACH TO RESUSCITATION OF THE ILL CHILD

The approach to the ill child differs minimally from the ill adult. Airway and breathing require immediate assessment because respiratory failure typically precedes circulatory insufficiency. Cardiopulmonary resuscitation (CPR) is performed at 100 compressions per minute with a depth of one-third of the anteroposterior diameter (single-provider ratio, 30:2; 2-provider ratio, 15:2). Ventilation in addition to compressions results in better outcomes in children during initial bystander CPR.[1] For pulseless electrical activity or asystole, the provider must perform high-quality CPR, treat underlying causes, and give epinephrine (0.01 mg/kg, 1:10,000, max 1 mg) every 3 to 5 minutes. For ventricular fibrillation-related arrest, the algorithm of shock (2 J/kg), a 2-minute cycle of CPR, shock (4 J/kg), CPR with epinephrine, shock (4 J/kg), CPR with amiodarone (5 mg/kg) is recommended. Extracorporeal life support should be considered in patients with a potentially reversible cause.

Following resuscitation, oxygen can be titrated to saturations of 94% or greater. Hypothermia for return of spontaneous circulation without neurologic function is only

Disclosure: None.

Department of Emergency Medicine, Keck School of Medicine, University of Southern California, Health Sciences Campus, Los Angeles, CA 90089, USA
* Corresponding author.
E-mail address: iaclaudius@gmail.com

Emerg Med Clin N Am 32 (2014) 939–954
http://dx.doi.org/10.1016/j.emc.2014.07.013 emed.theclinics.com
0733-8627/14/$ – see front matter

recommended by Pediatric Advanced Life Support (PALS) for adolescents with ventricular fibrillation-related arrest.[2] Consideration of family presence during resuscitation is also recommended.[2]

Common Sources of Severe Illness

Ill neonate

Subtle manifestations of early illness are difficult to recognize in neonates. Therefore, most critically ill babies present late with poor oral intake and lethargy, giving the clinician few clues to the cause. Top differential diagnoses include sepsis/infection, metabolic disease, ductal-dependent cardiac disease, and gastrointestinal disasters. The septic neonate is subject to unique pathogens, including *Escherichia coli*, group B *streptococcus*, and *Listeria monocytogenes*, and thus, antibiotic treatment includes ampicillin and either cefotaxime or an aminoglycoside.

The list of metabolic diseases is lengthy and arduous. For the neonate who arrives crashing within the first week of life, inborn errors of protein metabolism (urea cycle defects, organic acidemias) or congenital adrenal hyperplasia (CAH) are of concern. Gap acidosis and hyperammonemia (3–5 times normal) are expected with urea cycle defects and organic acidemias, respectively. Hypoglycemia, thrombocytopenia, and leukopenia may occur as well.[3] Definitive diagnosis is made from serum organic and plasma amino acids. For these patients, it is best to minimize protein available to the patient, by stopping both oral intake of protein (including breast milk and/or formula) and any starvation-related intrinsic protein catabolism with the administration of 10% dextrose with one-fourth the normal saline (D10.25NS) at 1.5 times maintenance, with concurrent correction of dehydration and hypoglycemia. Hyperammonemia can be treated with a combination of sodium benzoate and sodium phenylacetate (0.25 g/kg over a period of 90–120 min followed by an infusion of 0.25 g/kg over a period of 24 hours)[4] or by dialysis. Bicarbonate is controversial[5] but often given for pH less than 7.0–7.2. CAH, although a part of the neonatal screening, can present symptomatically before those results are available with emesis, shock, and, in female neonates, virilization. Hyponatremia, hyperkalemia, and metabolic acidosis are the hallmark laboratory triad in the CAH patient, and hypoglycemia is common. 17-Hydroxyprogesterone must be sent for definitive diagnosis before the initiation of therapy. Although these patients tolerate hyperkalemia well,[6] correction of glucose, electrolytes, and dehydration is important initial management. Hydrocortisone (25 mg intravenously [IV] or intramuscularly) should be given quickly, followed by a continuous drip or subsequent doses every 6 hours (50 mg/m^2/d).[7]

Malrotation and midgut volvulus typically present with poor oral intake and bilious emesis. Up to 60% of patients with volvulus can have no abnormalities on abdominal palpation.[8] Upper gastrointestinal test is the study of choice, with a sensitivity of 96% for malrotation.[9] The primary treatment is surgical, after placement of a nasogastric tube and fluid resuscitation. Any suspicion of necrosis or perforation should prompt use of broad-spectrum antibiotics.

Ductal-dependent heart disease presents with the functional closure of the ductus arteriosus, usually within the first few days of life. Prenatal ultrasound misses more than half of the cases[10] and up to 56% of children with structural heart disease may not have a murmur auscultated.[11] In the case of the cyanotic lesions, patients present with tachypnea and decreased oxygen saturation, whereas in the obstructive lesions, they present with systemic shock, often preferentially affecting the lower extremities. Chest radiographs and electrocardiograms each have sensitivity around 75%, and an echocardiogram is definitive. For cyanotic congenital heart disease, a hyperoxia test can be performed in the Emergency Department (ED), in which the patient is placed on 100% FiO_2 for 10 minutes and then an arterial blood gas test is obtained. A post-oxygen PaO_2 less than 150 mm Hg is highly suspicious for CCHD. Treatment with prostaglandin E_1 should be started through any intravenous access at a dose of 0.05 μg/kg/min. Side effects include apnea, hypotension, and hyperpyrexia. Correction of anemia, glucose, and acidosis (1 mEq/kg of 4.2% bicarbonate) is appropriate.

Septic child

Approximately 42,000 cases of sepsis in children occur in the United States annually with a mortality of 2% to 10%.[12,13] Diagnostic criteria for SIRS differ minimally from adults, but hypotension is a late finding in ill pediatric patients and is not required for the diagnosis of septic shock. Rather, evidence of cardiovascular dysfunction is diagnostic. Lactate is poorly studied in the pediatric population.[14]

Many children have poor cardiac output with normal-high systemic vascular resistance. The intrinsically high resting heart rate of a child limits the ability to compensate by increasing heart rate, making them highly dependent on stroke volume.[15] In addition, children are often dehydrated due to preceding poor oral intake, making aggressive fluid resuscitation essential. Crystalloid boluses of 20 mL/kg over a period of 5 to 10 minutes should be given and repeated until either evidence of significant fluid overload or shock is reversed. Most patients require 40 to 60 mL/kg in the first hour. After shock reversal, D10NS should be given at a rate to preserve perfusion and urine output. In patients with fluid-refractory shock, inotropes and vasopressors can be initiated through a peripheral line if central access in unavailable. Dopamine is a first-line option. Epinephrine is a first-line or second-line choice for cold shock (narrow pulse pressure, delayed capillary refill, poor perfusion), and norepinephrine is first or second line for warm shock (flash capillary refill, widened pulse pressure). Dobutamine is used with normal blood pressure but poor cardiac output.[16] Up to 25% of children with septic shock have adrenal insufficiency, and hydrocortisone administration should be considered in the catecholamine-resistant patient.[17] Up to 40% of cardiac output can be required to support ventilation in a septic patient and intubation is often necessary, particularly in fluid-resistant and catecholamine-resistant shock. As a sedative for intubation, ketamine avoids adrenal suppression seen with etomidate in septic patients.[16] $ScvO_2$ is an indicator of cardiac output and $ScvO_2$ greater than 70% is associated with better outcomes.[16,18]

Seizures

Seizure activity greater than 5 minutes requires urgent treatment.[19] Fever/infection is the most common cause of status epilepticus (SE) in children,[20] with nearly 20% of patient with febrile SE having meningitis/encephalitis.[21]

Benzodiazepines are first-line abortive therapy. Lorazepam (0.05–0.1 mg/kg) is first choice with IV access due to a longer duration of action. Intranasal midazolam (0.2 mg/kg), intramuscular midazolam (0.2 mg/kg), buccal midazolam (0.5 mg/kg), and rectal diazepam (0.5 mg/kg) are options without IV access.[22] The IV formulation can be given via these alternative routes. Two benzodiazepine doses 5 minutes apart followed by initiation of a second-line medication are recommended. Second-line options include phenytoin (20 mg/kg), fosphenytoin (20 phenytoin equivalents/kg), phenobarbital (20 phenytoin equivalents/kg), valproate, and levetiracetam. Valproate (20 mg/kg IV) causes no respiratory or cardiovascular depression and has comparable efficacy to phenytoin, phenobarbital, and diazepam with minimal side effects.[23–26] It is avoided age in less than 2 years (possible hepatotoxicity). Levetiracetam (20 mg/kg IV) is as safe and effective as lorazepam,[27,28] without risk of respiratory or cardiovascular depression. If ineffective after 10 minutes, a second medication from this group is selected.

Failure of 2 to 3 medications constitutes refractory SE,[20] at which point the airway should be secured, if the patient is not already intubated. Treatments for refractory SE include midazolam infusion (0.05–2 mg/kg/h), pentobarbital (or high-dose phenobarbital) coma, propofol (2 mg/kg IV bolus, then 1–15 mg/kg/h infusion), and ketamine.

Trauma

Approximately 14,000 children and adolescents die annually of injuries, more than all other causes of deaths combined. More than half are due to motor vehicle collisions.[29–31]

The predisposition to respiratory failure and ability to maintain blood pressure despite ongoing blood loss (secondary to better sympathetic tone) are unique features to managing a child after traumatic injury. Tachycardia may be the only initial sign of hemorrhage.

Poor perfusion requires 20 mL/kg crystalloid bolus, followed by 10 to 20 mL/kg packed red blood cells if unresponsive or suspected continued hemorrhage. Limited literature exists in children for transfusion of 1:1:1 ratio of packed red blood cells, platelets and fresh frozen plasma.[32,33] In addition to hemorrhage, the differential diagnoses of shock in trauma includes tension pneumothorax, pericardial tamponade, neurogenic shock, hypoxemia, metabolic derangement, and toxidromes.

One fatal cancer occurs per 1000 pediatric computed tomographic (CT) scans and one scan may triple the risk of leukemia or brain tumor.[34,35] It is recommended to maintain the "ALARA concept" (as low as reasonably achievable) regarding radiation exposure.[36]

Head injury accounts for approximately 80% of injury-related deaths in children, although less than 1% of all head-injured patients have significant intracranial pathologic abnormality. Low-risk features for intracranial injuries are listed in **Box 1**.[37–40] Management of severe head injury is focused on rigorous supportive care to prevent secondary injury.

Cervical spine injuries (CSI) occur in 1% to 2% of severe pediatric trauma[41–43] and approximately 40% occur with concomitant head injury.[41,44,45] Young children have a higher fulcrum for motion (C2-C3 vs C5-6 in adults), and 87% to 100% of injuries occur at C3 or higher in less than 8 year olds. Young children can sustain injury without bony involvement because of ligamentous laxity and horizontally aligned facet joints. No well-established decision tools exist in young children for clinical clearance, but they can be clinically cleared with low likelihood of injury.[46–52] Consider imaging if

Box 1
Prediction rule for low risk of clinically important brain injuries after head trauma

Children younger than 2 years: Normal mental status, no scalp hematoma (except frontal), no loss of consciousness (LOC)/LOC less than 5 seconds, nonsevere injury mechanism,[a] no palpable skull fracture, acting normally per parents. Negative predictive value of 99.99%.

Children 2 years or over: Normal mental status, no LOC, no vomiting, nonsevere injury mechanism,[a] no signs of basilar skull fracture, and no severe headache. Negative predicative value of 99.95%

[a] Severe mechanism: motor vehicle crash with patient ejection, death of another passenger, or rollover; pedestrian or bicyclist without helmet struck by a motorized vehicle; falls of more than 1.5 m (5 feet) for children aged 2 years and older and more than 0.9 m (3 feet) for those younger than 2 years; or head struck by a high-impact object.

Data from Kuppermann N, Holmes JF, Dayan PS, et al. Identification of children at very low risk of clinically-important brain injuries after head trauma: a prospective cohort study. Lancet 2009;374:1160–70.

National Emergency X-Radiography Utilization Study (NEXUS) low-risk criteria are not met (**Box 2**), with significant mechanism of injury, neurologic symptoms (on examination or per history), physical evidence of significant trauma to the head/neck, or if the child is altered or inconsolable.[53–55]

Plain films are insensitive for CSI in children and mimics of injury are common.[31,56,57] MRI is recommended in addition to CT in patients with neurologic symptoms to evaluate for acute spinal cord injury or ligamentous damage and could potentially be used in lieu of CT scan for evaluation of pediatric CSI.[58]

Blunt trauma accounts for greater than 90% of pediatric injuries. Increased chest wall compliance allows for significant transmission of force to underlying organs without rib fractures. Pulmonary contusions occur in 50% to 70% of children with significant thoracic injuries and may impair respiratory function. Pneumothorax, cardiac contusion, great vessel, or tracheal/bronchial injuries may also occur. Children are higher risk for pneumothorax because of hypermobility of the chest. Cardiac tamponade, penetrating trauma and arrest, chest tube output 20 mL/kg, or greater than 3 to 4 mL/kg/h are indications for surgery.[59]

Children are predisposed to abdominal injury because of their relatively larger solid organs, thinner abdominal musculature, and less subcutaneous fat. Concerning features in patients with abdominal trauma include hypotension, abnormal abdominal examination (pain, ecchymosis), abnormal laboratory values (AST, lipase, low hematocrit), or hematuria.[60] Solid organ injury is most common, but hollow viscus and mesenteric injuries may occur with a direct blow.

Solid organ injury may occur without free fluid on the Focused Assessment with Sonography for Trauma examination.[61] Less than 15% of children have intra-abdominal injury on imaging after blunt trauma and most are managed nonoperatively with good outcomes.[59,62–64] Safe discharge may occur with a normal abdominal CT after trauma if no other indication exists for admission.[60,65]

Penetrating injuries are uncommon in children.[66,67] Surgical consultation, CT imaging, and operative exploration are often required. Penetrating trauma below the nipple line and posteriorly below the tip of the scapula may involve the abdominal cavity.

PROCEDURES

Airway

Respiratory arrest accounts for approximately 95% of cardiac arrests in pediatric patients. Children are predisposed to respiratory failure because of increased airway resistance (small/compressible airway), low functional residual capacity, high oxygen

Box 2
NEXUS criteria for low probability of CSI

- No midline cervical tenderness
- No focal neurologic deficit
- Normal alertness
- No intoxication
- No painful, distracting injury

Data from Hoffman JR, Wolfson AB, Todd K, et al. Selective cervical spine radiography in blunt trauma: methodology of the National Emergency X-Radiography Utilization Study (NEXUS). Ann Emerg Med 1998;32(4):461–9.

metabolism, which leads to quicker fatigue, and shorter safe apnea time with precipitous hypoxia.

Bag-valve mask (BVM) is as effective as endotracheal intubation for temporary respiratory support.[68] The mask should cover the child's mouth and nose for a proper seal. Visible chest rise should be apparent (goal tidal volume of 6–8 cc/kg, but 10 cc/kg accounts for equipment dead space). Appropriate rates for neonates are 30 breaths per minute, infants 10–20 breaths per minute, and children 8–10 breaths per minute (saying "squeeze, release" in infants and "squeeze, squeeze, release" in children while bagging provides appropriate timing). The little finger, ring finger, and long fingers of one hand are spread (forming an "E") to lift the jaw and pull the face into the mask (to avoid compressing the neck and causing airway collapse/obstruction). The thumb and forefinger are placed over the top of the mask in a "C" shape to form a seal between the mask and face. All pediatric BVM units should have a safety pop-off valve and manometer to limit peak inspiratory pressures 35 to 40 cm H_2O per breath, but higher pressures may be required to achieve visible chest rise in some resuscitations.[69] Superior bag-mask ventilation is achieved with 2 persons, particularly in the scenario of airway obstruction or poor lung compliance.

Noninvasive Positive Pressure Ventilation

Noninvasive positive pressure ventilation is useful as a bridge to intubation or support in reversible causes of respiratory failure. Nasal devices, face masks, or helmets may be used in children with continuous or bi-level support and supplemental humidified oxygen greater than or equal to 4 L/min. Settings and mode depend on cause of respiratory failure. In the apprehensive or young child, initially placing the mask without flow, then increasing pressures in 2 cm H_2O increments to clinical improvement, may be helpful. Young children may require sedation with ketamine (0.5–1 mg/kg/bolus, then 0.25 mg/kg/h).[70–73]

Intubation/Rapid Sequence Intubation

The pediatric airway is more cephalad (more 'anterior') during visualization. Aligning the oral, tracheal, and pharyngeal axes may require a towel rolled under the infant's shoulders.

Preoxygenation is essential due to a child's intolerance for apnea. A high-flow nasal cannula (15 L in adolescents, up to 8 L in toddlers) can be used for preoxygenation in addition to the face mask and while intubating.[74,75] Two-person manual in-line stabilization can be used for C-spine immobilization.[76]

Profound bradycardia can occur during laryngoscopy because of vagal stimulation, because of hypoxemia, or with succinylcholine. Prophylactic atropine (0.02 mg/kg with a maximum dose of 0.5 mg and minimum dose of 0.1 mg) in infants younger than 1 year and those younger than 5 years who are receiving succinylcholine is widely recommended despite little supporting evidence.[77,78]

Higher success rates and fewer complications occur when rapid sequence intubation is used.[79–81] Induction agents include etomidate (0.2–0.4 mg/kg),[82–84] ketamine (1–2 mg/kg),[85] propofol (1.5–3 mg/kg), thiopental (2–5 mg/kg),[86] and midazolam (0.1–0.3 mg/kg).[79,86] Etomidate has no direct hemodynamic effect but causes transient adrenal suppression. Its use is not recommended in the septic patient. Paralytic agents include depolarizing agents, such as succinylcholine (1.5–3 mg/kg, onset of action 20–60 seconds with 3–5 minutes duration), and nondepolarizing agents, such as rocuronium (0.6–1.2 mg/kg, 30- to 90-second onset, and duration up to 40 minutes).[87] A *Cochrane Review* concluded that succinylcholine creates better intubating conditions.[88] However, it contains a US Food and Drug Administration "black box warning" due to cardiac arrest in children with undiagnosed myopathies.[89,90]

A straight blade is recommended in young children because it better elevates the base of the tongue to expose the glottic opening (**Table 1**). Cuffed endotracheal tubes (ETTs) are used in children older than 1 month, provided the cuff pressure can be maintained at less than 20 cm H_2O to avoid tracheal mucosal ischemia (**Box 3** for sizing).[76] Cuffed tubes may decrease aspiration risk and need for tube exchange and are endorsed as an acceptable alternative by PALS, American Heart Association, and the International Liaison Committee on Resuscitation.[2,76] Depth of insertion is roughly estimated at 3 times the ETT size (ie, a 5.0 ETT is inserted at approximately 15 cm). ETT placement is confirmed by visible chest wall rise, breath sounds in both axillae, continuous pulse oximetry, mist in ET tube, and end-tidal CO_2 with either colorimetric device or capnography.

Difficult Airway

The unanticipated difficult airway is rare in children. However, complications and intubation attempts may occur more commonly than perceived.[91] Passive nasal oxygenation during all stages of management may help prevent hypoxia should a delay in securing the tube occur. A gum elastic bougie may be used (standard fits 6.0 ETT, pediatric bougie 4.0), although young children's tracheal rings are not sufficiently calcified to help confirm location. Laryngeal mask airways (LMA; **Table 2**) are essential rescue devices. The LMA is inserted into the mouth and blindly passed along the palate and posterior pharynx until resistance is met. A partial seal around the larynx is formed with cuff inflation. The rotational technique where the device is initially placed with the cuff facing the palate then simultaneously advanced and rotated may improve successful placement in children younger than 7 years.[92–94] Partial mask inflation also improves placement success (inflate the device to the smooth edges of the mask before insertion). LMAs are also successfully used in neonatal resuscitation.[95,96]

Video laryngoscopy devices are important airway adjuncts in the difficult airway algorithm. However, preparation and practice must occur before the difficult airway scenario. Their use is an acquired skill and may, in children, increase time of intubation particularly in inexperienced users and during cervical spine immobilization.[97–99]

"CANNOT INTUBATE, CANNOT VENTILATE" SCENARIO

Surgical cricothyrotomy is not recommended in children less than 8 to 10 years of age because the larynx is high and the cricothyroid membrane is small and difficult to locate. Needle cricothyrotomy is alternatively used, but significant CO_2 retention limits its effectiveness. Commercial percutaneous transtracheal ventilation kits may be purchased but "homemade" kits can be created from tools readily available in the ED. A

Table 1
Simplified intubation blade sizing

Blade	Age
Miller 0	Premature/newborn
Miller 1	1 mo–2 y
Wis-Hipple 1.5	2 y
Miller 2	3–8 y
Macintosh 2	3 y
Macintosh 3	>8–10 y

Mnemonic: use a size 2 at 2 and 3 in third grade.

Box 3
ETT size calculation

Uncuffed: (Age/4) + 4

Cuffed: (Age/4) + 3.5 or uncuffed − 0.5

14- to 18-gauge angiocatheter is inserted in the cricothyroid membrane and connected to a 3-cc syringe (without the plunger) into which a 7.5 ETT adaptor is inserted (alternatively, a 3.0 ETT connector can be inserted directly into the angiocatheter). Unfortunately, this setup is rigid and may easily become dislodged. Alternatives include using IV tubing (attach IV tubing to the angiocatheter, cut the tubing, and attach a 2.5-ETT connector), or directly connecting oxygen tubing to the catheter with a Y connector or 3-way stopcock.

Once needle cricothyrotomy has been established, BVM (recommended in <5 years) can be performed slowly through the ETT adaptor (10–12 breaths/min) to minimize barotrauma by allowing for passive exhalation. Alternatively, percutaneous transtracheal ventilation can be administered with a 1:4 I:E (inspiratory:expiratory) ratio. Adults should receive oxygen from the wall source at 15 L/min (50–58 psi) and children at 10–12 L/min (25–35 psi).

Complete airway obstruction (eg, foreign body) does not allow for passive exhalation and necessitates a reduction of BVM to 5 to 6 breaths/min or I:E ratio of 1:8 to 1:10 as a temporizing measure. Furthermore, a hole should be made in the tubing that is covered during inspiration and uncovered during exhalation to allow passive exhalation of air. Complications of needle cricothyrotomy include barotrauma and damage to adjacent structures.[100–105]

Intraosseous

Intraosseous (IO) lines are quick[106–109] and easy to learn[110] and can be used in any age patient.[106,111,112] Manually inserted needles may be used, but mechanical devices such as the EZ-IO drill (Vidacare, San Antonio, TX, USA) facilitate placement. A fractured bone is the only absolute contraindication (**Box 4**) for common placement locations. To insert, cleanse skin with bactericidal solution. With EZ-IO, apply gentle downward pressure with the needle perpendicular to the bone while pulling back on the trigger. A pop or decrease in resistance is felt once the needle passes the bony cortex to the marrow. Correct placement is confirmed with bone marrow aspiration (although may not always occur), or if infusion occurs without evidence of extravasation and if the needle stands alone firmly. Gauze, tape, or a Styrofoam cup overlying

Table 2
Laryngeal mask airway sizing

LMA Size	Weight (kg)
1	≤5
1.5	5–10
2	10–20
2.5	20–30
3	30–50
4	50–70
5	70–100
6	>100

Box 4
Common IO line locations

- Proximal tibia: 1 cm below the tibial tuberosity on medial tibial plateau
- Distal femur: midline, 2–3 cm above the external femoral condyles
- Malleoli sites: midline, 1 cm superior to the malleoli (medial is easier to penetrate than lateral)
- Humerus: greater tubercle (best location in obese patients). Place patient's hand on abdomen and insert at most prominent aspect of greater tubercle. Use the 45-mm needle with EZ-IO system.

may be used to secure the needle and prevent dislodgement. A hemostat or needle driver clamped on the needle and secured distally may improve the ability to assess for extravasation. Bone marrow infusion is painful, and conscious children should receive cardiac lidocaine via the IO before fluid infusion (0.5 mg/kg). A pressure bag/infusion pump improves infusion speed. Any fluid, medication, or blood product may be given IO. Use of the line for less than 24 hours decreases complications.

Central Venous Lines

Central venous lines (CVL) are less commonly used in the ED but may be indicated in ill children requiring vasopressors and/or multiple medications (**Table 3**). The femoral vein is used most commonly because of the distance from the airway and chest during resuscitation efforts. Landmarks and technique are similar to adults. Gentle pressure should be used to avoid vessel collapse in the young child.

Umbilical vein catheterization is used in young neonates (<7–10 days) for emergency resuscitation. To place, cleanse with bactericidal solution and place the loop of umbilical tape/purse-string suture at the base of the cord. Cut the cord approximately 1 cm from the skin. The single umbilical vein with the large lumen is typically located in the 12 o'clock position. Insert and secure a flushed catheter (3.5 Fr if premature and 5 Fr in a term baby) into the lumen 1 to 2 cm past the point where blood flow is returned (typically 4–5 cm in a term baby). The catheter should be secured at this point, as deeper insertion may result in complications unless the position of the catheter is carefully monitored.

Thoracostomy Tubes

Thoracostomy tubes are typically required with pneumothorax or hemothorax. The most commonly used location is the anterior to midaxillary line at the fourth to fifth intercostal space (at the level of the nipple). Avoid the midclavicular approach to

Table 3
Central venous line sizing

Age	Weight (kg)	CVL Size (Fr)	CVL Length[a]
Newborn	4–8	3	5–12
Infant	5–10	3–3.5	5–12
1–3 y	10–15	4	5–15
3–8 y	15–30	4–5	5–25
≥8 y	30–70	5–8	5–30

[a] Longer lengths used for femoral lines. Ideal high line catheter position: before vessel junction with right atrium.

Table 4
Approximate pediatric tube thoracostomy sizing

Weight (kg)	Chest Tube (Fr)
<3	8–10
3–5	10–12
6–10	12–16
11–15	17–22
16–20	22–26
21–30	26–32
>30	32–40

prevent future breast deformity. Immediate needle aspiration or tube placement is indicated in tension pneumothorax. Traditional teaching recommends larger tube sizes to drain a hemothorax (**Table 4**). However, there is some evidence to suggest that blood may drain via a 7-Fr tube that is regularly flushed.[113] Seldinger technique with pigtail catheters allows easier placement between the small ribs of young children.

SUMMARY

Care of the ill and injured child requires knowledge of unique pediatric anatomic and physiologic differences. Respiratory arrest typically precedes circulatory arrest in the child. Noninvasive positive pressure ventilation, rapid sequence intubation, and high flow oxygenation during preintubation and peri-intubation are all reasonable options in children needing ventilator support. Cuffed ETTs may be used in children older than 1 month of age. LMA is an important rescue device. Surgical cricothyrotomy is not recommended in children less than 8 to 10 years of age and should be replaced by percutaneous transtracheal ventilation in this age group. Children tend to retain a normal blood pressure until peri-arrest and subtle signs of poor perfusion should be taken seriously and treated aggressively. Particularly in the neonate, it is important to appreciate subtle cues and cast a wide net, as critical illnesses present nonspecifically. In sepsis, aggressive fluid resuscitation in sepsis is essential. IO lines should be used immediately in a coding patient or after 90 seconds of attempting access in a critically ill child. Dopamine and norepinephrine are first-line vasopressors in fluid-refractory shock. Similarly, aggressive treatment of SE algorithm should be begun with 5 minutes of seizure activity. Benzodiazepines are first-line abortive therapy. Second-line agents include phenytoin/fosphenytoin, phenobarbital, valproate, and levetiracetam. Trauma accounts for more childhood deaths than all other causes combined. Head injury is the most common cause of death, although less than 1% of pediatric head injuries have significant intracranial pathologic abnormality. Most pediatric head trauma does not require imaging and the ALARA concept should be maintained to decrease radiation exposure in children. The pediatric C-spine may be clinically cleared if there is low suspicion for injury on history and physical examination. MRI is indicated to evaluate for acute spinal cord injury or ligamentous damage.

REFERENCES

1. Kitamura T, Iwami T, Kawamura T, et al. Conventional and chest-compression-only cardiopulmonary resuscitation by bystanders for children who have out-

of-hospital cardiac events: a prospective, nationwide, population-based cohort study. Lancet 2010;375(9723):1347–52.

2. Kleinman ME, de Caen AR, Chaneides L, et al. Pediatric basic and advanced life support: 2010 international consensus on cardiopulmonary resuscitation and emergency cardiovascular care science with treatment recommendations. Circulation 2010;122(16 Suppl 2):S466–515.
3. Claudius I, Fluharty C, Boles R. The emergency department approach to newborn and childhood metabolic crisis. Emerg Med Clin North Am 2005;23(3):843–83.
4. Enns GM, Berry SA, Berry GT, et al. Survival after treatment with phenylacetate and benzoate for urea-cycle disorders. N Engl J Med 2007;356(22):2282–92.
5. Claudius I. An evidence-based review of neonatal emergencies. Pediatr Emerg Med Pract 2010;7(8):1–20.
6. Kwon KT, Tsai VW. Metabolic emergencies. Emerg Med Clin North Am 2007; 25(4):1041–60.
7. Agus M. Endocrine emergencies. In: Fleisher GR, Ludwig S, Henretig FM, editors. Textbook of pediatric emergency medicine. 5th edition. Philadelphia: Lippincott Williams & Wilkins; 2006. p. 1180.
8. Bonadio WA, Clarkson T, Naus J. The clinical features of children with malrotation of the intestine. Pediatr Emerg Care 1991;7(6):348–9.
9. Sizemore AW, Rabbani KZ, Ladd A, et al. Diagnostic performance of the upper gastrointestinal series in the evaluation of children with clinically suspected malrotation. Pediatr Radiol 2008;38(5):518–28.
10. Mahle WT, Newburger JW, Matherne GP, et al. Role of pulse oximetry in examining newborns for congenital heart disease: a scientific statement from the American Heart Association and American Academy of Pediatrics. Circulation 2009;120(5):447–58.
11. Ainsworth S, Wyllie JP, Wren C. Prevalence and clinical significance of cardiac murmurs in neonates. Arch Dis Child Fetal Neonatal Ed 1999;80(1):F43–5.
12. Odetola FO, Gebremariam A, Freed GL. Patient and hospital correlates of clinical outcomes and resource utilization in severe pediatric sepsis. Pediatrics 2007;119(3):487–94.
13. Watson RS, Carcillo JA. Scope and epidemiology of pediatric sepsis. Pediatr Crit Care Med 2005;6:S3–5.
14. Scott HF, Donoghue AJ, Gaieski DF, et al. The utility of early lactate testing in undifferentiated pediatric inflammatory response syndrome. Acad Emerg Med 2012;19(11):1276–80.
15. Aneja RK, Carcillo JA. Differences between adult and pediatric septic shock. Minerva Anestesiol 2011;77(10):986–92.
16. Brierly J, Carcillo JA, Choong K, et al. Clinical practice parameters for hemodynamic support of pediatric and neonatal septic shock: 2007 update from American College of Critical Care Medicine. Crit Care Med 2009;37(2):666–8.
17. Dellinger RP, Levy MM, Rhodes A, et al. Surviving sepsis campaign: international guidelines for the management of severe sepsis and septic shock. Intensive Care Med 2013;39:15–228.
18. deOliveira CF, deOliveira DS, Gottschald AF, et al. ACCM/PALS haemodynamic support guidelines for paediatric septic shock: an outcomes comparison with and without monitoring central venous oxygen saturation. Intensive Care Med 2008;34:1065–75.
19. Michael GA, O'Connor RE. The diagnosis and management of seizures and status epilepticus in the prehospital setting. Emerg Med Clin North Am 2011;29(1): 20–39.

20. Shearer P, Riviello J. Generalized convulsive status epilepticus in adults and children: treatment guidelines and protocols. Emerg Med Clin North Am 2011; 29(1):51–64.
21. Chin RF, Neville BG, Scott RC. Meningitis is a common cause of convulsive status epilepticus with fever. Arch Dis Child 2005;90:66–9.
22. McMullan J, Sasson C, Pancioli A. Midalozam versus diazepam for the treatment of status epilepticus in children and young adults: a meta-analysis. Acad Emerg Med 2010;17(6):575–82.
23. Agarwal P, Kumar N, Chandra R, et al. Randomized study of intravenous valproate and phenytoin in status epilepticus. Seizure 2007;16(6):527–32.
24. Mehta V, Singhi P, Singhi S. Intravenous sodium valproate versus diazepam infusion for the control of refractory status epilepticus in children: a randomized controlled trial. J Child Neurol 2007;22(10):1191–7.
25. Brigo F, Storti M, DelFelice A, et al. IV valproate in generalized convulsive status epilepticus: a systematic review. Eur J Neurol 2012;19(9):1180–91.
26. Malamiri RA, Ghaempanah M, Khosroshahi N, et al. Efficacy and safety of intravenous sodium valproate versus pentobarbital in controlling convulsive status epilepticus and acute prolonged convulsive seizures in children: a randomized trial. Eur J Paediatr Neurol 2012;16(5):536–41.
27. Khan O, Chang E, Wright C, et al. Use of intravenous levetiracetam for management of acute seizures in neonates. Pediatr Neurol 2011;44(4):265–9.
28. Misra UK, Kalita J, Maurya PK. Levetiracetam versus lorazepam in status epilepticus: a randomized open labeled pilot study. J Neurol 2012;259(4): 645–8.
29. Kenefake ME, Swarm M, Walthall J. Nuances in pediatric trauma. Emerg Med Clin North Am 2013;31(3):627–52.
30. Junkins EP, O'Connell KJ, Mann NC. Pediatric trauma systems in the United States: do they make a difference? Clin Pediatr Emerg Med 2006;7:76–81.
31. Fatal injury reports, national and regional, 1999-2010. Centers for Disease Control and Prevention. Available at: http://webappa.cdc.gov/sasweb/ncipc/mortrate10_us.html. Accessed 10 January, 2013.
32. Hendrickson JE, Shaz BH, Pereira G, et al. Implementation of a pediatric trauma massive transfusion protocol: one institution's experience. Transfusion 2012; 52(6):1228–36.
33. Nosanov L, Inaba K, Okoye O, et al. The impact of blood product ratios in massively transfused pediatric trauma patients. Am J Surg 2013;206(5):655–60.
34. Muratore CS. Pediatric abdominal CT scans: do it correctly. Better yet, don't do it at all. J Surg Res 2013;185(2):533–4.
35. Pearce MS, Salotti JA, Little MP, et al. Radiation exposure from CT scans in childhood and subsequent risk of leukaemia and brain tumours: a retrospective cohort study. Lancet 2012;380(9840):499–505.
36. Strauss KJ, Kaste SC. The ALARA (as low as reasonably achievable) concept in pediatric interventional and fluoroscopic imaging: striving to keep radiation doses as low as possible during fluoroscopy of pediatric patients–a white paper executive summary. Pediatr Radiol 2006;36(Suppl 2):110–2.
37. Fabbri A, Servadei F, Marchesini G, et al. Analysis of different decision aids for clinical use in pediatric head injury in an emergency department of a general hospital. J Trauma Inj Infect Crit Care 2011;70(5):E79–83.
38. Simon B, Letourneau P, Vitorino EC, et al. Pediatric minor head trauma: indications for computed tomographic scanning revisited. J Trauma Inj Infect Crit Care 2001;51(2):231–8.

39. Cuff S, DiRusso S, Sullivan T, et al. Validation of a relative head injury severity scale for pediatric trauma. J Trauma Inj Infect Crit Care 2007; 63(1):172–8.
40. Kuppermann N, Holmes JF, Dayan PS, et al. Identification of children at very low risk of clinically-important brain injuries after head trauma: a prospective cohort study. Lancet 2009;374:1160–70.
41. Polk-Williams A, Carr BG, Blinman TA, et al. Cervical spine injury in young children: a National Trauma Data Bank review. J Pediatr Surg 2008;43(9): 1718–21.
42. Kreykes NS, Letton RW Jr. Current issues in the diagnosis of pediatric cervical spine injury. Semin Pediatr Surg 2010;19(4):257–64.
43. Kokoska ER, Keller MS, Rallo MC, et al. Characteristics of pediatric cervical spine injuries. J Pediatr Surg 2001;36(1):100–5.
44. Rush JK, Kelly DM, Astur N, et al. Associated injuries in children and adolescents with spinal trauma. J Pediatr Orthop 2013;33:393–7.
45. Garton HJ, Hammer M. Detection of pediatric cervical spine injury. Neurosurgery 2008;62(3):700–8.
46. Hoffman JR, Wolfson AB, Todd K, et al. Selective cervical spine radiography in blunt trauma: methodology of the National Emergency X-Radiography Utilization Study (NEXUS). Ann Emerg Med 1998;32(4):461–9.
47. Mower WR, Hoffman JR, Pollack CV Jr, et al. Use of plain radiography to screen for cervical spine injuries. Ann Emerg Med 2001;38(1):1–7.
48. Mower WR, Hoffman J. Comparison of the Canadian C-Spine rule and NEXUS decision instrument in evaluating blunt trauma patients for cervical spine injury. Ann Emerg Med 2004;43:515–7.
49. Stiell IG, Lesiuk H, Wells GA, et al. Canadian CT head rule study for patients with minor head injury: methodology for phase II (validation and economic analysis). Ann Emerg Med 2001;38(3):317–22.
50. Viccellio P, Simon H, Pressman BD, et al. A prospective multicenter study of cervical spine injury in children. Pediatrics 2001;108(2):E20.
51. Chung SM, Mikrogianakis AM, Wales PW, et al. Trauma Association of Canada Pediatric Subcommittee National Pediatric Cervical Spine Evaluation Pathway: consensus guidelines. J Trauma Inj Infect Crit Care 2011;70(4):873–84.
52. Pieretti-Vanmarcke R, Velmahos GC, Nance ML, et al. Clinical clearance of the cervical spine in blunt trauma patients younger than 3 years: a multi-center study of the American Association for the Surgery of Trauma. J Trauma Inj Infect Crit Care 2009;67(3):543–50.
53. Easter JS, Barkin R, Rosen CL, et al. Cervical spine injuries in children, part I: mechanism of injury, clinical presentation, and imaging. J Emerg Med 2011; 41(2):142–50.
54. Lee SL, Sena M, Greenholz SK, et al. A multidisciplinary approach to the development of a cervical spine clearance protocol: process, rationale, and initial results. J Pediatr Surg 2003;38(3):358–62 [discussion: 358–62].
55. Brown RL, Brunn MA, Garcia VF. Cervical spine injuries in children: a review of 103 patients treated consecutively at a level 1 pediatric trauma center. J Pediatr Surg 2001;36(8):1107–14.
56. Nigrovic LE, Rogers AJ, Adelgais KM, et al. Utility of plain radiographs in detecting traumatic injuries of the cervical spine in children. Pediatr Emerg Care 2012; 28(5):426–32.
57. Kriss VM, Kriss TC. Imaging of the cervical spine in infants. Pediatr Emerg Care 1997;13(1):44–9.

58. Booth TN. Cervical spine evaluation in pediatric trauma. Am J Roentgenol 2012; 198(5):W417–25.
59. Streck CJ Jr, Jewett BM, Wahlquist AH, et al. Evaluation for intra-abdominal injury in children after blunt torso trauma: can we reduce unnecessary abdominal computed tomography by utilizing a clinical prediction model? J Trauma Acute Care Surg 2012;73(2):371–6 [discussion: 376].
60. Kerrey BT, Rogers AJ, Lee LK, et al. A multicenter study of the risk of intra-abdominal injury in children after normal abdominal computed tomography scan results in the emergency department. Ann Emerg Med 2013;62(4): 319–26.
61. Scaife ER, Rollins MD, Barnhart DC, et al. The role of focused abdominal sonography for trauma (FAST) in pediatric trauma evaluation. J Pediatr Surg 2013;48(6):1377–83.
62. Nance ML, Lutz N, Carr MC, et al. Blunt renal injuries in children can be managed nonoperatively: outcome in a consecutive series of patients. J Trauma Inj Infect Crit Care 2004;57:474–8.
63. Christiano JG, Tummers M, Kennedy A. Clinical significance of isolated intraperitoneal fluid on computed tomography in pediatric blunt abdominal trauma. J Pediatr Surg 2009;44:1242–8.
64. Jacobs MA, Hotaling JM, Mueller BA, et al. Conservative management vs early surgery for high grade pediatric renal trauma–do nephrectomy rates differ? J Urol 2012;187:1817–22.
65. Hom J. The risk of intra-abdominal injuries in pediatric patients with stable blunt abdominal trauma and negative abdominal computed tomography. Acad Emerg Med 2010;17(5):469–75.
66. Vick LR, Islam S. Adding insult to injury: neck exploration for penetrating pediatric neck trauma. Am Surg 2008;74(11):1104–6.
67. Easter JS, Vinton DT, Haukoos JS. Emergent pediatric thoracotomy following traumatic arrest. Resuscitation 2012;83:1521–4.
68. Gausche M, Lewis RJ, Stratton SJ, et al. Effect of out-of-hospital pediatric endotracheal intubation on survival and neurological outcome: a controlled clinical trial. JAMA 2000;283(6):783–90.
69. Santillanes G, Gausche-Hill M. Pediatric airway management. Emerg Med Clin North Am 2008;26(4):961–75.
70. Akingbola OA, Hopkins RL. Pediatric noninvasive positive pressure ventilation. Pediatr Crit Care Med 2001;2(2):164–9.
71. Najaf-Zadeh A, Leclerc F. Noninvasive positive pressure ventilation for acute respiratory failure in children: a concise review. Ann Intensive Care 2011;1(1):15.
72. Essouri S, Chevret L, Durand P, et al. Noninvasive positive pressure ventilation: five years of experience in a pediatric intensive care unit. Pediatr Crit Care Med 2006;7(4):329–34.
73. Basnet S, Mander G, Andoh J, et al. Safety, efficacy, and tolerability of early initiation of noninvasive positive pressure ventilation in pediatric patients admitted with status asthmaticus: a pilot study. Pediatr Crit Care Med 2012;13(4):393–8.
74. Lee JH, Rehder KJ, Williford L, et al. Use of high flow nasal cannula in critically ill infants, children, and adults: a critical review of the literature. Intensive Care Med 2013;39(2):247–57.
75. Weingart SD, Levitan RM. Preoxygenation and prevention of desaturation during emergency airway management. Ann Emerg Med 2012;59(3):165–75.
76. Kleinman ME, Chameides L, Schexnayder SM, et al. 2010 American Heart Association guidelines for cardiopulmonary resuscitation and emergency cardiovascular care science: part 14: pediatric advanced life support: 2010 American

Heart Association guidelines for cardiopulmonary resuscitation and emergency cardiovascular care. Circulation 2010;122:S876–908.
77. Fastle RK, Roback MG. Pediatric rapid sequence intubation: incidence of reflex bradycardia and effects of pretreatment with atropine. Pediatr Emerg Care 2004;20(10):651–5.
78. Bean A, Jones J. Atropine: re-evaluating its use during paediatric RSI. Emerg Med J 2007;24(5):361–2.
79. Sagarin MJ, Chiang V, Sakles JC, et al. Rapid sequence intubation for pediatric emergency airway management. Pediatr Emerg Care 2002;18(6):417–23.
80. Zelicof-Paul A, Smith-Lockridge A, Schnadower D, et al. Controversies in rapid sequence intubation in children. Curr Opin Pediatr 2005;17(3):355–62.
81. Norman E, Wikstrom S, Hellstrom-Westas L, et al. Rapid sequence induction is superior to morphine for intubation of preterm infants: a randomized controlled trial. J Pediatr 2011;159(6):893–9.e1.
82. Zuckerbraun NS, Pitetti RD, Herr SM, et al. Use of etomidate as an induction agent for rapid sequence intubation in a pediatric emergency department. Acad Emerg Med 2006;13(6):602–9.
83. Oglesby AJ. Should etomidate be the induction agent of choice for rapid sequence intubation in the emergency department? Emerg Med J 2004;21(6):655–9.
84. Sokolove PE, Price DD, Okada P. The safety of etomidate for emergency rapid sequence intubation of pediatric patients. Pediatr Emerg Care 2000;16(1):18–21.
85. Gerardi MJ, Sacchetti AD, Cantor RM, et al. Rapid-sequence intubation of the pediatric patient. Ann Emerg Med 1996;28(1):55–74.
86. Sivilotti ML, Filbin MR, Murray HE, et al. Does the sedative agent facilitate emergency rapid sequence intubation? Acad Emerg Med 2003;10(6):612–20.
87. Ching KY, Baum CR. Newer agents for rapid sequence intubation: etomidate and rocuronium. Pediatr Emerg Care 2009;25(3):200–7 [quiz: 208–10].
88. Perry J, Lee J, Wells G. Rocuronium versus succinylcholine for rapid sequence induction intubation. Cochrane Database Syst Rev 2003;(1):CD002788.
89. Larach MG, Rosenberg H, Gronert GA, et al. Hyperkalemic cardiac arrest during anesthesia in infants and children with occult myopathies. Clin Pediatr (Phila) 1997;36(1):9–16.
90. Gronert GA. Cardiac arrest after succinylcholine: mortality greater with rhabdomyolysis than receptor upregulation. Anesthesiology 2001;94(3):523–9.
91. Kerrey BT, Rinderknecht AS, Geis GL, et al. Rapid sequence intubation for pediatric emergency patients: higher frequency of failed attempts and adverse effects found by video review. Ann Emerg Med 2012;60(3):251–9.
92. Nakayama S, Osaka Y, Yamashita M. The rotational technique with a partially inflated laryngeal mask airway improves the ease of insertion in children. Paediatr Anaesth 2002;12(5):416–9.
93. Ghai B, Makkar JK, Bhardwaj N, et al. Laryngeal mask airway insertion in children: comparison between rotational, lateral and standard technique. Paediatr Anaesth 2008;18(4):308–12.
94. Ghai B, Wig J. Comparison of different techniques of laryngeal mask placement in children. Curr Opin Anaesthesiol 2009;22(3):400–4.
95. Zhu XY, Lin BC, Zhang QS, et al. A prospective evaluation of the efficacy of the laryngeal mask airway during neonatal resuscitation. Resuscitation 2011;82(11):1405–9.
96. Zanardo V, Weiner G, Micaglio M, et al. Delivery room resuscitation of near-term infants: role of the laryngeal mask airway. Resuscitation 2010;81(3):327–30.
97. Kim JT, Na HS, Bae JY, et al. GlideScope video laryngoscope: a randomized clinical trial in 203 paediatric patients. Br J Anaesth 2008;101(4):531–4.

98. Vlatten A, Litz S, MacManus B, et al. A comparison of the GlideScope video laryngoscope and standard direct laryngoscopy in children with immobilized cervical spine. Pediatr Emerg Care 2012;28(12):1317–20.
99. Cui XL, Xue FS, Cheng YM, et al. Comparative performance of GlideScope video laryngoscope and macintosh laryngoscope in children with immobilized cervical spine. Pediatr Emerg Care 2013;29(5):690.
100. Sims C, von Ungern-Sternberg BS. The normal and the challenging pediatric airway. Paediatr Anaesth 2012;22(6):521–6.
101. Mace SE, Khan N. Needle cricothyrotomy. Emerg Med Clin North Am 2008; 26(4):1085–101.
102. Gaufberg SV, Workman TP. New needle cricothyroidotomy setup. Am J Emerg Med 2004;22(1):37–9.
103. Kofke WA, Horak J, Stiefel M, et al. Viable oxygenation with cannula-over-needle cricothyrotomy for asphyxial airway occlusion. Br J Anaesth. 107:642–643.
104. Langvad S, Hyldmo PK, Nakstad AR, et al. Emergency cricothyrotomy–a systematic review. Scand J Trauma Resusc Emerg Med 2013;21:43.
105. Stothert JC Jr, Stout MJ, Lewis LM, et al. High pressure percutaneous transtracheal ventilation: the use of large gauge intravenous-type catheters in the totally obstructed airway. Am J Emerg Med 1990;8(3):184–9.
106. Paxton JH, Knuth TE, Klausner HA. Proximal humerus intraosseous infusion: a preferred emergency venous access [article]. J Trauma Inj Infect Crit Care 2009;67(3):606–11.
107. Glaeser P, Losek J, Nelson D, et al. Pediatric intraosseous infusions: impact on vascular access time. Am J Emerg Med 1988;6:330–2.
108. Leidel BA, Kirchhoff C, Bogner V, et al. Is the intraosseous access route fast and efficacious compared to conventional central venous catheterization in adult patients under resuscitation in the emergency department? A prospective observational pilot study. Patient Saf Surg 2009;3(24):1–8.
109. Ngo AS, Oh JJ, Chen Y, et al. Intraosseous vascular access in adults using the EZ-IO in an emergency department. Int J Emerg Med 2009;2:155–60.
110. Orlowski JP. Comparison study of intraosseous, central intravenous, and peripheral intravenous infusions of emergency drugs. Am J Dis Child 1990;144(1):112–7.
111. Horton MA, Beamer C. Powered intraosseous insertion provides safe and effective vascular access for pediatric emergency patients. Pediatr Emerg Care 2008;24(6): 347–50.
112. Kanter R, Zimmerman J, Strauss R, et al. Pediatric emergency intravenous access. Evaluation of a protocol. Am J Dis Child 1986;140(2):132–4.
113. Fysh ET, Smith NA, Lee YC. Optimal chest drain size: the rise of the small-bore pleural catheter. Semin Respir Crit Care Med 2010;31:760–8.

End of Life/Palliative Care/ Ethics

Ashley Shreves, MD[a,*], Evie Marcolini, MD[b]

KEYWORDS

• End of life care • Palliative care • Bioethics

KEY POINTS

- Palliative and end-of-life care, once the purview of oncologists and intensivists, has also become the responsibility of the emergency physician.
- As our population ages and medical technology enables increased longevity, it is essential that all medical professionals know how to help patients negotiate the balance between quantity and quality of life.
- Specific communication strategies can improve patient and caregiver understanding of the medical options available at the end of life, minimizing the risk that patients receive burdensome and futile treatments.

INTRODUCTION

Although most dying patients have a strong preference to be at home, many patients visit the emergency department (ED) near the end of life (EOL).[1–3] Overwhelming symptoms, inadequate social support, poor communication, and regional factors, like an overabundance of hospital beds, have all been cited as variables associated with increased hospital utilization at the EOL.[4–6] Given the significant time constraints and resource limitations of the ED environment, it can be challenging to both elicit and then address all the needs of patients and families at the EOL. Not surprisingly, the experience of dying patients in the ED has typically been poor.[7,8] Nonetheless, understanding the factors that families and patients have endorsed as most important can help physicians prioritize care that best promotes patient-centered goals. Management of pain and symptoms, preparation for death, achieving a sense of completion, being involved in treatment decisions, and being treated as a whole person have been rated highly by families and patients with life-limiting conditions. In a study of hospice enrollees, the most important goals endorsed were control of symptoms and being

Disclosure: None.
[a] Department of Emergency Medicine and Brookdale Department of Geriatrics and Palliative Medicine, Icahn School of Medicine at Mt. Sinai, One Gustave L. Levy Place, New York, NY 10029, USA; [b] Divisions of Neurocritical Care and Emergency Neurology and Surgical Critical Care, Departments of Emergency Medicine and Neurology, Yale University School of Medicine, 464 Congress St. Suite 260, New Haven, CT 06519, USA
* Corresponding author.
E-mail address: ashley.shreves@mssm.edu

Emerg Med Clin N Am 32 (2014) 955–974
http://dx.doi.org/10.1016/j.emc.2014.07.010 **emed.theclinics.com**
0733-8627/14/$ – see front matter

with family.[9] Ultimately, it has been recognized that emergency physicians should have some basic competency in meeting the needs of dying patients.[10,11] With a general understanding of dying trajectories, communication strategies helpful in determining the goals of care, the bioethical framework that guides EOL decision making, and symptom management, the emergency physician can improve the care of patients presenting to the ED with life-limiting conditions.

DIAGNOSING DYING

It can be challenging to define when a patient is dying. Even so, it can be useful for emergency physicians to recognize when someone has entered this final stage of life, as there are unique needs in this population. The goals of care often transition at this time, and the resources available to patients at the EOL are unique.[9,12–14] There are 4 main dying trajectories that have been described: terminal disease, organ failure, frailty, and sudden death. Each of these trajectories is characterized by a unique pattern of functional decline that occurs at the EOL. Familiarity with these trajectories enables emergency physicians to contextualize acute illness presentations and even recognize when someone is at the EOL.

The classic terminal disease is metastatic cancer. Patients with cancer tend to maintain relatively good function until the very end of life. Multiple studies have demonstrated that once patients with cancer become disabled and weakened by their disease, there is a relatively predictable decline toward death.[15] Those classified as having a poor performance status, meaning that they are significantly disabled by their illness and are spending more than half of their waking hours in bed, have a prognosis of 2 months or less.[16–19] Other clinical variables that suggest patients with cancer are approaching the EOL include dyspnea, dysphagia, dry mouth, anorexia, and cognitive impairment.[15] In a cohort of patients with cancer presenting to the ED with dyspnea, about one-third of those with a history of uncontrolled metastatic disease died within 2 weeks.[20]

Congestive heart failure (CHF) and chronic obstructive pulmonary disease (COPD) are common organ failure diagnoses. In patients with these conditions, the final year of life is marked by sharp declines in function and health, often followed by surprising recoveries.[21] In the ED, it is notoriously challenging to generate accurate short-term prognoses in this population; it can be difficult to predict which patients will respond to conventional life-prolonging therapies, like noninvasive or mechanical ventilation and intravenous (IV) medications.[22–25] Furthermore, the introduction of devices like the left ventricular assist device for CHF can dramatically alter the clinical course of patients who would otherwise be in the end-stages of their illness.[26] For this reason, unless goals have been clearly defined before the ED arrival (ie, patients have enrolled in hospice or only wish to prioritize quality of life), diagnosing dying may be beyond the scope of emergency provider practice.

Patients with advanced dementia residing in long-term care typify the frailty category. These patients are profoundly disabled for the months to years preceding death and are less likely to have dramatic declines in function at the very EOL.[21,27] Patients on this trajectory succumb to the complications of their underlying illness rather than the illness itself.[6] For emergency providers, these complications, like acute infections and feeding difficulties, are familiar as they are common reasons for patients with advanced dementia to be transitioned to the acute care setting.[28] Once patients with advanced dementia develop an acute illness, such as pneumonia, the 6-month mortality is high (approximately 50%).[6,29] A recent study suggests that in patients with moderate to advanced dementia, 2 or more hospitalizations for the diagnoses of pneumonia, urinary tract infection, sepsis, and malnutrition/dehydration are correlated with a median survival of 3 months, 5 months, 3 months, and 3.5 months, respectively. Accordingly, patients meeting the aforementioned criteria should be presumed to be dying, particularly in light of the progressive and incurable nature of their underlying disease.[6]

The last dying trajectory, sudden death, is the subject of intense focus and interest to the emergency physician. These patients are presumably independent and in relatively good health until the moment when a sudden and devastating illness or event, like a massive myocardial infarction or motor vehicle accident, ends their life.[21] Observations in the ED have suggested that these patients receive a massive outpouring of resources, with emergency physicians prioritizing their resuscitation efforts above all other functions in the ED.[7] These patients, however, are not typically classified as dying until efforts to resuscitate them have been exhausted, at which point the time to death is brief.[7,30] Furthermore, death for these patients often follows the withdrawal of life-sustaining therapies.[30]

SYNDROME OF IMMINENT DEATH

Most of the available information about the dying process is based on observations of patients with terminal cancer.[31–33] For many of these patients not receiving life-sustaining measures, the last hours to days of life are characterized by a somewhat predictable pattern of symptoms and signs.[34] Familiarity with these patterns allows emergency physicians to both anticipate the needs of dying patients and offer counseling to family members about the dying process. A decline in mental status is one of the most consistent changes that patients experience at the EOL; most are either very drowsy or comatose in their last hours.[31,32] As patients move closer to death, respiratory abnormalities become pronounced, with dyspnea, alterations in breathing patterns, and noisy respirations common.[31–33] Patients moving through this process show marked derangements in vital signs, with low blood pressure and hypoxia often coinciding with physical signs of hypoperfusion, like mottled skin and cyanosis.[31,32] One study demonstrated that weakness, anorexia, dry mouth, confusion, and constipation were the most commonly experienced symptoms of patients with cancer in the last week of life.[13]

UNDERSTANDING PATIENTS' AND FAMILIES' PREFERENCES: COMMUNICATION AT THE EOL

When dying patients present to the ED, there are often important, time-urgent decisions that need to be made about the use of medical interventions. Specifically, emergency physicians seem to struggle with the issue of withholding potentially life-sustaining treatments (LST).[35] The approach taken in discussing goals of care with such patients and/or their families needs to be tailored to the acuity of patients.

GOALS OF CARE IN CRASHING PATIENTS

When patients are perceived to be unstable, meaning that there is an immediate threat to one of the ABCs, a streamlined approach is recommended for determining which treatments should be initiated. There are essentially 2 critical actions that emergency physicians should perform in all unstable patients before initiating life-sustaining interventions: (1) identifying advance directives (AD) when present and (2) determining patients' appropriate surrogate decision maker. An AD is any instructional device used to inform a patient's future medical care and can be either oral or written. Not surprisingly, up to 70% of patients lose decision-making capacity near the EOL, so previously completed AD can prove particularly useful.[36] The types of AD that exist vary by state; but examples of potentially relevant AD include a living will, out-of-hospital do-not-resuscitate (DNR) order, and physician orders for life-sustaining therapies (POLST). Most helpful, the POLST form includes instructions about the LST most commonly considered at the EOL, like medical resuscitation, intubation, noninvasive ventilation, artificial fluids, artificial nutrition, and antibiotics.[37] These directives are designed to be portable, maintaining their legal integrity across health care settings.

When written directives are not available, previously expressed wishes about invasive interventions should be sought. Although any member of the patients' family or community can contribute to this discussion, it is essential that the patients' legal surrogate be included in this process, if patients lack decision-making capacity. Some patients have appointed a decision maker, ideally the person who best understands the patients' goals and preferences about medical care. Depending on the state, this person is called either a health care proxy (HCP) or health care power of attorney. A study of community-dwelling elderly individuals in New York revealed that more than 30% had assigned an HCP.[38] An HCP takes precedence over patients' so-called natural surrogate. For example, if a patient appoints a close friend to be his HCP, and he is also legally married, his friend actually takes precedence over his spouse in regard to medical decision making.

The appropriate surrogate decision maker should then be engaged in a brief discussion with 2 specific goals: (1) elucidate clear, previously expressed wishes patients may have about the use of LST and (2) provide information about the risks and benefits of proceeding with LST. Although multiple studies have demonstrated that improved communication about the use of interventions, like cardiopulmonary resuscitation (CPR), in the context of a serious illness dramatically influences care choices,[6,39–42] there is no one validated approach to conversations about the use of LST. Regardless, because health literacy, more than any other patient factor, predicts choices about the use of LST, care should be taken to remove all medical jargon from such discussions and present information in a clear, accessible manner.[43,44]

If time permits, some information about the patient-centered outcomes most likely to occur with the use of invasive LST should be offered. For CPR, general survival statistics are important to convey; but patients consider functional and cognitive outcomes as critical when weighing the use of EOL treatments, so this information should also be communicated.[45] In patients with a recognized terminal illness, such as cancer or advanced dementia, survival after a cardiac arrest, even with full resuscitative efforts, is rare.[46] One study examined the rates of survival in inpatients with cancer and found that no patients with an anticipated cardiac arrest, meaning that the arrest followed a gradual clinical deterioration, survived.[47] Furthermore, a resuscitation that results in the return of spontaneous circulation rarely translates to a meaningful recovery in this population, with few of these patients returning home, and most survivors receiving what could be considered burdensome care in the intensive care unit (ICU) at the EOL.[48] In patients who are already critically ill, less than 5% of patients both survive a cardiac arrest and return home functionally independent.[49] Besides being unlikely to achieve meaningful outcomes in dying patients, CPR carries significant risks for this population. The use of CPR can result in a prolonged dying process in the ICU setting. It can also lead to survival but in a markedly dependent state necessitating institutional-level care indefinitely. These outcomes are often incompatible with patients' values and preferences.

For these reasons, it has been proposed that the physician make a strong recommendation against the use of CPR in patients with an advanced terminal illness, as they are at a low likelihood of benefit and high risk of harm with the procedure.[50] Physicians might consider framing their recommendation using positive language, offering patients the opportunity to have a natural death rather than using language that focuses on the withholding of resuscitation, as studies of patients who opt to be full code suggest that fears of being euthanized or being given substandard care influence their decision making.[51]

When considering intubation and the use of mechanical ventilation for patients with respiratory failure, it is important to consider that, in patients on a dying trajectory, the underlying cause of the patients' dyspnea may not be reversible. In a cohort of patients with cancer presenting to the ED with dyspnea, one-third of those with uncontrollable cancer died within 2 weeks.[20] In contrast, patients who have a noncancer diagnosis, like COPD, may respond well to brief trials of mechanical ventilation and critical care.[52] Regardless, patients and families have serious misconceptions about what a ventilator is and what life on one is like.[53] In one study, 20% of patients thought a mechanical ventilator was the same device as an oxygen tank.[53] For this reason, using clear language that allows patients and families to imagine the experience of mechanical ventilation, specifically that patients will be fully dependent on a machine for life support, often sedated, and unable to communicate with loved ones, is essential (eg, I understand your point). Helpful language is included in **Table 1**.

Table 1
Helpful phrases to use when considering the use of life-sustaining therapy in patients *on a clear dying trajectory*

Do Not	Do
Do you want us to intubate her?	Did she have any thoughts or preferences about the use of life support at the end of her life? This procedure would involve inserting a tube into her lungs and attaching her to a machine that would breathe for her. We are concerned that placing her on this machine may only prolong her dying process. There is a strong possibility that she will die, attached to this machine in the ICU. As an alternative plan, we can refocus our efforts toward maximizing her comfort and treat her shortness of breath with medications.
Do you want us to resuscitate her? Is she full code? Is she DNR?	Your loved one is dying, and we expect that at some point soon her heart will stop. Given her severe illness, it is our recommendation that we allow her to have a natural death, rather than trying to restart her heart when it stops. It is very unlikely that an attempted resuscitation would be successful; in the rare chance that we could restart her heart, she would most likely have a prolonged dying experience in the ICU. If you agree with our recommendation, we will place an order in the chart so that other members of the team know to allow for your loved one to have a natural death.

GOALS OF CARE IN HEMODYNAMICALLY STABLE BUT DYING PATIENTS

For patients who are dying, but in whom immediate life threats are not detected, a more deliberate, structured approach to the goals-of-care discussion should be undertaken. The overarching purpose of this conversation is to ensure that patients receive medical care that has the potential to help them meet their goals. Various approaches have been investigated in the ICU setting, including the use of palliative care specialists and/or ethics consultants to facilitate discussions, printed information about prognosis and treatment options, and standardized family meetings in which specific communication strategies are emphasized.[54,55] For the purposes of the emergency physician, outside resources such as these may not be readily available, so the responsibility for determining GOC often rests on the ED staff.

A guide proposed by Buckman and Kason[56] has gained wide-spread acceptance as an ideal model for delivering bad news to patients, and it proves particularly helpful in breaking the news that someone is dying. Furthermore, it can also be a useful roadmap for determining goals of care (**Table 2**). Although it might feel overly laborious to proceed through each of these steps, unnecessary and avoidable conflict may be generated by rushing to a question about goals before, for instance, patients really understand that they are dying.

In the ED, there is often limited time to prepare for EOL conversations. High-yield actions may include a quick review of the patients' medical chart and a call to the patients' PMD and/or oncologist to ensure an accurate understanding of the medical facts. The next step, establishing what patients know about their illness, is critical. It should never be assumed that patients have been told and/or understand the terminal nature of their disease. A recent study of patients with terminal cancer revealed that more than two-thirds of patients think their chemotherapy is potentially curative.[57] Only 18% of the HCPs of patients with advanced dementia, an incurable and progressive disease, report being given prognostic information from their physician; only one-third have received counseling about the expected complications of this disease, including repeated infections, feeding problems, and pressure ulcers.[6]

If the clinician detects a large gap between the patient/family perspective and the medical reality, assessing readiness and openness to hearing what is likely to be bad and surprising news is a useful next step. If there seems to be resistance or discomfort with the direction of the conversation, it may be appropriate to defer further discussions to the inpatient setting.

In this situation, step 4 would involve disclosing the news that patients are, in fact, dying. This process can be stressful and uncomfortable for medical providers[58]; yet, it is an essential skill, as patients and families have endorsed physician willingness to discuss dying as highly important to them.[59] It also empowers patients and families to make fully informed medical decisions. Multiple studies have demonstrated that when patients and/or families understand the terminal nature of their disease, they make different choices about medical care.[6,60]

Strong and varied emotional responses commonly follow news about dying. Step 5, responding to emotions, often falls just after this news has been delivered, particularly if this is the first time that patients and families are hearing the word dying. Silence may be the best device here. When confronted with the overwhelming sadness and disappointment patients often experience at this point, physicians can be tempted to retreat from the clinical reality and make unrealistic promises or statements about the patients' condition. Again, this is an unhelpful strategy, as it deprives patients and families of the honest and clear communication that they need to move forward.[61]

Table 2
Seven-step process for breaking bad news and determining goals of care

Step	Helpful Phrases	Do Not Say
1. Preparation	Would it be ok if we all sat down and discussed your wife's condition so that we can make the best medical plan for her?	We need to talk about your wife's code status.
2. Establish what patients/ families know	What have the doctors told you about your wife's illness? How have things been going lately at home?	Do you understand what is going on with your wife?
3. Assess willingness to hear information	We have some serious news to share about her condition. Is that something you are ready to talk about?	
4. Deliver medical information	I am afraid we have some bad news. Her illness has progressed despite our best efforts to control it. At this point, I think that she is dying. I wish things were different. I wish we had better treatments for your wife's disease.	There is nothing more we can do.
5. Respond to emotions	This must be hard to hear. I can only imagine how scary this must be. You seem angry. Can you tell me what is on your mind?	I am so sorry.
6. Establish goals of care	Knowing that time is short, what would your wife say is most important to her? What are your hopes for her when you look into the future? Are there any particular worries you have when you look into the future?	Would she want to be resuscitated? Would she want chest compressions? Does she want everything done?
7. Make medical recommendations/ summarize plan	Based on what you have told me, I recommend that we… We will refocus our efforts toward maximizing her comfort. We will aggressively manage her symptoms We will make sure we use all our resources to support her and all of you through her dying process. We will allow her to have a natural, peaceful death. We will not artificially prolong her dying process.	Let us just keep her comfortable.

Patients and families may then make specific requests about life expectancy in the face of a terminal diagnosis. Prognostication is a challenging skill. Physicians have proved notoriously inaccurate in their prognostic predictions, typically erring on the side of being overly optimistic.[62] Of relevance to emergency providers, the longer the physician-patient relationship is, the less accurate prognostic estimates tend to be, suggesting that a fresh, unbiased perspective from the emergency physician may be helpful.[63] When delivering information about life expectancy, it is best to suggest ranges of time, like hours to days, days to weeks, or weeks to months, as there is no tool available to generate a more precise estimate.

Establishing goals of care, step 6, comes next. Although there can be substantial nuance to patients' hopes and goals, it can be helpful for emergency physicians to consider goals as broadly falling into one of the following 3 categories: (1) life prolongation regardless of patient quality of life, burdens of treatments, and likelihood of benefit; (2) mostly comfort but interested in some life-prolonging therapies, like antibiotics if the burdens of treatment are low and potential benefits exist; and (3) comfort-focused care only, meaning that all treatments should have a comfort-oriented goal, and efforts to prolong the dying process are not desired. A good transitional question, to determine which category patients will fall into, would be an open-ended one, exploring the patients' hope for the future, given the new information about their disease and prognosis.

The last step, recommending a medical plan, will largely be the responsibility of the emergency physician. Patients and families do not typically have the health literacy to navigate the large array of medical treatments available in a modern health care system.[53] It is the doctor's job to determine which treatments make sense, given the clinical realities of the case, combined with patients' stated goals, and to then make a recommendation based on these factors.[64] This process can actually be complicated and may necessitate involvement of a palliative care specialist. Regardless, it should be clearly stressed that no matter what plan is pursued, patients and families will not be abandoned and will continue to receive high-quality care. Well-intended physician statements that can cause emotional harm to patients and families are included (see **Table 2**).

For some patient encounters, proceeding through these steps will be linear and relatively uncomplicated, with a meaningful plan generated as a result. For others, enormous conflict emerges when death and dying are discussed; this serves as a barrier to any forward movement in terms of medical decision making. Sources of conflict at the EOL are common and well described.[65] Examples include denial, anger, guilt, overwhelming grief, mistrust, and fear.[65,66] Occasionally, just recognizing and acknowledging the emotional conflict proves therapeutic in allowing patients and families to move past it. In many situations, however, addressing and resolving such conflict is a lengthy, complicated process beyond the scope of the emergency physician. Patients and families struggling with significant conflict often benefit from involvement of the palliative care team, including members of an interdisciplinary team of social workers, chaplains, art therapists, and massage therapists.

BIOETHICS

Bioethics has a rich history and background in medicine. Biomedical advances, such as the ventilator, organ transplant, and chronic hemodialysis, have simultaneously created medical opportunity and ethical dilemmas.[67] Medical technology that can prolong life (or death), immense overcrowding, and increasing utilization of EDs have essentially changed the practice of emergency medicine. The emergency physician should have a basic understanding of the ethical framework that informs his or her practice, particularly for patients at the EOL.[68–70] Code of ethics documents specific to the specialty of emergency medicine exist and should be reviewed for more information on the topic.[71,72]

Ethical issues commonly encountered with care of patients at the EOL include (1) autonomy, (2) justice, (3) futility, and (4) organ donation and declaration of death.

Bioethics has been historically dominated by the use of 4 basic principles: autonomy (patient self-determination), beneficence (do what is best for patients), nonmaleficence (do no harm), and justice (resource allocation). There are no universally accepted rules associated with these principles, and many ethicists and/or physicians will have different views of their application for any particular case. Many societies and cultures will also prioritize principles differently.[73,74] Typically in the United States, as differentiated from other countries, autonomy takes precedence over all other principles, which creates a potential for conflict if patients are not able to communicate and the families are unclear as to the patients' wishes at the EOL.[75] This can also create discord if patients or families are from a culture that places a higher premium on community and/or religion than autonomy.

Autonomy/Patient Self-determination

Autonomy plays a prominent role in biomedical ethics, focusing on each person's right to individual choice. In order to exercise autonomy, a person must have capacity, which implies knowledge of his or her medical condition and options, consequences and risks/benefits of each decision, and the ability to clearly communicate a decision without coercion.[76] Historically, there has been a distinction between capacity, which is determined by medical providers (typically psychiatrists), and competence, which is determined by a court. Since the 1990s, many states have been revising their statutes relating to competency to more closely align with the practical capacity definition. Thus, the distinction is no longer as relevant in clinical practice. Ethical issues arise when patients have lost capacity and have neither documented their EOL goals nor appointed a proxy to represent their wishes. In the case of surrogate decision makers, whether they have been appointed by patients or are established by default in the case of no prior designation, the most important principle is to attempt to make decisions that would be consistent with the patients' known values. Narrative ethics is a method of determining what patients would have wanted in a situation by interviewing the patients (if possible) as well as the families and those close to the patients to ascertain these values.[77] In this way, decisions can be made that are consistent with the way patients have lived their life and, it is hoped, represent what they would have chosen in an EOL situation. The Patient Self-Determination Act was enacted in 1991 by the US Congress in 1990 to ensure that persons admitted to extended care facilities were informed of and had discussions regarding their advance health care directives. In the case of ambiguity, it is expected that the EP will institute medically appropriate measures, acknowledging that, in terms of ethics, it is acceptable and permissible to withdraw life-supporting treatments if it is later determined that patients would not have wanted such measures.[71,76]

In some cases, patients' expressed (by self or surrogate) wishes run contrary to the medical team's opinion. Patients have the right to request therapy, refuse therapy, or even to relinquish their own EOL decisions to benefit a loved one's feelings.[78]

Justice

The question of responsible stewardship of ICU beds is a growing problem, evidenced by critically ill patients boarding in the ED. Many argue that futile therapies are being delivered in the ICU, taking up resources that would otherwise be used by other patients.[79] The distribution of scarce resources, such as extracorporeal membrane oxygenation, dialysis, transplantable organs, and even ICU beds with access to a ventilator, has proven to be ethically challenging.[76]

ICUs are generally populated by 3 types of patients: those who are severely critically ill and depend on life support for their survival, those who are being monitored because of anticipated problems, and those who are on life support but with no reasonable expectation of survival to an acceptable quality of life.[76] In the United States, the concept of rationing creates great public discord; it is currently unacceptable to discontinue life support for one patient in order to initiate it on another. Regardless, given the anticipated increase in critically ill patients in the future, there will likely come a time when demand for critical care exceeds supply.[80] Now, however, many argue that resource allocation is an issue best negotiated at a macro level, within the realm of government and policy making instead of by individual physicians at the bedside.[79]

Futility

The concept of futility in medicine is difficult to clarify, and even medical professionals do not agree on its definition.[67,81–87]

Typically, discussions of futility surface when a family or proxy request a therapy or procedure, such as continuation of life support, that the medical team thinks is not medically indicated, will not contribute toward the patients' goals of care, or is unethical. Optimal outcome in these cases occurs when there is clear and open communication and trust between the family and the medical team. Infrequently, there is impasse caused by a lack of family trust in the medical professionals' ability to prognosticate and/or religious or other beliefs that are not in line with medical standards of care.

Many hospitals have a conscientious practice policy, which is a tiered-step process such as the following: The medical team engages family in a discussion regarding the patient's medical status, prognosis, and available treatment options. If the family and medical team are unable to reach an agreement on a treatment plan or family is requesting therapy that the physicians think is futile, the family is given ample time to seek a second opinion and/or transfer patients to another accepting facility. If this is not accomplished, the case is referred to the ethics committee and/or chief of staff and a recommendation is made with respect to actions on the patient's behalf. In rare cases, the courts are called on to mediate. When issues of futility arise in the ED, the best course of action may be to consult palliative care and/or the ethics teams. It is helpful for the emergency physician to be aware of existing hospital policy and resources surrounding futility issues.

Most hospitals have an ethics committee, ideally composed of a diversified membership including ethicists, physicians, nurses, social workers, care coordinators, clergy, legal representatives, administrators, and community members.[88] Consults provided by ethics teams can address a variety of issues that arise when values or expectations of treatment options differ between patients/families and health care providers. For many consults, the issue is not strictly an ethical question and is resolved through inclusive communication with the patients, families, and medical team. Infrequently, a true ethical dilemma arises, such as the request for futile medical treatment by the family against the medical team's advice. Ethics consults are rarely placed from the ED, mostly because of time constraints; but this may be an underused resource.

Organ Donation and Declaration of Death

There are more than 100,000 individuals awaiting organ transplant in the United States, and less than one-third of them will get an organ each year.[89]

Organ donation typically occurs by one of 2 processes: (1) after brain death (which in most states equals death) but before ventilator and supportive medications have been discontinued (more common) or (2) by donation after cardiac death (DCD). DCD can proceed when the patients' brain still has minimal function, but the injury is such that patients would not have wanted to be kept alive, and the plan (separate from organ donation consideration) is to withdraw life support. Through this method, if the patients' heart stops within a proscribed period of time after life support is withdrawn, then the organs can then be procured and transplanted.[90] The ethics of this method are debated, mostly around the question of interpretation of the dead donor rule, which simply states that organs may not be procured from a living person and includes the caveat of irreversibility of cardiac arrest.[91–95] Some emergency medical services systems advocate out-of-hospital uncontrolled donation after circulatory determination of death.[96]

It is not uncommon for an EP to pronounce circulatory death in a patient. Brain death is typically more involved, requiring testing beyond the scope of practice of emergency medicine (eg, an apnea test).[97] In the ED setting, when patients present who may be appropriate for organ donation, it is preferable to find a representative from the organ procurement organization to talk with the families in order to separate the role of treating physician from that of organ procurement.[89] However, it is not always timely and/or possible, so the EP must act in accordance with what he or she feels is right for the patients, the families, and the situation.[98]

EOL SYMPTOM MANAGEMENT

It is common for patients at the EOL to seek care in the ED.[2,3,7] Often, the symptom burden that accompanies the dying process overwhelms patients and their caregivers at home and drives them into the acute care setting.[5,8] It is increasingly recognized that providing these patients with high-quality symptom relief is a basic competency within the scope of emergency medicine.[11,99] Dyspnea and dehydration occur commonly in dying patients, and the ideal management strategies differ from traditional emergency medicine pathways.

DYSPNEA

The American Thoracic Society has described dyspnea as the "subjective experience of breathing discomfort that consists of qualitatively distinct sensations that vary in intensity."[100] Regardless of the underlying disease process, many dying patients experience dyspnea near the EOL.[101–103] Furthermore, it is one of the most common reasons that patients with cancer present to the ED at the EOL.[2] Although the underlying cause may vary, treatment of dyspnea at the EOL tends to be rather uniform and symptom focused.[104–106] In awake patients, dyspnea can be assessed by simply inquiring about the presence of shortness of breath or feelings of air hunger. Unfortunately, many dying patients lose the ability to communicate, so physicians must rely on physical examination findings, like gasping or retractions, to infer that patients are experiencing discomfort.

Pharmacologic agents to consider when treating dyspnea include opiates and benzodiazepines. Opiates are the recommended first-line agents. Multiple studies have demonstrated both their efficacy and safety.[107–111] The goal with opiate use is either patient-reported relief of symptoms or a decrease in the appearance of labored breathing in nonverbal patients. There is limited clinical evidence to support the use of specific agents within the opiate class; therefore, physicians should select an opiate that is familiar and available to them. A general rule to follow when using opiates for dyspnea relief is start low and go slow. Initial doses of morphine 1 mg IV and hydromorphone 0.2 mg IV have been recommended.[112] In those without an initial clinical response, a stepwise algorithm should be followed in which the medication is administered every 10 to 15 minutes, with dosing increases of 50% to 100% with each injection.[112] In patients requiring large doses of opiates to maintain comfort, a continuous infusion may be preferable. If patients have needed a total of 12 mg of morphine over a 4-hour period, a morphine infusion would be ordered to run at a rate of 3 mg/h. Benzodiazepines may have a role in the management of dyspnea precipitated by anxiety, but the evidence to support their use is weak **Fig. 1**.[113,114]

Supplemental oxygen is routinely administered to dying patients with dyspnea. Clinical evidence does not support this practice.[115] At the EOL, hypoxia and the sensation of dyspnea are often unrelated, so it is not surprising that the only large-scale randomized trial to investigate the use of supplemental oxygen in dying patients did not show a benefit to this intervention.[111,116] Regardless, as long as the delivery device is not burdensome, a time-limited trial of oxygen may have value in select patients.

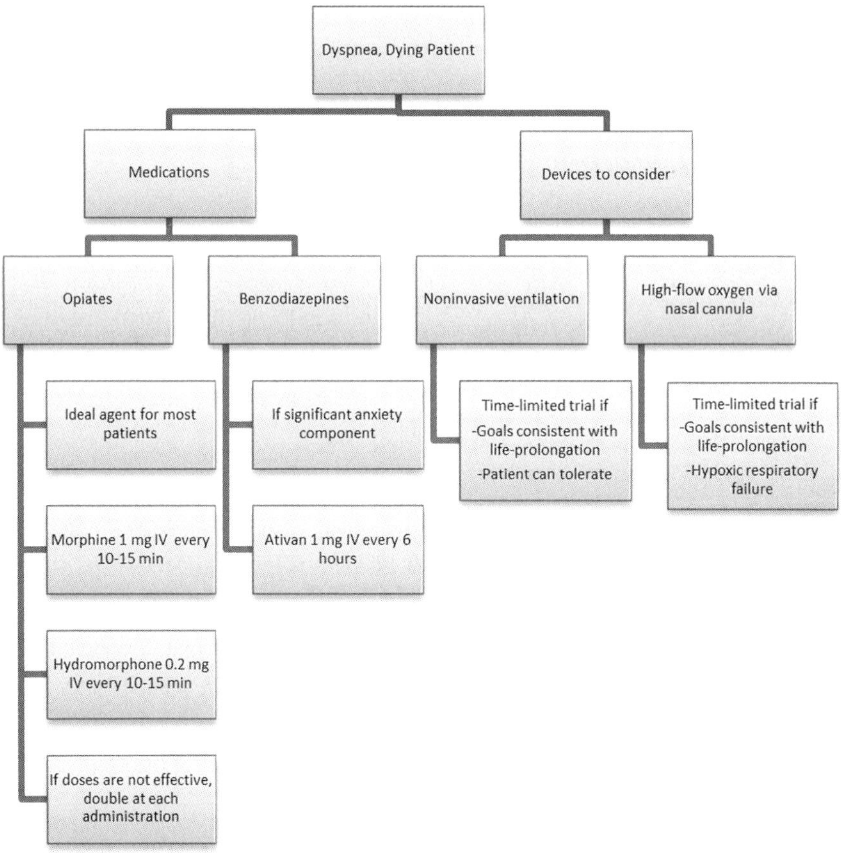

Fig. 1. Management of dyspnea at the EOL.

Noninvasive ventilation (NIV) is a familiar tool to emergency physicians, with its efficacy well-demonstrated in patients with CHF and COPD.[117,118] For those at the EOL, it may have a role in select patients.[119] Studies of patients who have chosen to forgo intubation suggest that many patients recover from episodes of respiratory failure with the use of NIV.[120] A cohort of terminally ill patients with cancer receiving NIV suggests that although about half benefit in terms of meaningful symptom relief and life-prolongation, others simply experience a prolongation of their dying process.[121] For this reason, before initiation of NIV, the patients' goals and the risks and benefits of an NIV trial should be carefully considered.

High-flow humidified oxygen, delivered via nasal cannula (HFNC) has been proposed as an alternative strategy to NIV in patients in respiratory distress who do not wish to pursue mechanical ventilation. With this device, oxygen is delivered at rates up to 40 L/min. Limited data suggest that HFNC may improve dyspnea in select patients.[122] Furthermore, in patients with underlying lung disease, like pulmonary fibrosis, this tool may allow for the reversal of hypoxemic respiratory failure.[123] If prolongation of life is consistent with the patients' goals, this relatively noninvasive device may be an appropriate adjunct. For many dying patients, however, the sensation of dyspnea and hypoxia are unrelated, so this tool would have minimal opportunity for improving symptom relief beyond opiates.

DEHYDRATION

Most patients lose interest in eating and drinking at the EOL; this is a normal part of the dying process and may even be protective in terms of symptom relief.[13,124] Regardless, families often struggle with this issue, expressing concerns about dehydration and its effect on symptoms and life expectancy.[125] Accordingly, they see artificial hydration as a way of providing both comfort and hope to their loved one.[125] A recent randomized trial of patients with cancer in the last weeks of life revealed no benefit with the use of IV hydration compared with placebo for any measured outcome, including dehydration symptoms, quality of life, and survival.[126] Although another study suggests that some patients experience improvement in dehydration symptoms, like sedation and myoclonus, with IVF, those benefits must be weighed against the adverse effects of artificial hydration also observed in dying patients, including increased edema, ascites, and bronchial secretions.[127,128] In appropriate patients, a time-limited trial of IVF may be considered; but there should be clear goals in place before initiation of this therapy.

DISPOSITION

When and where available, involvement of palliative care and/or hospice services is recommended to ensure that dying patients receive high-quality EOL care.[129] Palliative medicine is a relatively new specialty, focused on improving the quality of life of patients with serious illnesses. Hospice care, considered within the domain of palliative care, is specifically focused on those patients with a prognosis of 6 months or less. For the patients discussed here, the distinction between the two services is less important.

Initiating a palliative care consult may be one of the most important steps the emergency physician can take in improving the overall care of patients at the EOL.[129] These specialists can be particularly helpful at ensuring dying patients' transition from the ED to an appropriate care setting. For an increasing number of hospitals, this would be an inpatient palliative care or hospice unit.[130] For those patients with well-controlled symptoms, good social support, and a desire to be at home, hospice referral in the

ED is increasingly recognized as a viable option.[131] Hospice services can often be provided in the home within 24 to 48 hours of referral. For many patients, this is timely enough to meet their needs, allowing for a safe ED discharge.

SUMMARY

Palliative and EOL care, once the purview of oncologists and intensivists, has also become the responsibility of the emergency physician. As our population ages and medical technology enables increased longevity, it is essential that all medical professionals know how to help patients negotiate the balance between quantity and quality of life. Specific communication strategies can improve patient and caregiver understanding of medical options available at the EOL, minimizing the risk that patients receive burdensome and futile treatments. As emergency physicians, we have the opportunity to both educate patients and their loved ones on how to best accomplish their goals while also enhancing quality of life through the treatment of symptoms. In these endeavors, ethical questions and issues occasionally arise; and the emergency physician must be aware of the ethical and medicolegal parameters that govern decision making. When ethical principles are in conflict and beyond resolution in the ED, involvement of both palliative care and ethics consultation services can help patients, families, and physicians find the common ground needed to move forward.

REFERENCES

1. Higginson IJ, Sen-Gupta GJ. Place of care in advanced cancer: a qualitative systematic literature review of patient preferences. J Palliat Med 2000;3(3): 287–300.
2. Barbera L, Taylor C, Dudgeon D. Why do patients with cancer visit the emergency department near the end of life? Can Med Assoc J 2010;182(6):563–8.
3. Smith AK, McCarthy E, Weber E, et al. Half of older Americans seen in emergency department in last month of life; most admitted to hospital, and many die there. Health Aff 2012;31(6):1277–85.
4. Gomes B. Factors influencing death at home in terminally ill patients with cancer: systematic review. BMJ 2006;332(7540):515–21.
5. Wallace EM, Walsh J, Conroy M, et al. Why do palliative care patients present to the emergency department? Avoidable or unavoidable? Am J Hosp Palliat Care 2013;30(3):253–6.
6. Mitchell SL, Teno JM, Kiely DK, et al. The clinical course of advanced dementia. N Engl J Med 2009;361(16):1529–38.
7. Bailey C, Murphy R, Porock D. Trajectories of end-of-life care in the emergency department. Ann Emerg Med 2011;57(4):362–9.
8. Smith AK, Schonberg MA, Fisher J, et al. Emergency department experiences of acutely symptomatic patients with terminal illness and their family caregivers. J Pain Symptom Manage 2010;39(6):972–81.
9. Kumar G, Markert RJ, Patel R. Assessment of hospice patients' goals of care at the end of life. Am J Hosp Palliat Care 2011;28(1):31–4.
10. Quest TE, Marco CA, Derse AR. Hospice and palliative medicine: new subspecialty, new opportunities. Ann Emerg Med 2009;54(1):94–102.
11. Todd KH. Practically speaking: emergency medicine and the palliative care movement. Emerg Med Australas 2012;24(1):4–6.
12. Grudzen CR, Richardson LD, Morrison M, et al. Palliative care needs of seriously ill, older adults presenting to the emergency department. Acad Emerg Med 2010;17(11):1253–7.

13. Conill C, Verger E, Henriquez I, et al. Symptom prevalence in the last week of life. J Pain Symptom Manage 1997;14(6):328–31.
14. DeVader TE, Jeanmonod R. The effect of education in hospice and palliative care on emergency medicine residents' knowledge and referral patterns. J Palliat Med 2012;15(5):510–5.
15. Lamont EB, Christakis NA. Complexities in prognostication in advanced cancer: "to help them live their lives the way they want to". JAMA 2003; 290(1):98–104.
16. Morita T, Tsunoda J, Inoue S, et al. Validity of the palliative performance scale from a survival perspective. J Pain Symptom Manage 1999;18(1):2–3.
17. Llobera J, Esteva M, Rifa J, et al. Terminal cancer. Duration and prediction of survival time. Eur J Cancer 2000;36(16):2036–43.
18. Maltoni M, Pirovano M, Scarpi E, et al. Prediction of survival of patients terminally ill with cancer. Results of an Italian prospective multicentric study. Cancer 1995; 75(10):2613–22.
19. Reuben DB, Mor V, Hiris J. Clinical symptoms and length of survival in patients with terminal cancer. Arch Intern Med 1988;148(7):1586–91.
20. Escalante CP, Martin CG, Elting LS, et al. Identifying risk factors for imminent death in cancer patients with acute dyspnea. J Pain Symptom Manage 2000; 20(5):318–25.
21. Lunney JR, Lynn J, Foley DJ, et al. Patterns of functional decline at the end of life. JAMA 2003;289(18):2387–92.
22. Lee DS, Austin PC, Rouleau JL, et al. Predicting mortality among patients hospitalized for heart failure: derivation and validation of a clinical model. JAMA 2003;290(19):2581–7.
23. Fonarow GC, Adams KF Jr, Abraham WT, et al. Risk stratification for in-hospital mortality in acutely decompensated heart failure: classification and regression tree analysis. JAMA 2005;293(5):572–80.
24. Fox E, Landrum-McNiff K, Zhong Z, et al. Evaluation of prognostic criteria for determining hospice eligibility in patients with advanced lung, heart, or liver disease. Support Investigators. Study to understand prognoses and preferences for outcomes and risks of treatments. JAMA 1999;282(17):1638–45.
25. Nevins ML, Epstein SK. Predictors of outcome for patients with COPD requiring invasive mechanical ventilation. Chest 2001;119(6):1840–9.
26. Rose EA, Gelijns AC, Moskowitz AJ, et al. Long-term use of a left ventricular assist device for end-stage heart failure. N Engl J Med 2001;345(20): 1435–43.
27. Chen JH, Chan DC, Kiely DK, et al. Terminal trajectories of functional decline in the long-term care setting. J Gerontol A Biol Sci Med Sci 2007;62(5):531–6.
28. Gozalo P, Teno JM, Mitchell SL, et al. End-of-life transitions among nursing home residents with cognitive issues. N Engl J Med 2011;365(13):1212–21.
29. Morrison RS, Siu AL. Survival in end-stage dementia following acute illness. JAMA 2000;284(1):47–52.
30. Lamba S, Nagurka R, Murano T, et al. Early identification of dying trajectories in emergency department patients: potential impact on hospital care. J Palliat Med 2012;15(4):392–5.
31. Morita T, Ichiki T, Tsunoda J, et al. A prospective study on the dying process in terminally ill cancer patients. Am J Hosp Palliat Care 1998;15(4):217–22.
32. Hwang IC, Ahn HY, Park SM, et al. Clinical changes in terminally ill cancer patients and death within 48 h: when should we refer patients to a separate room? Support Care Canc 2013;21(3):835–40.

33. Mercadante S, Valle A, Porzio G, et al. How do cancer patients receiving palliative care at home die? A descriptive study. J Pain Symptom Manage 2011; 42(5):702–9.
34. Weissman D. Syndrome of imminent death. Fast facts and concepts. 2005. Available at: http://www.eperc.mcw.edu/EPERC/FastFactsIndex/ff_003.htm.
35. Smith AK, Fisher J, Schonberg MA, et al. Am I doing the right thing? Provider perspectives on improving palliative care in the emergency department. Ann Emerg Med 2009;54(1):86–93.e1.
36. Silveira MJ, Kim SY, Langa KM. Advance directives and outcomes of surrogate decision making before death. N Engl J Med 2010;362(13):1211–8.
37. Fromme EK, Zive D, Schmidt TA, et al. POLST registry do-not-resuscitate orders and other patient treatment preferences. JAMA 2012;307(1):34–5.
38. Morrison RS, Meier DE. High rates of advance care planning in New York City's elderly population. Arch Intern Med 2004;164(22):2421–6.
39. Volandes AE, Paasche-Orlow MK, Mitchell SL, et al. Randomized controlled trial of a video decision support tool for cardiopulmonary resuscitation decision making in advanced cancer. J Clin Oncol 2013;31(3):380–6.
40. McCannon JB, O'Donnell WJ, Thompson BT, et al. Augmenting communication and decision making in the intensive care unit with a cardiopulmonary resuscitation video decision support tool: a temporal intervention study. J Palliat Med 2012;15(12):1382–7.
41. Volandes AE, Paasche-Orlow MK, Barry MJ, et al. Video decision support tool for advance care planning in dementia: randomised controlled trial. BMJ 2009;338:b2159.
42. Volandes AE, Barry MJ, Chang Y, et al. Improving decision making at the end of life with video images. Med Decis Making 2010;30(1):29–34.
43. Volandes AE, Paasche-Orlow M, Gillick MR, et al. Health literacy not race predicts end-of-life care preferences. J Palliat Med 2008;11(5):754–62.
44. Volandes AE, Ferguson LA, Davis AD, et al. Assessing end-of-life preferences for advanced dementia in rural patients using an educational video: a randomized controlled trial. J Palliat Med 2011;14(2):169–77.
45. Fried TR, Bradley EH, Towle VR, et al. Understanding the treatment preferences of seriously ill patients. N Engl J Med 2002;346(14):1061–6.
46. Larkin GL, Copes WS, Nathanson BH, et al. Pre-resuscitation factors associated with mortality in 49,130 cases of in-hospital cardiac arrest: a report from the National registry for cardiopulmonary resuscitation. Resuscitation 2010;81(3): 302–11.
47. Ewer MS, Kish SK, Martin CG, et al. Characteristics of cardiac arrest in cancer patients as a predictor of survival after cardiopulmonary resuscitation. Cancer 2001;92(7):1905–12.
48. Hwang JP, Patlan J, de Achaval S, et al. Survival in cancer patients after out-of-hospital cardiac arrest. Support Care Canc 2010;18(1):51–5.
49. Gershengorn HB, Li G, Kramer A, et al. Survival and functional outcomes after cardiopulmonary resuscitation in the intensive care unit. J Crit Care 2012;27(4): 421.e9–17.
50. Blinderman CD, Krakauer EL, Solomon MZ. Time to revise the approach to determining cardiopulmonary resuscitation status. JAMA 2012;307(9):917–8.
51. Downar J, Luk T, Sibbald RW, et al. Why do patients agree to a "do not resuscitate" or "full code" order? Perspectives of medical inpatients. J Gen Intern Med 2011;26(6):582–7.

52. Seneff MG, Wagner DP, Wagner RP, et al. Hospital and 1-year survival of patients admitted to intensive care units with acute exacerbation of chronic obstructive pulmonary disease. JAMA 1995;274(23):1852–7.
53. Fischer GS, Tulsky JA, Rose MR, et al. Patient knowledge and physician predictions of treatment preferences after discussion of advance directives. J Gen Intern Med 1998;13(7):447–54.
54. Scheunemann LP, McDevitt M, Carson SS, et al. Randomized, controlled trials of interventions to improve communication in intensive care: a systematic review. Chest 2011;139(3):543–54.
55. Campbell ML, Guzman JA. Impact of a proactive approach to improve end-of-life care in a medical ICU. Chest 2003;123(1):266–71.
56. Buckman R, Kason Y. How to break bad news: a guide for health care professionals. Baltimore (MD): Johns Hopkins University Press; 1992.
57. Weeks JC, Catalano PJ, Cronin A, et al. Patients' expectations about effects of chemotherapy for advanced cancer. N Engl J Med 2012;367(17):1616–25.
58. Christakis NA, Iwashyna TJ. Attitude and self-reported practice regarding prognostication in a national sample of internists. Arch Intern Med 1998;158(21):2389–95.
59. Wenrich MD, Curtis JR, Shannon SE, et al. Communicating with dying patients within the spectrum of medical care from terminal diagnosis to death. Arch Intern Med 2001;161(6):868–74.
60. Temel JS, Greer JA, Admane S, et al. Longitudinal perceptions of prognosis and goals of therapy in patients with metastatic non-small-cell lung cancer: results of a randomized study of early palliative care. J Clin Oncol 2011;29(17):2319–26.
61. Apatira L, Boyd EA, Malvar G, et al. Hope, truth, and preparing for death: perspectives of surrogate decision makers. Ann Intern Med 2008;149(12):861–8.
62. Glare P, Virik K, Jones M, et al. A systematic review of physicians' survival predictions in terminally ill cancer patients. BMJ 2003;327(7408):195–8.
63. Christakis NA, Lamont EB. Extent and determinants of error in doctors' prognoses in terminally ill patients: prospective cohort study. BMJ 2000;320(7233):469–72.
64. Lamas D, Rosenbaum L. Freedom from the tyranny of choice–teaching the end-of-life conversation. N Engl J Med 2012;366(18):1655–7.
65. Quill TE, Arnold R, Back AL. Discussing treatment preferences with patients who want "everything". Ann Intern Med 2009;151(5):345–9.
66. von Gunten CF, Ferris FD, Emanuel LL. The patient-physician relationship. Ensuring competency in end-of-life care: communication and relational skills. JAMA 2000;284(23):3051–7.
67. Johnson DH. Helga Wanglie revisited: medical futility and the limits of autonomy. Camb Q Healthc Ethics 1993;2(2):161–70.
68. Iserson KV. Ethical principles–emergency medicine. Emerg Med Clin North Am 2006;24(3):513–45.
69. Iserson KV. Principles of biomedical ethics. Emerg Med Clin North Am 1999;17(2):283–306, ix.
70. Lyons RA, Wareham K, Hutchings HA, et al. Population requirement for adult critical-care beds: a prospective quantitative and qualitative study. Lancet 2000;355(9204):595–8.
71. ACEP. Code of ethics for emergency physicians. Ann Emerg Med 2008;52(5):581–90.

72. Larkin GL. A code of conduct for academic emergency medicine. SAEM Ethics Committee. Society for Academic Emergency Medicine. Acad Emerg Med 1999;6(1):45.
73. Parks SM, Winter L, Santana AJ, et al. Family factors in end-of-life decision-making: family conflict and proxy relationship. J Palliat Med 2011;14(2):179–84.
74. Bulow HH, Sprung CL, Baras M, et al. Are religion and religiosity important to end-of-life decisions and patient autonomy in the ICU? The Ethicatt study. Intensive Care Med 2012;38(7):1126–33.
75. Babgi A. Legal issues in end-of-life care: perspectives from Saudi Arabia and United States. Am J Hosp Palliat Care 2009;26(2):119–27.
76. Truog RD. Triage in the ICU. Hastings Cent Rep 1992;22(3):13–7.
77. MJ. Been there, done that: ethics consultation and the importance of "not knowing". Atrium Winter 2013;11:42–4.
78. Sudore RL. A piece of my mind. Can we agree to disagree? JAMA 2009;302(15):1629–30.
79. Crippen D, Burrows D, Stocchetti N, et al. Ethics roundtable: open-ended ICU care: can we afford it? Crit Care 2010;14(3):222.
80. Angus DC, Kelley MA, Schmitz RJ, et al. Caring for the critically ill patient. Current and projected workforce requirements for care of the critically ill and patients with pulmonary disease: can we meet the requirements of an aging population? JAMA 2000;284(21):2762–70.
81. Frick S, Uehlinger DE, Zuercher Zenklusen RM. Medical futility: predicting outcome of intensive care unit patients by nurses and doctors–a prospective comparative study. Crit Care Med 2003;31(2):456–61.
82. Asplund K, Britton M. Ethics of life support in patients with severe stroke. Stroke 1989;20(8):1107–12.
83. Laureys S. Science and society: death, unconsciousness and the brain. Nat Rev Neurosci 2005;6(11):899–909.
84. Burns JP, Truog RD. Futility: a concept in evolution. Chest 2007;132(6):1987–93.
85. Zier LS, Burack JH, Micco G, et al. Surrogate decision makers' responses to physicians' predictions of medical futility. Chest 2009;136(1):110–7.
86. Caplan AL. Odds and ends: trust and the debate over medical futility. Ann Intern Med 1996;125(8):688–9.
87. Siegel MD. End-of-life decision making in the ICU. Clin Chest Med 2009;30(1):181–94, x.
88. Fox E, Myers S, Pearlman RA. Ethics consultation in United States hospitals: a national survey. Am J Bioeth 2007;7(2):13–25.
89. Michael GE, Jesus JE. Treatment of potential organ donors in the emergency department: a review. Ann Emerg Med 2012;60(4):485–91.
90. Ethics Committee, American College of Critical Care Medicine, Society of Critical Care Medicine. Recommendations for nonheartbeating organ donation. A position paper by the Ethics Committee, American College of Critical Care Medicine, Society of Critical Care Medicine. Crit Care Med 2001;29(9):1826–31.
91. Robertson JA. The dead donor rule. Hastings Cent Rep 1999;29(6):6–14.
92. Boucek MM, Mashburn C, Dunn SM, et al. Pediatric heart transplantation after declaration of cardiocirculatory death. N Engl J Med 2008;359(7):709–14.
93. Truog RD, Fackler JC. Rethinking brain death. Crit Care Med 1992;20(12):1705–13.

94. Sade RM. Brain death, cardiac death, and the dead donor rule. J S C Med Assoc 2011;107(4):146–9.
95. Truog RD, Miller FG. The dead donor rule and organ transplantation. N Engl J Med 2008;359(7):674–5.
96. Wall SP, Goldfrank LR. Death on the waiting list: a failure in public health. Ann Emerg Med 2012;60(4):492–4.
97. Wijdicks EF, Varelas PN, Gronseth GS, et al. Evidence-based guideline update: determining brain death in adults: report of the Quality Standards Subcommittee of the American Academy of Neurology. Neurology 2010;74(23):1911–8.
98. Robey TE, Marcolini EG. Organ donation after acute brain death: addressing limitations of time and resources in the emergency department. Yale J Biol Med 2013;86(3):333–42.
99. Beemath A, Zalenski RJ. Palliative emergency medicine: resuscitating comfort care? Ann Emerg Med 2009;54(1):103–5.
100. Parshall MB, Schwartzstein RM, Adams L, et al. An official American Thoracic Society statement: update on the mechanisms, assessment, and management of dyspnea. Am J Respir Crit Care Med 2012;185(4):435–52.
101. Currow DC, Smith J, Davidson PM, et al. Do the trajectories of dyspnea differ in prevalence and intensity by diagnosis at the end of life? A consecutive cohort study. J Pain Symptom Manage 2010;39(4):680–90.
102. Reuben DB, Mor V. Dyspnea in terminally ill cancer patients. Chest 1986;89(2): 234–6.
103. Booth S, Silvester S, Todd C. Breathlessness in cancer and chronic obstructive pulmonary disease: using a qualitative approach to describe the experience of patients and carers. Palliat Support Care 2003;1(4):337–44.
104. Qaseem A, Snow V, Shekelle P, et al. Evidence-based interventions to improve the palliative care of pain, dyspnea, and depression at the end of life: a clinical practice guideline from the American College of Physicians. Ann Intern Med 2008;148(2):141–6.
105. Ben-Aharon I, Gafter-Gvili A, Leibovici L, et al. Interventions for alleviating cancer-related dyspnea: a systematic review and meta-analysis. Acta Oncol 2012;51(8):996–1008.
106. Viola R, Kiteley C, Lloyd NS, et al. The management of dyspnea in cancer patients: a systematic review. Support Care Canc 2008;16(4):329–37.
107. Bruera E, MacEachern T, Ripamonti C, et al. Subcutaneous morphine for dyspnea in cancer patients. Ann Intern Med 1993;119(9):906–7.
108. Jennings AL, Davies AN, Higgins JP, et al. Opioids for the palliation of breathlessness in terminal illness. Cochrane Database Syst Rev 2001;(4):CD002066.
109. Clemens KE, Klaschik E. Effect of hydromorphone on ventilation in palliative care patients with dyspnea. Support Care Canc 2008;16(1):93–9.
110. Clemens KE, Klaschik E. Symptomatic therapy of dyspnea with strong opioids and its effect on ventilation in palliative care patients. J Pain Symptom Manage 2007;33(4):473–81.
111. Clemens KE, Quednau I, Klaschik E. Use of oxygen and opioids in the palliation of dyspnoea in hypoxic and non-hypoxic palliative care patients: a prospective study. Support Care Canc 2009;17(4):367–77.
112. Shreves A, Pour T. Emergency management of dyspnea in dying patients. Emerg Med Pract 2013;15(5):1–19.
113. Simon ST, Higginson IJ, Booth S, et al. Benzodiazepines for the relief of breathlessness in advanced malignant and non-malignant diseases in adults. Cochrane Database Syst Rev 2010;(1):CD007354.

114. Clemens KE, Klaschik E. Dyspnoea associated with anxiety–symptomatic therapy with opioids in combination with lorazepam and its effect on ventilation in palliative care patients. Support Care Canc 2011;19(12):2027–33.
115. Uronis HE, Currow DC, McCrory DC, et al. Oxygen for relief of dyspnoea in mildly- or non-hypoxaemic patients with cancer: a systematic review and meta-analysis. Br J Cancer 2008;98(2):294–9.
116. Abernethy AP, McDonald CF, Frith PA, et al. Effect of palliative oxygen versus room air in relief of breathlessness in patients with refractory dyspnoea: a double-blind, randomised controlled trial. Lancet 2010;376(9743):784–93.
117. Quon BS, Gan WQ, Sin DD. Contemporary management of acute exacerbations of COPD: a systematic review and metaanalysis. Chest 2008;133(3):756–66.
118. Weng CL, Zhao YT, Liu QH, et al. Meta-analysis: noninvasive ventilation in acute cardiogenic pulmonary edema. Ann Intern Med 2010;152(9):590–600.
119. Curtis JR, Cook DJ, Sinuff T, et al. Noninvasive positive pressure ventilation in critical and palliative care settings: understanding the goals of therapy. Crit Care Med 2007;35(3):932–9.
120. Azoulay E, Demoule A, Jaber S, et al. Palliative noninvasive ventilation in patients with acute respiratory failure. Intensive Care Med 2011;37(8):1250–7.
121. Cuomo A, Delmastro M, Ceriana P, et al. Noninvasive mechanical ventilation as a palliative treatment of acute respiratory failure in patients with end-stage solid cancer. Palliative Med 2004;18(7):602–10.
122. Lenglet H, Sztrymf B, Leroy C, et al. Humidified high flow nasal oxygen during respiratory failure in the emergency department: feasibility and efficacy. Respir Care 2012;57(11):1873–8.
123. Peters SG, Holets SR, Gay PC. High-flow nasal cannula therapy in do-not-intubate patients with hypoxemic respiratory distress. Respir Care 2013;58(4):597–600.
124. Ganzini L, Goy ER, Miller LL, et al. Nurses' experiences with hospice patients who refuse food and fluids to hasten death. N Engl J Med 2003;349(4):359–65.
125. Cohen MZ, Torres-Vigil I, Burbach BE, et al. The meaning of parenteral hydration to family caregivers and patients with advanced cancer receiving hospice care. J Pain Symptom Manage 2012;43(5):855–65.
126. Bruera E, Hui D, Dalal S, et al. Parenteral hydration in patients with advanced cancer: a multicenter, double-blind, placebo-controlled randomized trial. J Clin Oncol 2013;31(1):111–8.
127. Bruera E, Sala R, Rico MA, et al. Effects of parenteral hydration in terminally ill cancer patients: a preliminary study. J Clin Oncol 2005;23(10):2366–71.
128. Nakajima N, Hata Y, Kusumuto K. A clinical study on the influence of hydration volume on the signs of terminally ill cancer patients with abdominal malignancies. J Palliat Med 2013;16(2):185–9.
129. Casarett D, Pickard A, Bailey FA, et al. Do palliative consultations improve patient outcomes? J Am Geriatr Soc 2008;56(4):593–9.
130. Binney ZO, Quest TE, Feingold PL, et al. Feasibility and economic impact of dedicated hospice inpatient units for terminally Ill ICU patients. Crit Care Med 2013;42(5):1074–80.
131. Lamba S, Quest TE, Weissman DE. Initiating a hospice referral from the emergency department #247. J Palliat Med 2011;14(12):1346–7.

Index

Note: Page numbers of article titles are in **boldface** type.

Emerg Med Clin N Am 32 (2014) 975–982
http://dx.doi.org/10.1016/S0733-8627(14)00093-5 emed.theclinics.com

O

P

R

S

United States Postal Service

Statement of Ownership, Management, and Circulation
(All Periodicals Publications Except Requestor Publications)

1. Publication Title	2. Publication Number	3. Filing Date
Emergency Medicine Clinics of North America	0 0 0 - 7 1 4	9/14/14
4. Issue Frequency Feb, May, Aug, Nov	**5. Number of Issues Published Annually** 4	**6. Annual Subscription Price** $315.00

7. Complete Mailing Address of Known Office of Publication (*Not printer*) (*Street, city, county, state, and ZIP+4®*)

Elsevier Inc.
360 Park Avenue South
New York, NY 10010-1710

Contact Person: Stephen R. Bushing
Telephone (Include area code): 215-239-3688

8. Complete Mailing Address of Headquarters or General Business Office of Publisher (*Not printer*)

Elsevier Inc., 360 Park Avenue South, New York, NY 10010-1710

9. Full Names and Complete Mailing Addresses of Publisher, Editor, and Managing Editor (*Do not leave blank*)

Publisher (*Name and complete mailing address*)

Linda Belfus, Elsevier Inc., 1600 John F. Kennedy Blvd., Suite 1800, Philadelphia, PA 19103-2899

Editor (*Name and complete mailing address*)

Patrick Manley, Elsevier Inc., 1600 John F. Kennedy Blvd., Suite 1800, Philadelphia, PA 19103-2899

Managing Editor (*Name and complete mailing address*)

Adrianne Brigido, Elsevier Inc., 1600 John F. Kennedy Blvd., Suite 1800, Philadelphia, PA 19103-2899

10. Owner (*Do not leave blank. If the publication is owned by a corporation, give the name and address of the corporation immediately followed by the names and addresses of all stockholders owning or holding 1 percent or more of the total amount of stock. If not owned by a corporation, give the names and addresses of the individual owners. If owned by a partnership or other unincorporated firm, give its name and address as well as those of each individual owner. If the publication is published by a nonprofit organization, give its name and address.*)

Full Name	Complete Mailing Address
Wholly owned subsidiary of	1600 John F. Kennedy Blvd, Ste. 1800
Reed/Elsevier, US holdings	Philadelphia, PA 19103-2899

11. Known Bondholders, Mortgagees, and Other Security Holders Owning or Holding 1 Percent or More of Total Amount of Bonds, Mortgages, or Other Securities. If none, check box → ☐ None

Full Name	Complete Mailing Address
N/A	

12. Tax Status (*For completion by nonprofit organizations authorized to mail at nonprofit rates*) (*Check one*)
The purpose, function, and nonprofit status of this organization and the exempt status for federal income tax purposes:
☐ Has Not Changed During Preceding 12 Months
☐ Has Changed During Preceding 12 Months (*Publisher must submit explanation of change with this statement*)

PS Form **3526**, August 2012 (Page 1 of 3 (Instructions Page 3)) PSN 7530-01-000-9931 **PRIVACY NOTICE**: See our Privacy policy in www.usps.com

13. Publication Title	14. Issue Date for Circulation Data Below
Emergency Medicine Clinics of North America	August 2014

15. Extent and Nature of Circulation		Average No. Copies Each Issue During Preceding 12 Months	No. Copies of Single Issue Published Nearest to Filing Date
a. Total Number of Copies (*Net press run*)		873	860
b. Paid Circulation (By Mail and Outside the Mail)	(1) Mailed Outside-County Paid Subscriptions Stated on PS Form 3541. (*Include paid distribution above nominal rate, advertiser's proof copies, and exchange copies*)	539	530
	(2) Mailed In-County Paid Subscriptions Stated on PS Form 3541 (*Include paid distribution above nominal rate, advertiser's proof copies, and exchange copies*)		
	(3) Paid Distribution Outside the Mails Including Sales Through Dealers and Carriers, Street Vendors, Counter Sales, and Other Paid Distribution Outside USPS®	121	130
	(4) Paid Distribution by Other Classes Mailed Through the USPS (e.g. First-Class Mail®)		
c. Total Paid Distribution (*Sum of 15b (1), (2), (3), and (4)*) ▶		660	660
d. Free or Nominal Rate Distribution (By Mail and Outside the Mail)	(1) Free or Nominal Rate Outside-County Copies Included on PS Form 3541	70	75
	(2) Free or Nominal Rate In-County Copies Included on PS Form 3541		
	(3) Free or Nominal Rate Copies Mailed at Other Classes Through the USPS (e.g. First-Class Mail)		
	(4) Free or Nominal Rate Distribution Outside the Mail (Carriers or other means)		
e. Total Free or Nominal Rate Distribution (Sum of 15d (1), (2), (3) and (4)		70	75
f. Total Distribution (Sum of 15c and 15e) ▶		730	735
g. Copies not Distributed (See instructions to publishers #4 (page #3)) ▶		143	125
h. Total (Sum of 15f and g)		873	860
i. Percent Paid (15c divided by 15f times 100) ▶		90.41%	89.80%
16. Total circulation includes electronic copies. Report circulation on PS Form 3526-X worksheet. ▶			

17. Publication of Statement of Ownership
If the publication is a general publication, publication of this statement is required. Will be printed in the November 2014 issue of this publication.

18. Signature and Title of Editor, Publisher, Business Manager, or Owner — Date

Stephen R. Bushing – Inventory Distribution Coordinator — September 14, 2014

I certify that all information furnished on this form is true and complete. I understand that anyone who furnishes false or misleading information on this form or who omits material or information requested on the form may be subject to criminal sanctions (including fines and imprisonment) and/or civil sanctions (including civil penalties).

PS Form **3526**, August 2012 (Page 2 of 3)